CLEANSING
THE
NATION

CLEANSING THE NATION

INDIA, THE HINDU MODERN, AND MEDIATIONS OF GENDER

RAKA SHOME

DUKE UNIVERSITY PRESS *Durham and London* 2025

© 2025 DUKE UNIVERSITY PRESS
All rights reserved
Project Editor: Ihsan Taylor
Designed by Matthew Tauch
Typeset in Arno Pro and Barlow by Westchester
Publishing Services

Library of Congress Cataloging-in-Publication Data
Names: Shome, Raka, [date] author.
Title: Cleansing the nation : India, the Hindu modern,
and mediations of gender / Raka Shome.
Other titles: India, the Hindu modern, and mediations
of gender
Description: Durham : Duke University Press, 2025. |
Includes bibliographical references and index.
Identifiers: LCCN 2025006509 (print)
LCCN 2025006510 (ebook)
ISBN 9781478032755 (paperback)
ISBN 9781478029311 (hardcover)
ISBN 9781478061519 (ebook)
Subjects: LCSH: Sanitation—Social aspects—India. |
Sanitation—Political aspects—India. | Hygiene—
Political aspects—India. | Hygiene—Social aspects—
India. | Hindutva—India. | Caste—Political aspects—
India. | India—Politics and government—21st century.
Classification: LCC RA567.5.I4 S485 2025 (print) | LCC
RA567.5.I4 (ebook) | DDC 353.9/3—dc23/eng/20250821
LC record available at https://lccn.loc.gov/2025006509
LC ebook record available at https://lccn.loc.gov/
2025006510

Cover art: People waving saffron flags during the festival
of Dussehra, October 19, 2022, Dehradun, Uttarakhand,
India. Rupendra Rawat / Alamy.

I dedicate this book to all those who are being violently excised today by the Hindu nationalist imagination.

The infrastructure of fascism is staring us in the face . . .
and yet we hesitate to call it by its name.
—ARUNDHATI ROY, *AZADI*

CONTENTS

PREFACE

Writing this book has been a journey in humility. When I conceived of this book, I was primarily interested in finding out what is going on with Hindu nationalism in contemporary India, with the ascent of the Bhartiya Janata Party to power in 2014; how Hindu nationalism has taken on such fascist colors; and why it is succeeding without much significant resistance—which marks a difference from its earlier avatars—and why more and more people in India today are consciously asserting their Hindu identity.

As I plunged into this study, I took a deep dive into issues that I knew something about: caste and the oppression of Muslim identities in India. But it is one thing to "know something" (and realize that it has been a very small knowing), quite another to dive into their everyday realities through research and engage the brutal exclusions that shape, and have shaped, the polity of India. As I spent months plunging into the writings of B. R. Ambedkar, Kancha Ilaiah, Jyotirao Phule, Dalit Panthers, Anand Teltumbde, Braj Mani, Gail Omvedt, Sharmila Rege, Yassica Dutta, and others, I was confronted again—as if I had received a sharp slap in the face ("sharp" because of the hard realization that so little has changed)—by how caste oppression is not only a fulcrum upon which the nation pivots but the violent structure that makes it *even possible*. These are not writers or thinkers whose works ever surface in the curricula of most Indian schools and colleges. Reading the works of these Dalit scholars or scholars committed to caste issues also led me to descend into the Hindu supremacist writings of Savarkar, M. S. Golwalkar, and others. You learn in such works, again and again, that "being Hindu" is deeply rooted not only in an ideology of supremacy but also hate—something that everyday liberal Hindus deny in their desire to distance themselves from such ideologies in order to appear "modern" in contemporary India. But rarely do they pause to see if the currents of those ideologies infiltrate their lives in some way or another. Thus, when Ambedkar said in 1936 that "there is no Hindu consciousness of kind. In every Hindu the consciousness that exists is the consciousness of his [sic] caste" (2014, 189), he was so very right.

Anyone paying attention to India today also cannot, and should not, ignore the brutal yet tragic ways in which the Muslim body is being excised from the national imagination. To some extent this has always been the case in India before and after Partition. But this time around, it is happening *without apologies* and *with pride*. Stuart Hall once said, "Against the urgency of people dying in the streets what in God's name is the point of Cultural Studies?" (1992, 284). Indeed, what is the point of being scholars and intellectuals studying India when Dalits, Muslims, and other minorities (including the poor) are symbolically and even materially dying or being abused in the streets of India? What does all this brutality demand of us, especially those who are Hindus and privileged? Do we stand by and watch a multireligious and multiethnic democracy crumble just because "our lives" are not that affected by the process? As scholars and intellectuals, what are our choices here? How do we make visible, in loud and unapologetic ways, the processes of purification and cleansing at work in the nation today? How do we refuse such processes?

Speaking out against all this in whatever way possible is definitely one way. But going back and learning about the (unacknowledged) histories of violence (especially of caste and Muslim oppression) that have made today's India possible is another. For one cannot challenge something whose history (small *h*) one does not fully understand or know. To that extent, this book has been a deep exercise in relearning. I tried to access—however and wherever I could (and it is increasingly hard to do so these days)—stories and voices of caste and Muslim oppression in India, before and since Partition and right into the present. The present in India is what it is today because these histories have not been made visible in any significant way in the media, in schools and colleges, in the publishing industry (with a few notable exceptions), in the entertainment industry, in government documents, and in legends and folklore. Yet their shadows are everywhere today, growing darker and longer every moment. Such historical relearning is important also because today in India history is being used (and denied) in particular ways by the state to cleanse the nation. In focusing on a signature development campaign in current India, this book tries to address (however imperfectly) how the past reemerges in current discourses of progress and modernity in the nation.

A few months ago (at the time of writing this preface) the nation exploded in outrage about the rape of a young female doctor in Kolkata's

R. G. Kar Medical Hospital. As with the 2012 Nirbhaya rape case, the nation (and diasporic Indians) cohered in outrage against the rape (and its attempted cover up) of a (Hindu) woman—nothing wrong in that. But in that clamor and outrage, I could only hear the resounding silence around the everyday rapes and molestation of Dalit women and the increasing violence toward Muslim women—including calls for their rape and abduction—that are at an all-time high today. These women can never be India's daughters: never a Nirbhaya or an Abhaya (the name given to the female victim of the R. G. Kar Medical Hospital case). The media does not cover the violence toward them. The nation does not organize around them. Celebrities do not create hashtags for them. There are no candlelight marches that light up their violated bodies. The global Indian diaspora does not explode in outrage. There is only silence. And ignorance. And prejudice. And fear.

This book is thus a small attempt to intellectually make some noise in this climate of silence and fear. Here, I join many other intellectuals, scholars, and writers whose courage is contagious and inspiring, and who are similarly trying to make some noise about the crumbling of democracy in India, while risking being silenced.

Through the process of writing this book, I found myself haunted by questions such as: How is "being Hindu" built on violence and exclusion? Has India really been a "free" nation since 1947? Free for whom? How is the democracy (however imperfect and incomplete) that India created in the post-Partition years disintegrating with such speed? And how is the silence of the upper and middle classes and castes in the nation, who proudly espouse the arrival of a "new India," entangled with this disintegration? While these are questions for and about India, they are also not just about India but about a larger global trend: the demise of democracy, the entrenchment of authoritarianism, the normalization of state violence, and the suppression of "other" imaginations that mark our times.

ACKNOWLEDGMENTS

No book is ever written in isolation. Academic projects are always indirectly collaborative. Conversations with thinkers throughout our intellectual journeys shape our imaginations, our ways of writing, our ways of asking questions about the social. So, a big thanks to everyone I have encountered on my intellectual journey and from whom I have learnt something—even if I may have unconsciously forgotten that learning.

Within my own community of scholars and friends, there are many who have supported me, directly or indirectly, from whom I have learned so much, and with whom I enjoy (or have enjoyed) various intellectual exchanges: Soyini Madison, Dana Cloud, Angharad Valdivia (my feminist support group), Raymie McKerrow, Kent Ono, Lawrence Grossberg, Radhika Parameswaran, Wendy Willems, Terhi Rantanen, John Erni, Herman Wasserman, Ted Striphas, and so many others I know I am forgetting. In the Philadelphia circle, I appreciate the connections with Fabienne Darling-Wolf and Aswin Punathambekar (as well as Rahul Mukherjee and Sarah Banet-Weiser). Our occasional chats and social meetings provide good intellectual energy.

Various parts of this project have been presented as keynote and plenary talks at conferences, and as lectures at various universities and forums: the "Gender, Mobility and Transformations in Asia" conference at University of Melbourne; the "Mapping Global Futures" conference at Ghent University, Belgium organized by the International Rhetoric Society; the Giles Wilkeson Gray Lecture at Louisiana State University; the Audrey Fisher Lecture at the University of Utah; the Annual Rhetorical Leadership Lecture at the University of Wisconsin–Milwaukee; the "Fire on the Mountain" conference at the Center for Media, Religion, and Culture at the University of Colorado–Boulder; the Rhetoric Speaker Series at Northwestern University; and the Graduate Speaker Series at Temple University, among others. Additionally, parts of this book have been presented at annual conferences of the International Communication Association, the

National Communication Association, the Association for Cultural Studies (their biennial Crossroads Conference), the Inter-Asia Cultural Studies Conference (Seoul), and the South Asia Conference at the University of Wisconsin–Madison. I thank the audiences at all these forums for their questions and comments, which have pushed my thinking in helpful ways.

At Villanova University, I thank the Dean of Liberal Arts and Sciences, Adele Lindenmeyer, for supporting this book with a research leave semester. The research funds available through the Harron Family Endowment supported many research trips to India and other needs of this project. The Waterhouse Family Institute and the Small Research Grant at Villanova University, as well as the university's 2025 subvention grant program, also provided funding in support of this project. Outside of Villanova University, I thank the Organization for Research on Women and Communication (ORWAC) for supporting this research with a grant in 2022.

Three graduate assistants worked on this project; their labor has been critical in finding and amassing the research materials I needed as well as the tedious task of checking and hunting down citations. Big thanks to Cheyenne Zaremba, Sofia Fazal, and Anna Levine. I also thank members of the Department of Communication at Villanova for their support. I must further thank Loretta Chiaverini, my department's staff member, for her constant help, always given with a smile. Laura Capriotti, my other department staff member, has also been a source of help in so many ways. The invisible labor of such staff members, which we often tend to take for granted, makes our lives as faculty members in our department homes so much easier.

Within the Villanova community I am grateful for the joyful camaraderie and support of Hibba Abugideiri and Elizabeth Kolsky, two women with great progressive politics. I also thank Bryan Crable (who departed for greener pastures), Heze Lewis, Billie Murray, Gabrielle Rockhill, and Terry Nance for their support and friendship at various stages of my life at Villanova.

Thanks to Ken Wissoker at Duke University Press for seeing something valuable in this project, for supporting it, and shepherding it through. Ken's invaluable advice has definitely sharpened the project. Thanks to Ryan Kendall for always answering email questions promptly and cheerfully, and providing information whenever I needed it. Thanks are also due to Ihsan Taylor, project editor, for his assistance. Three anonymous reviewers offered comments that pushed me in productive ways. I thank them for their time and wonderful suggestions. I also thank editor Shanon

Fitzpatrick for her excellent editorial support and assistance, which have been invaluable.

My community in Greater Philadelphia involves some wonderful, loving people who keep me grounded with their love, support, and hospitality: Thank you Sunanda Banerjee, Gabbu (Collin Banerjee), Ananda Banerjee, and Shanta Ghosh. You provide me with a family-like environment that sustains and nourishes me, and keeps my feet firmly planted on the ground. Thanks as well to Monisha Nayar-Akhtar, David Drum, and Curtis Key for their friendship, love, support, and humor. I cherish the times that we get together over food and drinks and drop into heated discussions about the state of the country (USA) and the world.

Last, but not least, I owe a debt of gratitude to my mother for her constant unconditional love, and to my loving sister, chef extraordinaire. She indulges me with food and a constant stream of gifts. And then there is Ebrahim, my kind of brother-in-law who has now become a part of my family; I am grateful for his positive presence in our lives. And to Seema: Thank you for decades of friendship and craziness. Thanks also to Sanjay and Jaba, part of my greater family in the United States and whose presence I cherish. Finally, a big thanks to my grandmother, my *Dida*, who I know is beaming with pride from the skies. You are always missed.

ONE

CLEANSING THE NATION

HINDU NATIONALISM, THE HINDU MODERN, AND GENDER

Our country is our Identity, so, keep Identity clean.
—@BPC RETAILGOA

Swachhata [cleanliness/purity] is a puja [a Hindu prayer] for me.
—NARENDRA MODI

May 2014 changed the political and cultural landscape of India, arguably forever. The Bhartiya Janata Party (BJP), the political arm of the Hindu supremacist organization Rashtriya Swayamsevak Sangh (RSS) gained power in a landslide victory. Narendra Modi, the former chief minister of the state of Gujarat, referred to by some critics as the "butcher of Gujarat" because of his alleged silent enablement of the massacre of scores of Muslims there in 2002, was inaugurated as prime minister.[1] Never before had a party with strong religious associations achieved such a huge victory by promising so much to the people—no less than a "new India" and *acche din* (good days) of which the people could be proud. Fatigued by the alleged corruption in the previously ruling Congress Party, whose image had been dented by scandal after scandal, and lured by the promise of a "new India" with global power, "the people" decided to take a chance on a Hindu nationalist party, despite awareness of the BJP's hard Hindu nationalist agenda and association with the RSS.

While the "saffron wave" (Hansen 1999), referring to the color associated with Hindu supremacist movements, had existed in India prior to this time, from 2014 onward something quite unique emerged. Hindutva—the ideology of Hindu supremacy that claims Hindus are the original people of India—entered the very fabric of statecraft and governance in new ways, resulting in what Thomas Blom Hansen and Srirupa Roy term "governmental Hindutva" (2022, 9). Going forward, Hindu nationalism became seamlessly attached to national development as visions of national progress frequently came to be expressed through the vocabulary and imagery of Hinduism—sometimes explicitly and sometimes in coded language. As Angana Chatterji, Thomas Blom Hansen, and Christophe Jaffrelot note, today, Hindu nationalism "is shifting the relations between the Indian state and its diverse people" in a way in which the state functions not just as a political organ but as a cultural organ for celebrating and protecting the (Hindu) majority (Chatterji et al. 2019a, 2). Meanwhile, in Hindutva discourse, minorities of all stripes—Muslims, Christians, Dalits—become a threat; or they are appropriated into a majoritarian framework (often to secure votes) that keeps alive only a hollow pretense of pluralism. Fittingly, Jaffrelot (2021) calls India today an "ethnic democracy." This explicit entrance of Hindutva into national governance today in India is what is being termed *majoritarianism* by scholars (e.g., Chatterji et al. 2019b)— which is the idea that it is the (Hindu) majority who need the nation's protection as its power has thus far been weakened by the various protections and rights given to minorities. Another idea underpinning this formation is that the past glories of Hinduism have been suppressed by Muslim cultures since the medieval era, when Muslim empires dominated and seemingly diluted ancient Hindu grandeur. The issue in today's political climate thus is less Hinduism and more, to use Partha Chatterjee's phrase, the "*nationalization* of Hinduism" (1992, 1, emphasis added).

The terms *Hindutva* and *Hindu nationalism* will often be used interchangeably in this book because the political and cultural project of Hindutva weaponizes Hinduism and conflates it with the nation and national belonging. While not all expressions of Hindu nationalism reflect the militant, culturally, and politically exclusionary aspects typical of Hindutva, which works in multiple ways, contemporary Hindu nationalism cannot be separated from Hindutva, for Hindu nationalism *is* the chief formation through which Hindutva secures itself today. It is through Hindu nationalism that Hindutva weaponizes the state so that the state—through its policies and instruments—functions to resecure the power of Hindus and relegates all others to second-class citizenship. Hindu nationalism, I emphasize, is not only manifest in nationalist performances and rhetorics at the formal state and government level. There is also a kind of everyday Hindu nationalism that is both mobilized by the state *and* circulates through the discourses of nonstate actors and institutions such as the media, popular art, education, social media, digital apps, and everyday interactions between people online and on the ground. Further, Hindu nationalism is not a hardened monolith; its strategies and logics often shift in response to contextual factors, such as the needs of the ruling party in different times, places, and political situations.

This book contributes to our understanding of this nationalization of Hinduism through identifying an important yet underexplored recent campaign that has contributed to the normalization of Hindutva—the Clean India campaign, or as it is known in India, Swachh Bharat Abhiyan (SBA). Through this campaign, state and nonstate actors mobilizing upper and upper middle-class and caste notions of hygiene have linked together national development and national sanitation to enable a program of Hindu nationalist governance through cleanliness. The case of SBA brings into relief particular *logics and governmentalities* of contemporary Hindu nationalism that constitute what I call (and elaborate later) the Hindu *modern*—where ideas, images, and values informing national development, progress, and governance often rely on a Hindu civilizational ethos while also becoming aligned with the project of Hindutva, overtly or covertly. One of the most important features of the Modi government is the manner in which it is rewriting modernity in new ways through (Hindu) religious and vernacular logics.[2] The governmentality of the Hindu modern, I posit, enables that rewriting. Rather than merely situating SBA under the umbrella of the Hindu modern, this book contends that the SBA campaign has served as an important crucible for the refinement and enactment of a vision of Hindu modernity as an intertwined state and popular project. Organized around the ostensibly politically neutral goals of hygiene and disinfection, hallmarks of global modernity, SBA, I argue, structures a cleaning agenda at home that echoes and mobilizes a more insidious project of national cleansing; simultaneously, it works to sanitize the violence that has accompanied the enactment of Hindu modern governmentality in SBA and beyond.

The SBA campaign has been the BJP's pet development program. It was inaugurated by Modi with much fanfare and media hype on October 2, 2014, the birthday of Mahatma Gandhi, to acknowledge his commitment to cleanliness and sanitation during the freedom struggle movement.

While SBA documents do not explicitly define "dirt" or "clean," its main goals are to forge a "clean" nation by discouraging people from dropping garbage, encouraging people to adopt hygienic habits, bringing about behavioral change through raising awareness about hygiene and health, and, most importantly, eliminating open defecation (especially in rural India) by 2019 in order to achieve universal sanitation (Parmar 2020). The latter goal was the rationale upon which the World Bank pledged $1.5 billion, a loan that by latest accounts has not yet been received due to questions about whether the program's stated goals have truly been achieved and whether *independent* verification of ground results has been done (Rajagopal 2017; Yadavar 2017).[3] The overall aim of the first phase of the SBA campaign (from 2014 to 2019) was to construct twelve crore (approximately 120 million) toilets across India, with a focus on poorer rural and urban areas. Union budget documents indicate that until 2020 approximately 67,000 crore rupees (approximately $8.046 billion) have been spent on SBA (Gulankar 2020), and in the first three years, roughly 530 crore rupees (approximately $63.7 million) have been spent on public campaigns (Deep 2017). This book primarily focuses on the first phase of the SBA campaign, since that has been the most spectacularly mediated phase of the program, where lots of publicity occurred and global attention—and funding—was secured or promised. Additionally, it is this phase that overtly in its rhetoric mobilized a (Hindu) nationalist imaginary. When it was originally announced, the SBA campaign was supposed to run until 2019. However, as this date approached, new phases were announced and now it is in the second phase, whose stated goal is to cement the aims of the first. (This second phase, which, among other issues, aims to focus more on technicalities around biodegradable waste management and wastewater treatment, is beyond the scope of this book.) Thus, instead of writing about SBA in the past tense, this book considers the campaign as ongoing, and uses the present tense in discussing the completed, and significant, first phase, which was also hypermediated in relation to the second.

The SBA campaign has two intersecting arms: SBA Urban and SBA Grameen (or rural). The former is under the Ministry of Housing and Urban Development and the latter under the Ministry of Drinking Water and Sanitation (now the Ministry of Jal Shakti). Sources of funding come from the central government; individual state governments (following a 60:40 ratio for most states); a 0.5 percent tax levied on all services, so citizens are also paying for it (this is in addition to the 14 percent service tax that is typically charged); the private sector (through corporate social responsibility programs); and other tax exempt donations to the SBA *kosh* (fund).[4] The government offers a financial incentive of 12,000 rupees to individual families under the SBA Grameen scheme to build in-home toilets. In the SBA Urban scheme, the central government offers a subsidy of 4,000 rupees and states are to contribute at least 2,667 rupees (PTI 2018c). This has been critiqued by many, for in urban India the subsidy is simply not enough for constructing private toilets.

Financially, SBA typically operates on a reimbursement model. The government subsidy is generally paid only after a household has made the initial investment toward toilet construction, but some reports state that this money does not always make its way to families due to bureaucratic hiccups or corruption at the local level.[5] The program is run by local states that operate with financial and technical support from the central government. The latter issues guidelines to states to be implemented. Although on the eve of the alleged completion of the first phase of SBA in October 2019 the prime minister declared that India is now "open defecation free" (ODF) because 109 crore toilets have been constructed, there is ongoing skepticism about this declaration (PIB 2022a). Some reports contest this claim because toilet construction does not equate to usage nor confirms the usability of the constructions. Independent agencies have not fully verified the government's tall claims.[6]

During the SBA campaign, especially in the first phase, there has been limited focus on solid and liquid waste management, which includes sewage cleaning issues as well. This is important to note for, as the following chapters will address, it raises questions about who cleans the waste from toilets. The Centre for Policy Research notes that only 374 crore rupees (approximately $43 million) were spent in the whole country on solid and liquid waste management from 2015–16 through December 2018 (Kapur and Deshpande 2019). This was less than 1 percent of the total of the government's share of SBA. In 2018–19 it was 4 percent, and in 2019–20 (until early July) it was, on average, 5 percent (Shekhar 2023). This is indeed a sorry state of affairs. In the second phase of the SBA campaign (2020 to 2025), there is some commitment signaled in the policy document about the guidelines for this phase, which signal initiatives that will be undertaken to secure the safety, health, and improved living conditions for sanitation workers, which it admits was ignored earlier (see Shekhar 2023). But as Shekhar notes, "nowhere in the document one finds mention of specific initiatives" that have "improved living conditions, ensuring safety and health, and providing dignity etc. to the sanitation workers" (2023, 140), who, as is well known, are primarily from Dalit communities. In other words, there still seems to be continued vagueness about whether the state will protect sanitation (Dalit) workers from the horrendous task of fecal waste management. Nor is there an indication of whether the state will fully recognize and acknowledge the interlinkage between a clean India, caste awareness, and structural issues relating to caste.

While these figures provide more context for the SBA program, in the end they are less important to the goal of this book, which is not to assess the "success" of SBA in the government's terms—for example, whether purported targets are being met—but rather to explore the Hindu cultural/nationalist logics that inform the narrativization of SBA and how they may offer insights into the governmentalities of the Hindu modern in contemporary India. In particular, this book analyzes the mediation of SBA in order to demonstrate how national development logics in India today advance notions of being (or becoming) modern that are anchored in a Hindu civilizational ethos. Such narrativization, I emphasize, has "on the ground" effects in terms of excluding Muslims, Dalits, Adivasis and other minorities from the developmental imaginary of the nation, and who, according to Hindu modern sensibilities promoted by SBA and other projects—often in unseen ways—require cleansing. Its impacts also, as we will see, have particular ramifications for differentially situated women and the hetero-gendered systems of power through which exclusions and marginalizations operate in India today.

On launch day in October 2014, Modi and a host of other BJP members appeared on national television with crisp new brooms cleaning up dirt and filth in Valmiki Colony, which houses sanitation workers, most of whom are Dalits (figure 1.1). Advertisements had been placed in major newspapers over preceding days asking people to come in large numbers and participate in the launch of SBA. The prime minister reminded the people of Gandhi's famous statement that "cleanliness is next to godliness," and that cleanliness and sanitation had been dreams of Gandhi, the father of the nation. He emphasized that "Mahatma Gandhi secured freedom for Mother India. Now it is our duty to serve Mother India by keeping the country neat and clean" (PM India 2014).

Valmiki Colony was a symbolic choice because Mahatma Gandhi had lived there for approximately two hundred days with Dalits (formerly "untouchables") who were and are (despite a law outlawing the practice) primarily manual scavengers. Although some Dalits have made advancements through higher education despite gross systemic obstacles, cleaning filth,

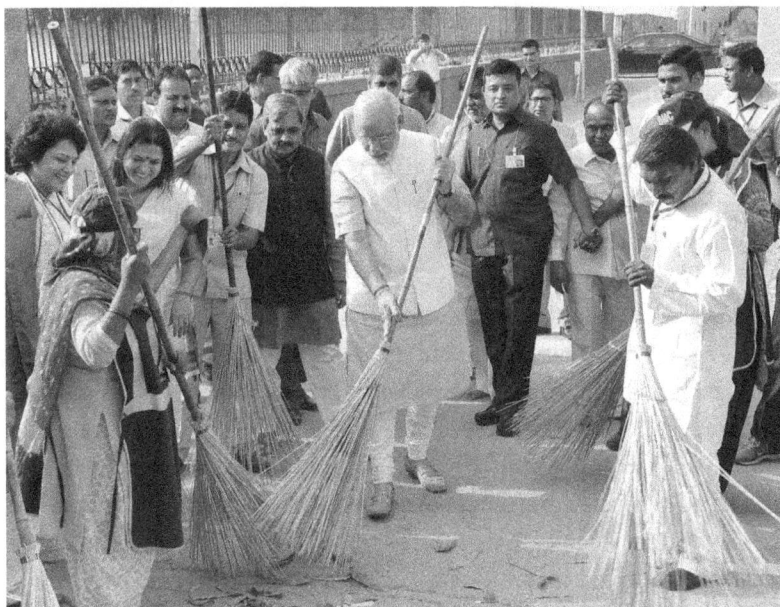

FIGURE 1.1 Modi at Valmiki Colony launching Swachh Bharat Abhiyan. This picture has gone viral and become emblematic of "clean patriotism." Photo: India Press Information Bureau, via European Pressphoto Agency.

sewers, and latrines has remained their primary occupation because of centuries of the dominance of the Hindu Brahmanical order. So, inaugurating the movement in Valmiki Colony was supposed to be a respectful but tokenistic nod to the labor of Dalits—yet, as we will see in this book, the Dalit body too often disappears from the screens of the Clean India spectacle which I argue functions to further entrench social and political hierarchies.

From its launch, Modi positioned SBA as a patriotic project devoid of politics: "this is beyond politics. This is inspired by patriotism not politics. . . . If we paint this again with a brush of politics, we will again do a disservice to mother India" (Srivastava 2014). The launch of the SBA campaign, with its contemporary usage of the term *Bharat Mata* (Mother India), set the stage for a broader project: a patriotic people's campaign, articulated through Hindu divine and familial frameworks, to cleanse the national space of filthy elements. Through centering Bharat Mata, a Hindu figure who has variously been imagined through different incarnations of Hindu goddesses in nationalist history, Modi positioned SBA as a freedom struggle *within* the nation—a struggle not against external colonizers but against filth and dirt that have subjugated Bharat Mata from inside the nation's borders. If Bharat Mata must be saved from dirt and filth, then, metaphorically, that saving also becomes linked to the excising of Muslim and Dalits, whose bodies can never be birthed by Bharat Mata and have historically been seen as "contaminating" her, given her situatedness in a Hindu symbolic order that this campaign modernizes through the rubrics of hygiene and development.

The media has framed SBA as one of the most popular movements in recent times to grip the imagination of the nation by inviting participation from everyday citizens to build a clean nation. It has invited behavioral change where people, especially in villages or poor areas of cities, are being taught the importance of using latrines and other hygienic habits. This movement, mobilized primarily through the media and social media, has been framed by the government as a "people's movement" (Jan Andolan) as it invites "the people" to do their bit to rid Bharat Mata of filth and dirt.[7] The movement has impressed global health leaders such as Bill Gates, whose foundation (with Melinda Gates) conferred the Global Goal Keeper Award to Modi for the SBA program despite criticism from many Indians—in India and globally—that Modi's government is turning India into an authoritarian Hindu nation. The Gates Foundation's award speaks to SBA's power, enabled by its associations with modernity, to sanitize Modi's reputation and attempt to legitimize Hindu modern governmentality not only at home but also on the wider global stage. In an effort to oppose such legitimations of ethnoreligious nationalism and authoritarian power, this book critiques the SBA campaign and the Hindu modern logics and governmentalities that it shores up. And importantly, it does so through foregrounding postcolonial feminist insights that explicitly challenge the government's framing of SBA as an arena of empowerment for women, the rural and urban poor, and even the nation itself.

HINDU MODERN

The SBA campaign evinces practices of governmentality that are anchored in a logic (or logics) of the Hindu modern that have become pervasive in Modi's India and through which visions of Hindu modernity are being institutionalized. Here I would like to make a distinction between the Hindu modern and Hindu modernity, categories that may sometimes bleed into each other. By Hindu modernity I am referring to a *project* that aims at

Hindu revivalism by suturing it to the idea of a "new India." It is a nationalist project that functions to secure a "developed" India that rests on Hindu values, and notions of a culturally/morally pure (and even sacred) Hindu self, while aligning that self to neoliberal ideologies, shallow notions of empowerment, and global ascendancy. With Hindu modern, a concept I develop through this study of SBA, I am referring to *a mode of governmentality or logic* (and I often use these terms—*governmentality* and *logic*—interchangeably in the book) through which citizens and noncitizens are being disciplined and regulated in manufacturing and institutionalizing a project of Hindu modernity—with its visions of a new and powerful Hindu India. Scholars such as Talal Asad have argued that modernity is neither a "coherent object" nor an entirely "bounded one" (2003, loc. 272 of 5724). Nor is modernity, as has been well argued, something that is found only in the West, and it is not only secular. Modernities can be religious in their manifestations, as contemporary India demonstrates.

Modi's 2022 Independence Day speech crystallized this project of Hindu modernity when he spoke about the aspirations of a coming Amrit Kaal, a phrase from Vedic astrology that signifies a golden time period when ambitious ventures can be taken up. Reminding the people of their already rich heritage (read: Hindu/Vedic), which will power them into the development aspirations of their future, he roused the people with these words: "We are those people who see Shiva in every living being. We are those people who see Lord Narayana in every man. We are people who call women 'Narayani'. . . . We are those people who see Shankar in every stone. This is our power" (Times Now 2022). That is, the people were/are already sacred (a Hindu sacred), and now they have to recover that sacrality to power neoliberal development aspirations, which happen to be coterminous with empowering Modi and his party. Recovering that sacrality relies on the governmentality of the Hindu modern. While the logic of the Hindu modern pervades many areas of governance, and particularly developmental governance today, this book addresses the ones that infuse and emerge from the SBA program because they not only elucidate the governmentalities of contemporary Hindu nationalism, but hint at the ultimate destructiveness—of communities, and of democracy—inherent in its "developmental" visions. By democracy, here, and elsewhere in the book, I do not simply mean the procedures of democracy (such as voting, mass elections, and so on) but the egalitarian outcomes—equalities and rights for all, especially the disenfranchised—that democracy is meant to deliver and protect. Many scholars observe that democracy today is being reduced merely to procedures of democracy instead of functioning as a "substantive democracy."[8] Hindu nationalist India today has emerged as an appropriate and troubling example of this. Thus, in using the term *democracy* in this book, my focus is on substantive democracy.

The logic of the Hindu modern does not simply marry a Hindu ethos to notions of being developed or modern. It is very much *a political logic*. In the name of crafting a "new India," it shores up caste and religious inequalities that constantly determine who is authentically Indian and who is not, and who belongs to the nation and who does not. While it is casteist and antiminority in its tenor, it also stretches itself when needed to assimilate minorities, sometimes violently, into its logics—often promising them development and upliftment that frequently rests on their deracination, which can be proven through participation.[9] It refuses to recognize minorities as *political subjects* with political/economic needs and agendas that are inherently incompatible with the neoliberal Hindu nationalist project. Rather, it treats minorities as cultural identities, bearers of cultural difference, that can be brought into (by conversion or, if need be, force) the folds of the Hindu nationalist project, thus flagging the project's seeming inclusionary potential. The recent appointment of Droupudi Murmu, an educated tribal woman, as India's president is a case in point, for the BJP has been hostile to tribal communities, not hesitating to contain their resistance to land grabs and polluting mining ventures while implementing draconian forest laws that allow forest guards to shoot with impunity.

Practices of gender and sexuality are centrally written into the logics and governmentalities of the Hindu modern. Because the governmentality of the Hindu modern disciplines subjects into new (but reworked from old) subject positions of being Hindu that cohere with new visions of being Indian, gender and sexuality are often evoked in apparently progressive ways that on careful scrutiny belie the deep privileging of a casteist and classist Hindu heteropatriarchal order. Murmu, for instance, is one of several high-ranking women in the BJP government; yet India today is ranked 126 out of 146 countries in gender parity, according to the 2023 Gender Gap Report of the World Economic Forum (PTI 2023).

The case of SBA helps us to identify some *specific features* of the Hindu modern. First, as indicated earlier, development aspirations in India today are being framed by Hindu values, categories, constructs, logics, assumptions, symbols, referents, and imagery in which ancient Hindu ideologies, gods, heroes, and traditions are actively employed in the construction of a sense of moral grandness and exceptionalism about a "new India" and being Indian.

This "new India" enlists ancient Hindu mythological pasts and projects and turns them into dreams and aspirations of a modern present and future.[10]

This offers explanations for why, in arguing for developments in science, BJP ministers and officials have made claims that: reproductive genetics and cosmetic surgery existed in ancient India, for how else could Karna (a character in the ancient Hindu epic the Mahabharata) have been born to virgin queen Kunti, or Lord Ganesh have had an elephant head attached to his body (this point was made by Modi); that the internet existed in ancient times, for how else could Sanjay (the charioteer) have narrated the Kurukshetra War to King Dhritarashtra in the Mahabharata; or that the cow is the only animal that inhales and exhales oxygen and cow urine cures cancer, thus the need for cow protectionism (the cow has a revered divine status in the Hindu religion). In the BJP's rhetoric, myths often take on the authority of facts, and Hindu mythological narratives and symbols charge up national dreams of advancement and global recognition. Meera Nanda terms this as manifesting a logic of "India first" (2016, 6)—that is, Hindus had already achieved x, y, or z (all traits of progress) several centuries ago, but the people seem to have forgotten that, so they need to recover and revive them.

We see this voluminously in how SBA discourse offers "clean citizen" as a national subject position that is frequently based on ideas of (Hindu) civilizationalism, bodily discipline, and purity. This is represented, for example, by an article in an online journal that chastised contemporary India by reminding readers that cleanliness and sanitation were an integral part of ancient Hindu practices (see Talukdar 2019). The author quotes from Hindu religious texts including the Vedas to claim this. Quotes such as "Do not disturb the sky and do not pollute the atmosphere," in the Yajur Veda (5:43), or a verse from the Manusmriti that says "Let him not throw urine or faeces into the water, nor saliva, nor clothes defiled by impure substances, nor any other impurity," or a reference to Kautiliya's Arthashastra are offered as evidence by Talukdar (2019) that cleanliness was an integral part of ancient Hindu civilizations. Thus, that ethos needs to be recovered.

A second feature is the sacralization of land (national territory), which is combined with the sacralization of forms of development. This has been a key characteristic of Hindutva discourses from the very inception of the Hindutva project (Jaffrelot 2019). It is prominently evident in the works of Savarkar, the father of Hindutva, who, in his book *Who Is a Hindu?* (originally published in 1923), claimed that a Hindu is one who sees the land from the Indus River to the sea not only as his country but as his holy land. Thus, he famously exhorted Hindus to "Hinduise all politics and militarise Hinduism" (quoted in Banerjee 2005, loc. 851 of 2549). Since the 1990s, and more aggressively in the Modi era, this sacralizing of land has moved to the center of political imaginations. It is mobilized not just by the BJP administration but by an increasing everyday culture of Hindutva vigilantes who terrorize national space by targeting those seen as engaging in non-Hindu activities, such as killing cows (which are sacred to the land and Hindu religion) and eating beef, or preventing the loud public reading of Muslim prayers in mosques on the grounds that it causes sound pollution in the environment (which has always occurred in mosques but has never been challenged as it is being today), thus polluting the land. Such hyper-sacralization of land of course makes perfect sense, for if "the people" were already civilized (and sacred) in ancient times and beyond, then their land is a blessed land. Modi, on the anniversary of Savarkar's birth in 2014, tweeted about Savarkar's "tireless efforts towards the regeneration of our Motherland" (Modi 2014).

Modi frequently refers to Bharat (he rarely uses the secular term India) as a *punyabhoomi* (holy land)—a word littered in ancient Hindu epics such as the Mahabharata and Ramayana, and utilized dangerously in Savarkar's work itself (see Savarkar 2022, loc. 998). If national territory is a *punyabhoomi*, then its development is not a political obligation but a sacred obligation. And since Bharat is a "sacred geography" (Eck 2013), that sacrality needs to be *visible* and *reclaimed*. Cultural cleansing thus becomes an easy rationale, and anything or anybody that threatens the sacrality of the land—even verbally—must be ousted or otherwise neutralized. Thus, the minister of culture, Mahesh Sharma, said in 2015, "We will cleanse every area of public discourse that has been westernized and where Indian culture and civilization need to be restored—be it the history we read, our cultural heritage or our institutes that have been polluted over years" (quoted in Gowda 2015). There is thus what Kajri Jain identifies as a new kind of "spatial emergence" in contemporary India (2021, 5). Cities are being renamed with Hindi names; statues of Hindu icons and gods are aggressively being built (Jain 2021); Muslims are being prevented from performing prayers in public spaces; Muslim (especially poor and lower middle-class) homes are being demolished; Muslim women are being banned from wearing hijab in some colleges, so that religion (that is, Islamic religion) does not contaminate public space, even though Hindu religion is always allowed to be public; Hindu prayer sites are being (re)developed with millions of dollars (for example, the Namami Gange project, the Kashi Vishwanath corridor in Varanasi, and the construction of the gigantic Ram Temple in Ayodhya);

mosques are being demolished, often based on claims of "illegal construction" (the destruction of Babri Masjid in Ayodhya in 1992 was just the beginning!); and national leaders, increasingly fashioning themselves to look like Hindu sages, dominate media spaces.[11]

This *visible* deification and marking of land as Hindu are a prominent part of SBA. During the implementation of the SBA program, the land that is to be cleaned up is figured in the prime minister's speeches as well as posts by everyday citizens on social media platforms as Bharat Mata[12]—a figure that in Indian nationalism has often been represented through Hindu goddesses, as addressed earlier. Currently, this figure can be activated to reference women's rights discourse that can be marked as modern. Once we are taught to see the land that is now seemingly dying under filth as Bharat Mata, we begin to see the land as Hindu, and SBA as a vehicle for women's protection and empowerment. As I discuss in chapter 2, Bharat Mata is frequently represented in many SBA media spaces, including Modi's own speeches, as an injured figure—that is, "the people" have damaged her by dirtying her. Figuring the nation's land as a divine Hindu gendered figure invites awe toward that land, and also calls for heteropatriarchal protection of, and attachment to, the land as the Hindu mother.

A third, and I would suggest a central, feature of the Hindu modern is security.[13] This directly follows from the notion that India is a sacred Hindu land. For if it is a *punyabhoomi*, then it needs to be fiercely protected as the original land of Hindus. Thus, heightened security emerges as a logic of national governance, and this logic is simultaneously hetero-gendered (while also spinning on the entangled axes of caste, class, and sexuality) as the nation reemerges as Bharat Mata, who needs protection, and Hindu majorities (especially men) reemerge as her protectors. Today, protecting Bharat Mata serves as a rallying cry in BJP quarters as well as in everyday spaces to shore up a national security framework. Unlike earlier, this security framework is not just operational in terms of "external" threats to the home/land but internal "enemies" as well. In fact, the line between external and internal enemies has blurred. The "threat" is frequently the Muslim body, dissenters of the government or (perceived) critics of Hinduism such as journalists/artists/intellectuals, who are seen as sullying Bharat Mata with their criticisms, or even Dalit bodies that dare to transgress the boundaries that keep the Hindu order alive. As an aside, I would not be surprised if I were "punished" for writing this book as it analyzes and critiques the BJP's pet development program, and one that has received considerable international praise.

Protecting Bharat Mata thus calls for a Hindu heteropatriarchal and militaristic call to arms, seen today most explicitly in relation to Kashmir. Kashmir represents the head of the geobody conceived as Bharat Mata (Ramaswamy 2010). Thus, it cannot be severed from the national body—anyone (typically Muslims) can be arrested and thrown in jail without trial for at least two years under the brutal Public Safety Act that operates in Kashmir. Religious gatherings of Hindus today increasingly call for the killing of Muslims or exhort other Hindus to pick up weapons for a large "cleansing" of Bharat Mata—this occurred for example in Hardiwar in 2021 (Al Jazeera 2021)—while other Hindu religious gatherings have called for impregnating Muslim women (via rape) by Hindu men if Muslim men dare to look at Hindu women. The raped Muslim women would then produce Hindu babies, and this would also prevent Muslim population increase (Asthana 2022). The potential rape of Muslim women becomes a security act!

This security logic today pervades spaces of intimacy—seen in the policing of "love jihad" and the implementation of anti-conversion laws, as well as in personal hygienic realms that will be discussed later in this book. Thus, security has become intimate and intimacy has become securitized (see chapter 3). Hindutva hardliners such as Yogi Adityanath (chief minister of the state of Uttar Pradesh) stated in 2021 that the National Security Act will be used against religious conversion. Although unstated, religious conversion in Yogi's statement particularly implies a Hindu (especially a woman) becoming Muslim through marriage (see Ali 2021)—although it can also include becoming Christian or other non-Hindu religions. As chapter 3 will elaborate, as a highly hetero-gendered logic, this security logic ultimately functions to protect the Hindu (upper/middle class) heterosexual woman as a symbol of the nation while ignoring assaults on other women's bodies—for example, caste-based rapes of Dalit women that are at an all-time high today. From the implementation of the National Register of Citizens (NRC) to Aadhar biometrics and the lockdown and heightened surveillance of Kashmir (and revocation of its semiautonomous status), India today has turned into what Chatterji terms a "majoritarian security state" (2019, loc. 7580 of 13123), gripped by the "fear of small numbers" (Appadurai 2006)—a fear that is not uncoincidentally compatible with germ metaphors.

In operating through spaces of intimacy, this security feature is significantly focused on morality—the policing of morality that produces moral panics that are gendered and sexualized with intersections of caste and religion—about the loss of culture and values that often find embodiment in the idealized figure of the heterosexual upper/middle class Hindu woman. In theorizing a new security governance in the Global South, Paul Amar (2013) argues that today security regimes play themselves out through, and secure, morality regimes—that is, we are witnessing a fusion of security and morality. While I depart from other observations by Amar—regarding what he calls "human security governance" (2013, 175) replacing neoliberal governance in the Global South—I am in agreement that at least in the Indian case, as security logics today operate through the intimate, security itself has become a feature of the moral and cultural aspects of the governmentality of the Hindu modern. Further, everyday security features also function to protect corporate power as contemporary Hindu nationalism reveals the alliance of Hindutva with corporatism, or what some call neoliberal Hindutva (Teltumbde 2018).[14]

The production of fear is a significant attribute of this security nexus. Ronald Inglehart and Pippa Norris argue that one of ways in which contemporary authoritarianism works is by whipping up fear: "The politics of fear drives the search for collective security for the tribe—even if this means sacrificing personal freedoms" (2019, 7). Dibyesh Anand further argues that security is "a productive discourse that *produces* insecurities to be operated upon, as well as defines the identity of the object to be secured" (2005, 206, emphasis added). This politics of fear invites subject positions (that also tend to be gendered) of "exceptional citizens" (Grewal 2017a, loc. 153). We can also add here *dutiful citizens*—those who are to save (and thus securitize) an exceptional nation.[15]

In India today, such security logics do not simply operate at the level of the state but percolate in everyday spaces, seen for example in quotidian acts of communal and caste violence performed by Hindutva vigilantes or even performed by otherwise ordinary Hindus in the name of duty to Bharat Mata.[16] Protecting Bharat Mata has emerged as an everyday duty of citizens, and Modi takes every opportunity to remind the people of this sacred duty. All this is matched by a muscling up of India's weapons and defense program, as the BJP government keeps buying sophisticated weaponry from foreign nations while also shoring up its own indigenous defense production at an unprecedented scale.[17]

The SBA campaign makes visible this security feature, especially the way in which it remains hetero-gendered, while frequently pivoting on religion/caste/class axes, even as it extends beyond military and state apparatuses and into more intimate realms of everyday life. In SBA discourse, cleaning Bharat Mata sometimes becomes attached to militaristic frameworks.

In 2016, before a Coldplay concert in Mumbai, Modi compared SBA with then recent military operations against Pakistan: "With the cleanliness in the streets, villages and cities of the country, the scope of the sanitation campaign has also increased. Nowadays cleanliness across the border [a reference to a surgical strike by the Indian army in Pakistani-occupied Kashmir] . . . everything is going forward in a grand way. In this second phase of the sanitation [Clean India] movement, I am getting your invaluable help" (quoted in Kapur 2018).[18] The military operations in Pakistani-occupied Kashmir were very much also a strike against Muslims (given the Muslim dominance in that region), as India's relation with Pakistan (and Kashmir) has been at the forefront of the Hindu nationalist agenda of the BJP. Guarding the nation against Pakistan, a Muslim-dominant country, becomes the same as guarding the nation against filth and dirt through SBA. This strengthens an ongoing Hindu nationalist discourse, prevalent since pre-independence days but one that has become more forceful now, where the Muslim body is seen as unclean, a national pollutant (that is, a pollutant to Hindu culture) and sexually deviant—a trope that has a long global history due to orientalist logics that came to India via European colonialism and influenced Hindutva attitudes toward Muslims. While positioning the Muslim body in national rhetoric as a terrorist contaminant has a long history in pre- and post-independence India, the "dirty Muslim" logic today powerfully undergirds Hindu nationalism's cultural imagination. It is seen in the emergence of cow vigilantism and beef bans; in attitudes toward Bangladeshi (Muslim) migrants, whom the current Home Minister Amit Shah recently called "termites" (Ghoshal 2019); in punitive measures against Muslims, many lacking documents due to post-Partition chaos, in the northeast, whose legal status of belonging in India is questioned under the NRC; in "love jihad" campaigns that construct the Muslim man as debauched and sexually licentious; and in attitudes toward Rohingya (Muslim) refugees in India who, my acquaintances tell me, are often referred to degradingly as Rohin-goo (goo is a lowly vernacular term for shit). During the COVID-19 pandemic, Muslims in India were framed as "corona jihadis"—a metaphor that captures precisely the twinning of dirt/contagion and violence in the framing of Muslims. Scholars have explored the ways in which the Muslim (especially male) body has been considered unclean including debauched, a threat and a pollutant to Hindus both in post-independence and pre-independence times (Anand 2017; Gupta 2000). By making Muslims and Muslim culture largely invisible in its mediated screens that advocate cleanliness, SBA reinforces this history.

The language of cleanliness made popular by the SBA campaign has now even exceeded the specific context of SBA itself and is being used by many everyday Hindus to express their desire to see the nation being cleansed of antinationals. Social media is rife with patriotic messages celebrating SBA. For example, one tweet implores the Prime Minster to "*clean* the decades of injury inflicted on Bharat Mata" in order to restore the seeming glorious cultural heritage of the nation (figure 1.2).[19] The image of the Hindu god Krishna blowing his conch at the start of Kurukshetra war (signifying a war between good and evil) in the grand Hindu epic the Mahabharata is one of the most powerful moments in the Bhagavad Gita (the most important verse in the epic). Here, it has become part of the tweeter's online identity. While the tweeter is unclear about what he means by "decades" of "injury" and what exactly is the nature of the injury, one can reasonably surmise based on other parts of the message that it is an "injury" to "the rich cultural heritage of our country"—that is to a Hindu order signified by Bharat Mata. This implicitly evokes the Muslim body, once again.

....

indiyanesan
@indiyanesan
Nov 17, 2018
Replying to
@narendramodi

Yes Sir We had India (Bharat) sceptic Govts for many years since British Raj and even after Independence. Nie the time has come to "Clean" the decades of injury inflicted on Bharat Mata and Restore the Glorious Rich Cultural Heritage of our country with Prosperity in All Areas. (Indiyanesan 2018)[20]

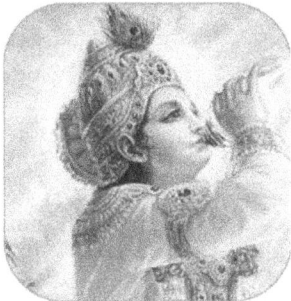

FIGURE 1.2

....

In chapter 3 I explore how security and the protection of the Hindu woman from assault that can occur due to open defecation is offered by SBA as a rationale for building toilets, especially, in rural and semirural areas. Invoking specters of women (primarily represented as Hindu heterosexual women) being assaulted by dangerous men when they go out to the fields to defecate, SBA shores up a logic of protecting women's honor and thus the home/land itself (where Hindu women's bodies and honor signify the home/land that is to be protected). Building toilets, as I explore later, becomes part of that same rhetorical assemblage that increasingly asks everyday Hindu men to protect the nation—Bharat Mata—except that in SBA narratives it is husbands/fathers who are to protect their Hindu wives (or Hindu daughters) through the construction of private toilets.

A fourth feature of the Hindu modern is its endless capacity for mediation, which is made possible by online spaces that SBA is also helping to turn into Hindu nationalist spaces. From grand publicity campaigns to carefully crafted images (such as of Modi) to the rise of Hindutva pop on social media that spreads pro-Hindu messages, the digital space of social media is populated by online volunteers of Hindutva (S. Mohan 2015; Udupa 2015). Hindu nationalism today would be unable to secure its dreams of a Ram Rajya (kingdom or state of the god Ram) without the sophisticated informational and mediated infrastructure that powers the nation today. This is what Basu terms "informational Hindutva" (2020, 157). It works through a heightened "regulation of signs and references" and is characterized by an "informational synergy" that combines a "Hindu sense of being and a neoliberal credo of development" (2020, 165). Indeed, as the scholars cited above have argued, the sophisticated architecture of informational space in India, which through its online reach exceeds the nation's literal borders, today makes possible the emergence of an online volunteer army of Hindus, many of whom through social media interactions find themselves recruited into a Hindu sensibility, and in ways not possible earlier (Udupa 2015). This enables the formation of an informational assemblage that defines the "ground rules of discursive and affective engagement" (Basu 2020, 157) that begin to dominate not just the online sphere but the larger public sphere. Digital media and its various streaming platforms and apps constitute what Ravi Sundaram calls a "distribution engine" (2020, 735). This engine amplifies the affects and effects of Hindu modern governmentality. As a distribution machine, digitally mediated Hindutva functions as a "crisis machine" (2020, 735). Via digital platforms, some kind of a crisis or anxiety about Hindu culture is generated (such as "love jihad" as a crisis, or "Bharat Mata" dying under filth in the case of SBA) through the viral spread of a video or an image posted by a Hindu nationalist. This digitally mobilizes other Hindus. The affective response to the crisis swells across different platforms, creating an expansive sensory apparatus that charges up contemporary Hindu nationalism while continuing to expand its base. With SBA, a crisis was generated via various media platforms that streamed Modi's SBA launch message about Mother India (Bharat Mata) needing to be saved from filth through a national cleansing campaign. This "crisis" and the expansive nationalist sentiments it digitally mobilized was possible as messages and images representing Bharat Mata's oppression by dirt and filth spread across different social (and traditional) media platforms. As these messages and images spread rapidly, the SBA campaign became framed largely by the media as a nationalist obligation in which citizens had to engage if they wished to save Mother India.

Further, any critique of Hindu nationalism today, or the BJP or the nation (and in today's climate the nation is equated with the government) is policed both by the government and nonstate actors. The new laws on internet freedom introduced by the BJP government that require owners of social media platforms to take down any post critical of the nation/government, to cleanse their platform of opposition, is a case in point.

Underlying all these features of the Hindu modern, however, is violence—both material and symbolic. Jaffrelot (2019, 54) makes the point that unlike Savarkar and his ilk, who wanted Hindutva ideologies to drive state power, the RSS—which so powerfully informs current Hindu nationalism—never had as it goal to just seize state power but rather to build a Hindu nation "from below" by persuading Hindus to adhere to the Hindutva worldview as well as impose Hindu cultural practices in the sphere of everyday life. Since the BJP came to power, everyday vigilantism, violence, and moral policing have been on rise in the nation. These are performed primarily by nonstate actors—what D. Jha refers to as the "shadow armies" of Hindutva (2017, 7)—whose actions are usually met by government silence (and thus sanction). From targeting Muslims (such as putting up Muslim women for sale online, an issue to which I shall return in chapter 3), Christians (burning churches, raping nuns), and Dalits (sexual assaults of Dalit women have risen in some BJP-dominant states such as Uttar Pradesh), to harassing liberals and dissenters, to expressions of vile and violent social media trolls even by everyday Hindus, there is now an emergent corresponding power structure that serves the increasingly Hinduized state.[21] Prathama Banerjee identifies this as a new type of "modern day violence" in postcolonial states (2017, 30), where the locus of violence is not always exactly the state (there is often no face-to-face encounter with the state in these instances), although it is also *not* not-the-state.[22] Rather, these "shadow armies"—private groups and Hindu mobs, often mobilized by social media—serve the state's violent agenda from a distance, and while not directly recruited by the state, they are sanctioned by the state in the form of impunity. For Banerjee, recognizing this calls for a new theory of the state that disrupts the traditional binary of state violence versus social violence, for state and social violence now mediate each other in complex ways. Although the goal of this book is not to advance a new theory of state violence, I address this issue to highlight the complex structure of violence that informs the mass-mediated, authoritarian-populist governmentalities of the Hindu modern.

While, for the most part, the SBA program has not been *overtly* mobilized by such "shadow armies," it has, however, spawned a coercive culture of cleanliness that reflects an ongoing muscular masculinization of the nation where all kinds of Swachh foot soldiers (local volunteers or motivators, known as *swachhagrahis*) and state-appointed officials monitor open defecation, especially but not only in rural towns. According to many reports (addressed in chapter 4), they frequently coerce families to construct toilets (even when they cannot afford the initial investment needed, only after which does the government subsidy kick in). The goal often is to meet the government's target for toilet construction hastily, which is connected to international loans, so boxes on forms have to be checked any way possible. The victims are often poor, or lower caste—people who are unable to push back. These *swachhagrahis* are typically upper-caste Hindu men. Evidence suggests that caste plays a significant role in determining who faces coercion (Gupta et al. 2019b). In a *panchayat* in the state of Madhya Pradesh, a billboard in 2017 carried messages threatening death to those caught defecating in the open, while in other states people have been threatened with "no ration" if they are seen to be violating cleanliness protocols–especially those related to open defecation—advocated by the SBA program. Chapter 4 will provide a detailed analysis of such coercive tactics, which challenge the idea that SBA is a "people's movement." The SBA campaign has opened another space for the assertion of aggressive and even vigilante (largely Hindu) masculinity that is hell-bent on purifying and protecting Bharat Mata.

The violence that characterizes the Hindu modern as a mode of governmentality is not just physical (or militaristic) or explicitly coercive. It simultaneously expresses itself as what Gyanendra Pandey might call "routine violence": "the *enabling* of conditions of what is commonly seen as violence" (2006, 1, emphasis added). These enabling conditions today are seen in online spaces that spew Hindutva hate, in education where textbooks are being revised to privilege a Hindu history of India, in the passing of laws that forbid or regulate interfaith marriages, in the erection of statues and monuments glorifying past Hindu leaders, and in development discourses such as SBA where cleaning the nation is equated with cleaning a Hindu goddess. The logic of the Hindu modern is shot through with violence that, as Amrita Basu correctly argues, has become "both routinized and normalized" (2021, 59). And in being normalized it is also becoming less visible and marked as it is becoming familiar; and even more so in the case of SBA, as it is given a stamp of approval by powerful international forces.

The SBA campaign constitutes one powerful example or case study of the workings of Hindu modern governmentality, offering particular insights into its gendered, racialized, and class/caste dimensions. Throughout this book, I often make brief references to other projects, programs, and discourses of contemporary BJP-driven Hindutva—such as "love jihad," the Beti Bachao Beti Padhao (lit. save daughters, educate daughters) campaign, and "women's empowerment," among others—to show how some of the same logics of the Hindu modern are evident in these other programs and discourses as well. In other words, it is through the various logics of Hindu modern governmentality that SBA articulates with other programs, projects, and discourses of contemporary Hindu (BJP-driven) nationalism—an articulation that calls attention to the widespread workings of Hindu modern governance in the BJP's various development practices and programs. For instance, in chapter 3 I discuss how the security ethos of the Hindu modern plays out in SBA by securitizing Hindu women's bodily (that is, toilet) intimacies in ways that leave out discussions of the security of Muslim or Dalit women. This is also seen, I indicate, in a different way in the "love jihad" campaigns that strive to securitize the body of the Hindu woman (but not other women). Similarly, in chapter 4 I address how cleanliness is often enforced in semirural towns and villages (as well as other sites) through coercive and violent acts performed by local volunteers who have signed up for SBA campaigns, or officials of SBA, against violators of cleanliness, which have sometimes led to the disappearance (or even proven death) of these "violators." I briefly refer to how this is similar to the kind of violence being enacted in various demolition programs in the nation where Muslim habitations are being demolished (and Muslim populations are being disappeared) by Hindus on the grounds that many of the habitations are illegal or simply because people want to remove them.

Significantly, it is also through the cleansing logic (and metaphor) that SBA articulates and connects with other BJP national programs and Hindutva discourses that purport to prioritize order (for cleanliness is about creating order). These include, along with the aforementioned demolition of Muslim properties, the NRC exercise, the suppression of any speech that signifies dissent, the frantic building of Hindu temples over Muslim mosques, the Citizenship Amendment Act, and so much more. Together they all cohere around the logic of cleansing, which is what the workings of Hindu modern governmentality in the nation attempt to enforce in its desire to create a *punyabhoomi*. It would be important for future research to analyze the other programs and projects of BJP-driven Hindutva in order to further understand how they articulate each other, something that would make an important contribution to the work of analyzing Hindu modern governmentality that I hope to have initiated in this book. Such an analysis, however, requires deep research into the numerous programs of the BJP and everyday Hindutva discourses. As such, this kind of cataloging of programs is beyond the scope of this book, but I hope that this study of the SBA campaign will provide a model of how this project might be expanded to other policy discourses, programs, and initiatives of the BJP.

In exploring how the Hindu modern as a mode of governmentality informs the SBA program, this book adopts three foci. First, it demonstrates how cleanliness operates as a practice of the postcolonial logic of Hindu modern governmentality that functions to secure a larger project of a Hindu modernity in contemporary India, and how, in the process, it classifies populations in ways that reinforce who belongs and does not belong to the nation. The SBA campaign reveals how non-secular versions of modernity are being constructed and operationalized through logics of development and sanitation in contemporary India that facilitate the linking of religious elements to otherwise secular notions of cleanliness.

Second, this book simultaneously explores how many of the BJP's development initiatives—such as SBA—are structured by gender politics that are informed by, and inform, logics of the Hindu modern. The BJP promotes its development agenda as being sensitive to the needs of women and focused on uplifting them. The various development initiatives that the BJP government has launched since coming to power—such as SBA, Ujjwala Yojana, Jan Dhan Yojana, Beti Bachao, Beti Padhao, Digital India and its Mahila e-Haat arm—are often touted by the BJP as evidence of its commitment to women's empowerment.[23] For example, on July 20, 2018, when the Modi government faced a motion of no confidence in parliament, it began its self-defense by highlighting its (seeming) record on women's empowerment. A BJP member argued that the Modi government's Ujjwala Yojana and SBA schemes have enhanced the lives of millions of mothers and sisters in India. Yet, while women's empowerment is evoked in such modernizing development initiatives, its underlying logics frequently reinforce traditional (hetero)normative gender boundaries that are etched through Hindu frameworks, thus excluding Muslim, Dalit, and many "other" women from the imaginaries of development. As I argue later, the "woman" in "woman's empowerment" is rather monolithic, as it ignores the intersecting caste/religious/sexual/trans axes that fracture this category. In other words, while many of the current development schemes such as SBA foreground a commitment to the nation's women, that commitment is emptied of any feminist critique that would interrogate heteropatriarchal Hindu structures that keep heterosexual Hindu women (and differently, Dalit, Muslim, queer, trans women) "in place." The image below (figure 1.3) is an example of how SBA is framed through the logic of "women's empowerment." Modi, the patriarchal father, is foregrounded against the background of shadowy anonymous female figures. The visual narrative centers on a heteropatriarchal rescue narrative (Sulabh Swachh Bharat 2017). This heteropatriarchal rescue narrative forms and is also formed by the structures of SBA.

In examining how developmental schemes such as SBA function as a Hindu nationalist/modernist discourse that exemplifies the workings of Hindu modern governmentality, this book also explores how the logic of *women's empowerment* and *protection* are coopted into larger Hindu heteropatriarchal casteist structures of nationalism. Given the focus on "women's empowerment" and "women's honor" in the BJP's Hindu nationalism—and its reverberations at an everyday level in various discourses—this book is concurrently interested in a larger question: How is right-wing (and often authoritarian) nationalism today employing notions of women's rights and empowerment in ways that are diluted of any feminist sentiment and are thus easily accommodated into structures of authoritarian nationalism? The SBA campaign offers a rich site through which to explore this question. Additionally, as indicated earlier, this book also explores some of the coercive practices through which clean citizenship is being enforced, and links these coercive practices to the rise of toxic and vigilante Hindu masculinity in India today.

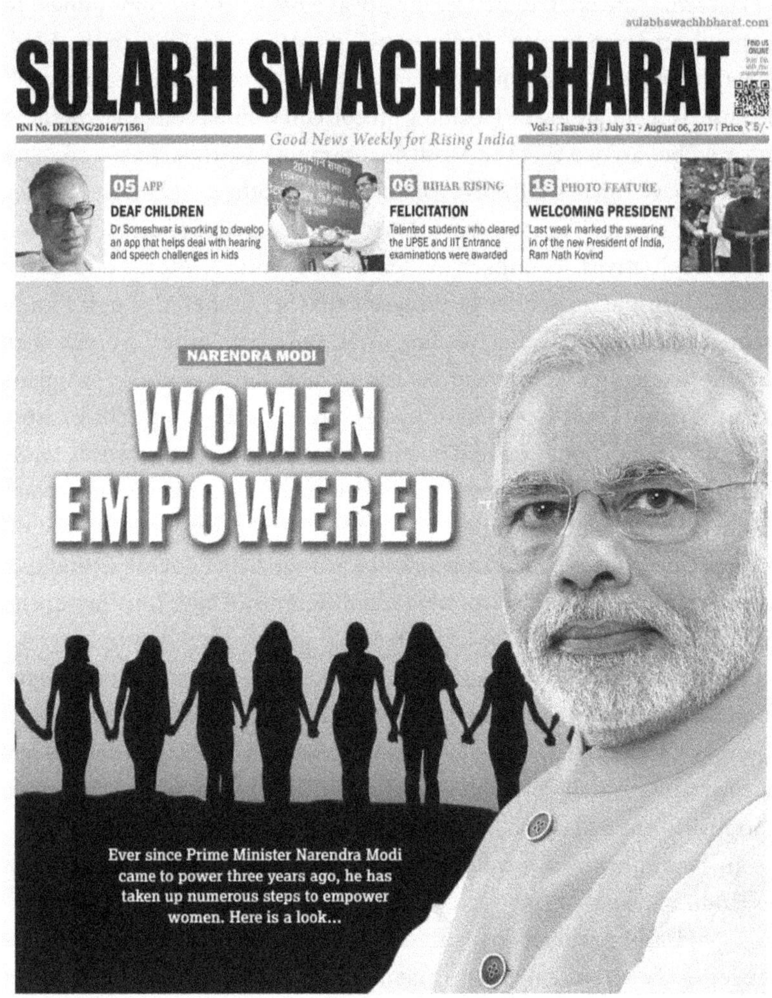

FIGURE 1.3 "Narendra Modi: Women Empowered," *Sulabh Swachh Bharat*, July 31–August 6, 2017.

Third, this book foregrounds the mediation of SBA, linking its mass-mediated cultural spectacle to everyday material practices of surveillance, violence, and intimidation. The messaging of the Clean India campaign occurs through traditional media, such as public televised advertisements and short films created by various production houses, with the active participation of Bollywood. It also occurs, more dominantly, through social media as referenced earlier, which is used by everyday citizens to discuss national cleanliness (for example, users creating and uploading videos celebrating a clean nation, or selfies capturing their neighborhood cleanliness activities); by the government (which has websites that are regularly updated with messages, events, and pictures of cleanliness activities in the nation); and media sponsors such as the New Delhi–based media group, NDTV. Functioning as a national media spectacle, SBA invites awe and devotion to the nation, and offers subject positions of clean citizenship—or one might call pure (or purified) citizenship—that links cleanliness/purity to the Hindu order, submission to which constitutes patriotism today.

Prior to the SBA scheme there existed, under a previous administration, the Nirmal Bharat Abhiyan, which was also a cleanliness initiative instituted in 1999. But this earlier program did not have the same level of popular support and enthusiasm as SBA, including from diasporic Indians, many of whom are strong Modi supporters and are lured by the thought of a "clean India" to which they can either return or visit temporarily with their family without being inconvenienced or embarrassed by public filth. This enthusiastic popular support has been made possible with SBA because of the ways in which the campaign has mobilized popular and media culture, including online culture. Billboards, radio jingles, television and social media advertisements; speeches by the prime minister and celebrities; cleanliness anthems created and uploaded on iTunes; social media updates on cleanliness by regular and celebrity citizens; short films produced and submitted by everyday citizens to the government's short film contests on cleanliness that are overseen by the prestigious National Film Development Corporation and where the best film carries a prize of 10 lakh rupees (approximately $11,000) and is showcased on government websites; video games (a significant gaming culture has evolved around SBA); Bollywood films such as *Toilet: Ek Prem Katha* (Toilet: A love story); the active involvement of Bollywood celebrities in the campaign; the digital tracking of unclean sites; and so much more attest to the spectacular nature of this initiative. The functioning of SBA as a mediated phenomenon, rife with imagery and symbolism that frequently center Hindu identity and referents and are based on neoliberal bourgeois notions of cleanliness, provides a fascinating case study of how populism, national development, media, and informational culture intersect powerfully to produce a desired (in this case Hindu) "modern" national culture. The SBA campaign exemplifies a *mediated pedagogy* of cleanliness, in which spectacular mediated messages about cleanliness often link to on-the-ground material enforcement of cleanliness by "the people" who are mobilized through them, and who in turn make such incidents viral for the whole nation (and world) to see.

The identity of SBA as a "people's movement" or a "mass movement" (as Modi and the media often like to call it) enabled through media and online space demonstrates how it is so much more than simply a cleanliness exercise. The BJP government and Modi in particular have always been astute about symbolism, image, and representations, and acutely aware of the power of mediation to mobilize the people with imaginings of the nation. This, as I discussed earlier, is a crucial part of contemporary Hindu nationalism. This book suggests that both the form and content of media—especially, but not only, social media and its online architecture—in the SBA campaign plays a central role in advancing narratives of national cleansing that, while playing out as an empowering citizens' movement, ultimately contributes to and solidifies an exclusionary *Hindu* national space in and through its mediation of cleanliness and purity.

While SBA is beginning to receive some scholarly attention—and some of this work has rightly begun calling attention to caste exclusion—there is to my knowledge no work yet that has engaged with SBA as an explicitly *Hindu nationalist discourse* (that also evinces a Hindu modern governmentality) that is entangled with gender politics and its mediation, while simultaneously informed by caste, class, heteronormativity, neoliberalism, and other intersecting power structures.[24] For instance, Doron and Jeffrey give a comprehensive cultural analysis of "beliefs and practices relating to waste" (2018, loc. 343 of 8878, 12) in India that also focuses on the SBA campaign. While this important work touches on caste and class issues related to waste in India, it does not focus on the entanglement of SBA with the current context of Hindu nationalism. While they briefly mention, albeit critically, that the "success" of the SBA campaign might lead one toward a "promised land of development under the banner of a Hindu nationalism aimed at purging India of its unruly elements" (2018, loc. 4947 of 8878, 255), Hindu-gendered nationalism is not the framework within which cleanliness and SBA is situated. My claim, on the other hand, is that the SBA campaign and its mediation cannot be sufficiently comprehended without seeing it as an integral part of contemporary Hindu nationalism and specifically the governmentality of the Hindu modern. In the nonscholarly realm, there is a lot of buzz around SBA both in India and in the Indian diaspora. However, this remains primarily celebratory of SBA, barring criticisms waged in a few online leftist magazines (which are themselves increasingly under attack). The problem is that where SBA is concerned, most ordinary people, including in the diaspora, do not see it as having anything to do with Hindu nationalism. Most seem happy that such cleanliness initiatives are being undertaken as though they are culturally neutral and as though social discourses and practices remain untouched by the currents of their times.

Thus, I found it quite ironic that it was ultimately a Hindu right-wing magazine, *Swarajya*, that lamented the fact that people have not noticed the connection between Hindutva and the SBA campaign. A 2019 article stated that, "While almost everyone, both positively and negatively, speak of the Hindutva connection to the surgical strikes [i.e., military operations in Kashmir], nobody speaks of the Hindutva connection to the phenomenal sanitary coverage that the Modi government has achieved" (Neelakandan 2019). The article emphasized how ideas around SBA draw from Hindu Upanishads and thus have Vedic authority—a claim that that once again reinforces how Hindu logics and Hindu civilizationalism are articulated in SBA. Thus, in focusing on SBA as a (hetero)gendered Hindu nationalist program, this book offers pioneering insights into the attempted institutionalization of cleanliness as a form of Hindu modern governmentality in contemporary India.

UNTANGLING CULTURAL NARRATIVES OF DEVELOPMENT AND CLEANLINESS

Development has always represented a primary logic through which nations forge articulations of modernity. In India, after independence, the Nehru government instituted five-year plans to modernize India during the post-independence years. These were national development initiatives geared toward building infrastructure for the new nation—in areas such as agriculture and industry—and alleviating poverty. However, there was nothing explicitly culturalist about it, as Nehru always endorsed secularism (although clearly there is no untainted secularism—secularism is always tainted by religious elements, but sometimes that tainting is latent and other times, as they are now in India, it is explicitly cultural). In Modi's fashioning of a "new India" since 2014, development has shifted explicitly to a culturalist realm. Narratives of development are now packaged through Hindu symbolism and authority.

Development, or *Vikas*, was a key signature through which Modi and the BJP conducted the 2014 election campaign. Since then, Modi has been labeled the *Vikas Purush* (the "development man"). His famous campaign slogan in 2014 was *Vikas, sab ki sath* ("development, with and for everyone"). Along with the promise of efficiency and transparency in governance, the development agenda resonated across the country, creating much excitement and hope. But this excitement obscured the fact that the theme of *Vikas* was frequently narrated through Hindu symbolism and sutured to Hindu frameworks (often invoking Hindu gods, epics, and mythologies). And for the few who might have objected to this, the following statement by Yogi Adityanath, the current BJP chief minister of the state of Uttar Pradesh and a Modi protégé, summed up well the BJP's response to such objections: "Hindutva and development are complementary to each other. . . . Those who are opposing Hindutva are in fact opposing development and *Bhartiya* (Indianness)" (PTI 2017a). What Arvind Rajagopal recently noted of contemporary India—that "something new is taking shape here" (Rajagopal 2015)—is indeed correct. That something new is the way in which Hindu symbolism has taken on a populist character, and overt or subliminal Hindu imagery has begun to inundate the language of national progress—both at the formal state/government level and also at an everyday level. Many evoke Hindu imagery and referents (such as in their X or Facebook feeds) to celebrate a new India.

Development narratives of a nation are first and foremost cultural narratives. Along with others such as Arturo Escobar, Akhil Gupta (1998) has suggested that development is centrally premised upon the ordering of identities in relation to some notion of the modern. Someone has to be seen as backward or not belonging to the aspirations of the nation for the logic of development to hold up—again reinforcing the notion that development is a cultural matter. Development is the arena in which "self-representations of modernity" (1998, 36) are given expression. As projects of the state at a particular time, development schemes evince an attempt to establish a logic of modernity—whatever that modernity may be in a particular national context and time. In contemporary India, as I am suggesting in this book, it is an attempt to forge a Hindu modernity, through the governmentality of the Hindu modern via projects such as SBA.

Development is also seen by many as not having anything to do with politics and ideology since it is seen as simply being to do with infrastructure or capacity building. James Ferguson addresses how development is typically seen as an "anti-politics machine" that depoliticizes everything "while performing, *almost unnoticed*, its own preeminently political operation of expanding bureaucratic state power" (Ferguson 1994, xv, emphasis added). Indeed, infrastructures are not apolitical (Anand 2017; Anand et al. 2018; Larkin 2013; Shome 2019). Nor are they, in a country such as India, secular. For example, as the SBA campaign pushes toilet construction, we know that the cleaning of public toilets—or the cleaning of the sewers where public shit flows into—are domains where Dalits work, for the most part. Dalits' intimate relations with sewers and excrement is a direct result of the age-old Hindu Brahminical order. Thus, toilet infrastructures in India are intimately caste ridden: they mediate and reinforce spatial boundaries between upper/middle class Hindus and the Dalit body, yet these infrastructures are rarely seen as Hindu. Asher Ghertner powerfully refers to toilet and sewage infrastructures in India as evincing "Hindu extrastatecraft"—that is, infrastructures such as pipes, drains, and so on that sit below the surface, unnoticed and lacking "superstructural symbolics," bear a "spatial disposition that facilitates Hindu socio-spatial divisions founded on caste hierarchy" (2018, 101).

Anthropologist James Ferguson reminds us that what is important in the analysis of a development program is not just what it does not do (although that is important) but "what it *does* do" (1994, 254, emphasis added)—for what it "does do" is intimately linked to what it "does not do" and the erasures informing that. As I demonstrate in this book, what the SBA campaign "does do" is institute an unmarked pedagogy of (Hindu) national cleanliness and regeneration of the Hindu body that metaphorically and literally ties development to a logic of national purification—the expunging of others who do not fit or subscribe to a Hindu national order. What it also does is normalize Hindu categories of purification and kinship in the name of health, cleanliness, national wellbeing, and national status on the global stage. And what it further does, is forge a vision of national progress by linking ideas of women's empowerment and honor to a clean nation in ways that reinforce traditional Hindu (hetero)gendered boundaries of belonging and that ascribe values of purity, domesticity, and morality to the (Hindu) female body through which, as we will see in later chapters, cleanliness is frequently imagined—while excluding Dalit, Muslim, and many other nonnormative women from this regime of morality.

The SBA campaign, as well as other development schemes of the BJP such as Ujjwala Yojana, or Beti Bachao, Beti Padhao, expresses what Harriss, Jeffrey, and Brown (2020) term "banal Hindutva." The idea of "banal Hindutva" (or "banal Hindu nationalism" [see Nanda 2011]) evokes Michael

Billig's notion of banal nationalism (Billig 1995). Unlike the in-your-face expressions of hard Hindutva, banal Hindutva or banal Hindu nationalism is often invisible and everyday, and circulated by nonstate actors and nonstate discourses—such as the media. Edward Anderson (2015, 47) similarly defines contemporary Hindutva dynamics through the term *neo-Hindutva*, which refers to expressions of Hindu nationalism that are not directly linked to the institutional framework of Sangh Parivar (the larger RSS affiliates that make up the Hindutva family). This neo-Hindutva, he argues, has two arms: soft Hindutva, which does not express itself as Hindutva and in fact denies and obfuscates direct connections to Sangh ideologies; and hard Hindutva, which expresses the more militant and unambiguous expressions of Hindutva. Soft Hindutva is more in line with banal Hindu nationalism, and in fact can be more dangerous in that it reflects a common sense that is continually naturalized and not seen as having anything to do with Hindu identity or a Hindu order. Thus, banal Hindu nationalism is far more ideologically pervasive and sedimented because its Hindu-ness is not seen. And in the current climate in India—as this book argues—it is expressed through development schemes such as SBA that further reinforce its power.

The emergence of SBA as a development scheme in 2014 is particularly striking. In India, spaces of dirt have always existed, so what is going on now? Why this current obsession with cleanliness? This is the question that first drew me into this project. Because the SBA campaign emerged at a time when the nation, fueled by the BJP's Hindutva trajectory, has been in the throes of all kinds of religious, ethnic, and caste cleansing through which a fascist Hindu order is being reinstated, it was impossible for me not to see the SBA cleansing project as overlapping with the cultural cleansing occurring in the broader public space, a cleansing that at times has been overtly owned by Hindu leaders. When we expand our scope of SBA beyond being just a literal cleanliness program, so much more comes into view about this development project, and development in India today more broadly. This book argues that it is imperative to read the SBA campaign within the larger context of excising minorities and the suppression of dissent that is going on in the nation, and shows how we might do so.

As a cultural studies scholar, I have always understood contexts not as closed, bounded phenomena but as existing in relation to other contexts, always acquiring meaning in relation to other contexts and the social relations that make up those other contexts. The relations that constitute various contexts often bleed into or link up with each other—what Stuart Hall differently called articulation (cited in Grossberg 1986)—to en-

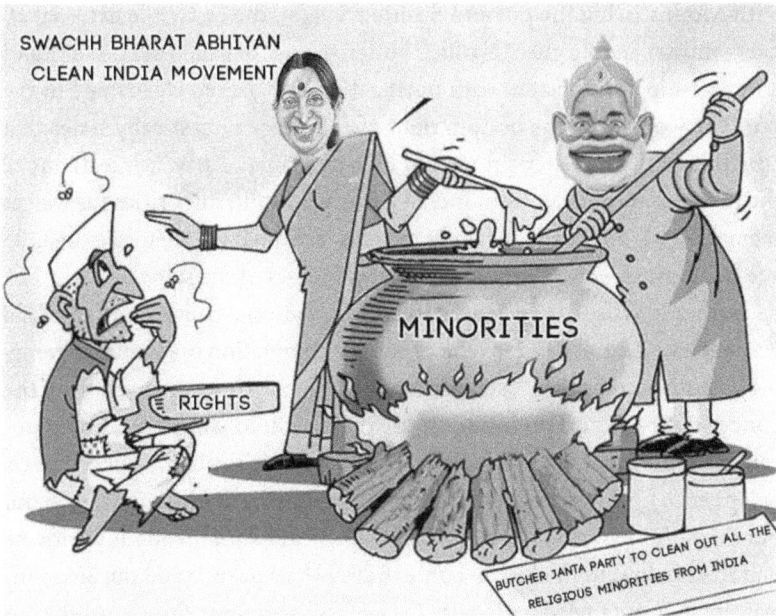

FIGURE 1.4 "Whitewashing India's religious freedom." *Muslim Mirror*, August 12, 2018.

able larger hegemonic (or even counterhegemonic) political moments to occur. As Grossberg writes, as a "study of contexts, cultural studies refuses all forms of reductions" and the idea that "any single context or event is all about one thing" (Grossberg 2019, 47). In a similar spirit, my assertion is that SBA is not simply about dirt and filth; instead, SBA functions as a mediated public screen through which we are witnessing a larger ongoing Hindu nationalist rhetoric of purifying the national body, which on the streets can become more than rhetoric. Thus, what *Hindu nationalist* work the logics and ideologies of development, cleanliness, and empowerment (especially women's empowerment) are doing in the SBA campaign, and what they reveal about governmentalities of the Hindu modern, is what this book attempts to untangle.

That many religious minorities, unlike Hindus, see the cleanliness logic of the SBA project in such a light—that is, as a Hindu nationalist initiative—is evident in a recent cartoon that was published in the *Muslim Mirror* (figure 1.4). I find this image rather telling. Cleaning, if we think of it, is often a form of burning; whether we burn garbage or clean our kitchen tops with disinfectant, there is an unseen burning of microbes and germs going on. This image links cleaning to the burning of minority rights with Modi stirring the pot and Sushma Swaraj, the erstwhile external affairs minister adding ghee (clarified butter, the use of which in Hindu rituals and worship is associated with purification and sacred cleansing) to the pot. The wording at the bottom right of the image sarcastically states that "the Butcher Janta Party [instead of Bhartiya Janata Party] to clean out all the religious minorities from India." Clearly, Muslim minorities (as well as many Dalits), unlike many Hindu citizens, are quickly able to see the linkage between SBA and national purification logics of the state.

Bezwada Wilson, a Dalit activist and the national convenor of the Safai Karmachari Andolan (a movement for the elimination of manual scavenging) astutely notes that "even the name of the movement comes from the concept of pure and pollution in the caste system. Why could they not call the movement Saaf Karo Bharat? It cannot be swachh" (quoted in Us Salam 2016). This is key. That the movement was not called Saaf Bharat but Swachh Bharat. *Saaf* just means "clean," but *swachh* is about purity. As I address below, in the Indian context, *swachh* as purity (and purification) is intimately entangled with caste (as well as the figure of the Muslim who renders impure the Hindu social order).

This book also illustrates how the staging of cleanliness as a national development program in SBA functions both as a biopolitical *and* necropolitical project. Not only are the bodies of citizens being managed and governed through Hinduized and neoliberal subject positions of "clean citizenship," the bodies of some (especially lower-caste and lower-class) citizens are also being terrorized and, in some cases, lynched or killed if their bodily practices are seen as violating the protocols of cleanliness and hygiene encouraged by the SBA program. In September 2019, two Dalit children were found defecating in the open in Bhavkedhi, a village in Shivpuri District, Madhya Pradesh. Shivpuri is an area that residents claimed had been declared "open defecation-free," but the home of the two Dalit children was the only one without a toilet. The children were beaten up by two Hindu men, and they later died in hospital. One of the attackers stated to the police that a god had ordered him to kill these "demons" (PTI 2019a). Such lynching in the name of cleanliness is not a lone example but indicative of a growing trend where vulnerable populations are frequently targeted or intimidated or lynched for being "unclean" or engaging in perceived "unclean" activities. The latter category today is also metaphorically applied to dissenting citizens such as journalists whose critiques of the nationalism of the current government are seen as impure acts toward the nation.

CLEANLINESS AS GOVERNMENTALITY

I began my research on the SBA program with the recognition that national obsession with cleanliness and hygiene emerges only in particular times and contexts in a nation's history. When cleanliness becomes a form of governmentality often other things are at work. This was the lesson we learned from the Nazis and the Third Reich. The Third Reich's obsession with cleanliness and waste was intimately linked to a logic of racial hygiene and national purity in which Jews, along with material waste—such as filth and dirt—were implicated. Hitler enthralled his audiences with talk of "cleanliness everywhere, cleanliness of our government, cleanliness in public life, and also this cleanliness in our culture . . . that will restore our [national] soul to us" (quoted in Koonz 2005, 22). Such rhetoric eerily echoes that of the current Indian government's Swachhata Hi Seva (cleanliness is service to the nation) campaign. In Hitler's Germany, cleanliness was also about making sacrifices for the nation in order to purify it. In a crematorium at the Dachau concentration camp, a sign stated "here cleanliness is a duty. Don't forget to wash your hands" (quoted in Sax 2013, 145). Further, on the roof of one of the buildings at Dachau was a painted slogan: "There is one way to freedom. Its milestones are: obedience, zeal, honesty, order, cleanliness, temperance, truth, sense of sacrifice and love for the Fatherland" (History Place 2001). This statement reminds us that nationalist cleanliness projects are rarely just that: they are often bound up with a host of other meanings and associations, all of which invite some kind of submission to a national sublime.

The cleanliness-obsessed Third Reich, with its racial hygiene project, reminds us that when cleanliness becomes a moral and national project we often witness a violent (re)ordering of social relations. As Gay Hawkins notes, "Waste doesn't just threaten the self in the horror of abjection, it also constitutes the self in the habits and embodied practices through which we decide what is connected to us and what isn't" (Hawkins 2006, 4). She further argues, echoing Mary Douglas (2015), that shit (and we can substitute other "dirty" things as well) is imbricated in *disturbance*—the disturbance of a desired social order (Hawkins 2006). The regulation of filth, dirt, and excrement is an important element in the constitution of a public self, or an appropriate orderly (and pure) modern national self. The desire for national purity was at the heart of the modernist Third Reich project, and this desire for national purity that is at the heart of Modi's SBA should, history entreats, command our attention today. Indeed, Norbert Elias's classic work on the civilizing process (Elias 1978) reminds us that it is often under conditions of heightened forms of state power that the obsession (metaphorical or literal) with cleanliness emerges (Singapore being a powerful case in point). Elizabeth Grosz's work offers a reason for why that may be the case. While discussing bodily fluids (shit, urine, spit, sweat), Grosz argues that because they "betray a certain irreducible materiality" they "assert the priority of the body over subjectivity," and thus "level differences" (Grosz 1994, 194). They remind us that we all exhibit bodily functions, we all possess waste matter on and in our bodies, we all leak waste. One person's shit is no different from another's. Thus, during times of heightened state power especially, it becomes important to *deny this sameness* of bodily dirt in order to keep alive, and even intensify, social hierarchies whereby some populations bear the burden of being seen as dirt or dirty—and hence to be regulated, exterminated or eradicated in various ways—and others not. We cannot forget how the construction of Jews as dirty—lice-infected and more—played a role in justifying their extermination in the Holocaust.

Tulasi Srinivas (2002) reminds us that in the Indian context, concepts of cleanliness have been historically and intrinsically tied to the ritual purity of Hinduism that simultaneously evokes caste. Unlike in Europe (for the most part at least), in India, cleanliness was never a secular notion. Thus, one cannot discuss cleanliness in India without recognizing its situatedness in rituals of Hindu purity in which both gender and caste intersect. Similarly, Louis Dumont's influential study of the caste system shows how the opposition between pure and impure has been integral to the separation and hierarchy of castes (Dumont 1981). While Dumont has been critiqued for evacuating issues of power and the political in his exploration of caste, his work is still central to recognizing how ideas of im/purity are woven into caste as well as gender. Anupama Rao, in contrast, explicitly emphasizes the political in understanding caste when she notes how, in pre-independence years, a compromise between the Congress radicals and nationalist social reformers—who refused to politicize caste—led to "defining untouchability as a matter of hygiene and personal cleanliness" (and *not* power and structural hierarchy) while at the same time this compromise undertook projects of religious inclusion (Rao 2009, 269–70).

An example from contemporary India under the BJP demonstrating that cleanliness and notions of Hindu purity are intrinsically linked in India is the recent 2019 Sabarimala protests. Sabarimala is a temple in south

India where female devotees of menstruating ages have been historically prevented from visiting as their bodies are seen as unclean. In 2018, the Supreme Court of India overturned the centuries-long ban on entry into Sabarimala of women aged ten to fifty (that is, of menstruating age and therefore "impure"), but priests and many locals fought hard to prevent women from entering the temple. Modi and the BJP government remained silent over this situation for a long time, causing a national outcry among many protesting women's groups. When the BJP did speak—against a crackdown by the Kerela government against those who defied the Supreme Court verdict—they issued a warning to the local left government against allowing women to enter the temple.

The Sabarimala incident reveals how women are forced to bear contradictory burdens in nationalism: they are seen as both unclean—due to menstruation (Grosz 1994) or because of their involvement with domestic labor, which is simultaneously classed—and expected to be pure embodiments of the nation/family.[25] This contradiction becomes complicated when refracted through the lenses of caste, class, and sexuality. In dominant Indian national culture, it is typically upper-middle-class heteronormative Hindu women who tend to be represented as clean and pure—although when menstruating they become unclean—while lower-class Hindu women's bodies (such as those of domestic servants engaged in cleanliness at home) are seen as filthy (in many homes in India, there is still a separate servant's entry). However, being Hindu, those lower-classed female bodies can *sometimes* be redeemed along the axis of cleanliness (or through a neoliberal striving to become richer). This assimilative mobility, however, is completely denied to Dalit women. Dalit women, however, can *never* be seen as clean and pure (menstruating or not) due to their caste outsider status that historically positions them as always "dirty." This reveals how their bodies ironically do not bear this contradiction, for this contradiction— while coercive in its own way—speaks more to the contradictory containment of the Hindu upper/middle class/caste woman's body.

On the other hand, Muslim women in India—historically associated with courtesans and prostitutes—represent "dirty" bodies polluting Hindu culture, for it is through them that the nation can slip into otherness. This has emerged as a powerful logic today, as referenced earlier, as calls for raping and impregnating Muslim women by Hindus are being heard openly in public. Trans and queer people, on the other hand, occupy a position that Bacchetta refers to as "queer ambiguity" (2019, 391). Trans and queer folks who are upper caste or Islamophobic are finding a space of acceptance today (however fraught that might be) in Hindu culture (and the supposed purity it signifies), while Dalit or Muslim or lower-caste queers and their trans populations continue to suffer as impure subjects, often triply impure—women, trans/queer, Dalit (or Muslim). Transgender demigoddess Laxmi Tripathi, a dominant caste Brahmin and hardened Hindu fundamentalist, is a case in point of this acceptance. This reveals how Hindu nationalism today, in order to signal its queer and trans-inclusive potential, sometimes relies on images of bigender or transgender divinity in ancient Hindu culture (Bacchetta 2019), which are not attached to any guarantees of health and safety for actual sexual minority communities.

My argument that SBA is, first and foremost, a Hindu nationalist modernist project, is indebted to many influential scholars who have, in various ways, examined the relationship between cleanliness/hygiene, the production of social distinctions, and the articulation of the sacred. Anthropologist Mary Douglas famously argues that dirt is matter out of place: "Dirt then, is never a unique, isolated event. Where there is dirt there is system. Dirt is the by-product of systematic ordering and classification of matter, in so far as ordering involves rejecting inappropriate elements. This idea of dirt takes us straight into the field of symbolism and promises a link-up with more obviously symbolic systems of purity" (Douglas 2015, 36). Similarly, Dominique Laporte notes that "civilization despises odor and will oust it with increased ferocity as power strives to close the gap between itself and *divine purity*" (Laporte 2002, 84, emphasis added). Others such as Michael Taussig (1999) remind us that defacement—the spoiling of something—reveals the thing that is being defaced as sacred, and thus imbues it with power. Not every act of defacement, however, is seen as defacement. If I go to a slum in Kolkata and deface something there, or someone urinates there, these acts may not cause a hue and cry, for the slum is already outside notions of purity and cleanliness. The concern with defacement then also expresses a concern with or a desire for the sacred. This is the logic that was probably in the mind of the painter who painted public government walls in the state of Uttar Pradesh with the image of the god Ram to discourage urination on the wall. You cannot deface the wall for Ram lives here!

Anne McClintock (1995) addresses how a logic of discrimination often emerges when those who are most empowered within a social order feel this order is being threatened. In her discussion of imperialism, she argues that soap in the British Empire did not flourish when imperialism was at its peak. Rather, its commercial emergence occurred when "the uncertain boundaries of class, gender and race identity in a social order felt to be threatened" by slums, social agitation, anticolonial resistance and economic upheavals (1995, 211). Serving as a fetish, soap as a "regime of domestic hygiene" was seen as something "that could restore the threatened potency of the imperial body politic" (1995, 211) by reconstituting the self through the reordering of distinctions.[26] Clearly, then, the distinctions afforded by cleanliness are not universal but derive their meanings often from the anxieties of a threatened social order and the rewriting of cultural boundaries that occurs because of those anxieties.[27] These anxieties are often tied to the production of an outside—and the bodies that inhabit that outside—that is seen as unruly and uncivilized in relation to that which has to be protected inside. In his widely cited essay on garbage, modernity, and the bazaar, Dipesh Chakrabarty makes this point cogently:

> In contrast to the ritually enclosed inside, then, the outside, for which we have used the bazaar as a paradigm, has a deeply ambiguous character. . . . It is not subject to a single set of (enclosing) rules and rituals defining a community. . . . All that do not belong to the "inside" (family/kinship/community) lie there, cheek by jowl, in unassorted collection, violating rules of mixing: from faeces to prostitutes. It is, in other words, a place against which one needs protection. (Chakrabarty 1992, 543)

Charu Gupta's important work has also noted how, in colonial India, Indian middle and upper classes who wanted their areas to be cleansed of filth campaigned to marginalize prostitutes—women who were seen as having gone astray and possessing dirty morals and bodies (Gupta 2002). For the Hindu bourgeois class, the attack on prostitutes (as unclean immoral bodies)—with their associations with courtesan culture during precolonial times—was another way of criminalizing and condemning the seeming lewdness of Muslim kings (and Muslim masculinity) of the late medieval period as well as "fallen" (sometimes Hindu) women—demonstrating how gender is differentially imbricated in the politics of cleanliness and purity.

Stallybrass and White's classic work has taught us that who (and which body) is seen as unseemly, lowly, or uncivilized always acquires meaning from the vantage point of who and which body is seen as superior; the grotesque designates "the marginal, the low, and the outside from the perspective of a classical body situated as high, inside and central by virtue of its very exclusions" (1986, 23).[28] Indeed, high and low—and I would even argue, the transcendental—are always written into logics of cleanliness, hygiene, and sanitation. Transcendental because, like Agamben's sovereign body that determines the law but remains outside it, there are bodies that regulate cleanliness and yet remain outside its regulations. These bodies occupy a transcendental position—outside regimes of dirt and filth and even cleanliness. They become the originary authority in relation to which cleanliness acquires meaning. In a nation such as India, these bodies are indeed upper-class/caste (and largely Brahmanical) Hindu bodies, and often also male. And, as we will see in later chapters, in SBA representations of cleanliness, celebrity bodies also emerge as highly clean bodies, as many celebrities go around instructing people on cleanliness and serve as ambassadors for the program. This celebrity phenomenon reinforces what many scholars—such as Richard Dyer, Sean Redmond, and others—who study celebrity culture note: that celebrities in contemporary culture function as transcendental ideal bodies on whom the aspirations, desires, and virtues of a society are often projected.

Bhaskar Mukhopadhyay, chastising the "privatization of excrement" that occurs in such "clean movements," invites us to put "shit and filth up for reconsideration" from subaltern perspectives in order to trouble the unmarked but always present normative body of cleanliness (2006, 227). He invites us to "engag[e] with popular or subaltern practices as *ethico political* responses" and reflect "on their sources of authority rather than simply denigrating them from the vantage point of some absolute wisdom" (2006, 227, emphasis mine). Indeed, instead of chastising or shaming "primitive" or "rural" or "poor, or "lower caste" bodies for their "unclean" habits, it is traveling a far more ethical path when we try to understand the sources of authority from which subaltern, Indigenous, or rural populations acquire their notions of cleanliness and inquire why those sources make sense to them. Could some of their practices related to cleanliness actually have the potential to subvert our (Hindu) modernist class- and caste-based taken-for-granted notions of cleanliness?[29]

At issue here in the SBA campaign and other such cleanliness movements is an epistemological (and political) struggle over the notion of cleanliness—a struggle in which some may (sometimes unintentionally) "refuse" to be a "clean citizen" by refusing the modernist, urbanist, caste-based, upper-middle-class protocols of cleanliness (Chakrabarty 1992). In his classic essay on filth and public space in Calcutta, Sudipta Kaviraj argues how such refusals really demonstrate different ways of "acting upon the world": the ways of the rich, the powerful, of those who own property, of legality and illegality, and the ways of those who defile such rules via "furtive evasion" (1997, 84). It is possible that such refusals—if attended to carefully—may reveal a space for a politics that challenges not only Hindu modernist bourgeois logics of cleanliness and their entanglement today with neoliberal logics—for instance producing a gleaming India that is attractive for recruiting overseas capital and returning nonresident Indians—but also the larger Hindu modern logics of national governmentality that prescribe in very narrow and suffocating ways how to be a citizen in contemporary India.

Assa Doron and Ira Raja (2015), in trying to throw light on alternative rationales for open defecation in subaltern classes, share a story that shook my Hindu upper-middle-class privilege. They note how Chamars (a particular section of Dalits) are *forced* to defecate in upper-class Jat fields so that their excrement will turn into fertilizer over time: "Not only is Dalit labor extracted in lieu of inadequate payment, even their bodily excretions are appropriated for the benefit of their landlords" (2015, 201). Here, "open defecation" is not a choice but *forced labor* without pay, conducted to fertilize upper-caste fields. It is these numerous alternative rationales for "open defecation"—a phrase that as Doron and Raja (2015) rightly note already naturalize certain toilet habits and criminalize others—that need to be explored and addressed in order to enable a more nuanced and complex understanding of what work "cleanliness" or its lack does in India and how caste/class are intrinsically written into it. Gatade, for instance, argues that we have to remember that millions in India "are condemned to live a subhuman life [referring to Dalits who are primarily sewer cleaners] in the second decade of the 21st century, so that the rest of the society looks 'clean'" (2015, 30). And sometimes, exploring gender issues provides alternative rationales for understanding the practice of open defecation, as when women in villages reportedly prefer to go out to the fields to escape the heteropatriarchal authority within their families and to socialize with other women, form support groups, or sometimes even meet a secret lover (typically these would be Hindu women as Muslim or Dalit women congregating in groups in rural villages would be threatening to villagers). Additionally, as Doron and Raja remind us, the SBA campaign, in reproducing a fixed binary between a healthy (read: clean, indoor—thus privatized—body) and a pathological body (an openly defecating body, as in poor rural villages), does not ask the question "who has the choice of retreating to a private arena which is clean and hygienic, and who, on the other hand, has perforce to live with the filth and/or stay back and clean up after" (Doron and Raja 2015, 195).

This, for instance, might speak to why even now in some cities we may see someone urinating in public. Part of the problem is that the SBA campaign has primarily focused on toilet construction as a *private activity*. While in cities a stated goal was to create more public toilets, reports have noted that when there *are* public toilets, they are not often maintained, or they lack water and sewer facilities, and thus remain so dirty that they quickly become unusable.[30] What occurs then is that a poor person or someone who is not middle or upper class cannot then access a usable toilet in the city while an upper-middle-class person can easily find the nearest decent hotel or restaurant in the city and use the toilets there. Hence, due to a lack of access to *usable* toilets, urinating at a sheltered spot on the side of road ends up being a more practical option for a poor or lower-middle-class man. This problem is also gendered, as women cannot engage in open urination in congested roadsides in city spaces. Clearly there are numerous reasons that may result in someone openly urinating on the side of a road in a city, but class issues are significant here. Thus, some are also *unable* to be a "clean citizen" due to public infrastructural inadequacy and associated class and caste barriers—a point explored in chapter 4—that make such inadequacy far more impactful for some than others.

Clearly, I am not advocating open defecation (or open urination) in a generalized way. I am aware of health and other risks that both can pose. Like Doron and Raja (2015) and Mukhopadhyay (2006), I am, however, concerned with *how* the use of "open defecation" (and its eradication as the state's goal) covers numerous heterogeneities that are linked to various social inequalities in contemporary India and how it stands in for a failed (Hindu) nation that must be restored to a pure order.[31]

This is also an opportune moment to refer to Appadurai's discussion of toilet festivals in Mumbai organized by the poor, which he sees as an expression of democracy from below, or "deep democracy" (Appadurai 2001, 40). The urban poor who often defecate without any proper sewage system, running water, ventilation and so on attempt to reverse this humiliating practice by building public toilets themselves that involve complex systems of maintenance including collective payments. The festivals associated with these—which are often timed to coincide with visits of World Bank officials, who are encouraged to discuss matters with the "shitters" themselves—constitute for Appadurai an instance of a politics of recognition from below and demonstrate the capacity of the poor to aspire (Appadurai 2004) to change their circumstances. While there is a lot that is useful in this argument, there is, however, a romanticization of the poor and a granting of significant agency to the poor to alter their conditions that diminishes structural issues and barriers. Additionally, as Mukhopadhyay

(2006) and Doron and Raja (2015) have pointed out, Appadurai's position reflects the "moral righteousness characteristic of global civil society" (Doron and Raja 2015, 196) and already assumes Western-style toilets to be normative or civilized and other practices of shitting as humiliating (Mukhopadhyay 2006).

But what could be wrong with cleanliness, one might ask. Nothing, really. On the face of it, it is highly desirable. We all desire cleanliness. And in a nation such as India, where public littering thus far has been quite common, creating an awareness is a good thing. I do not dispute the importance of raising civic awareness as long as *civic* does not only signify bourgeois upper-caste/class rationality. Nor do I dispute the importance of more cleanliness management in India, especially in public spaces. My interest, however, is in the *narrativization and mediation* of cleanliness in the SBA campaign and the cultural logics and related forms of political economy they shore up. On closer analysis, SBA narratives reveal a central problem: they do not connect issues of cleanliness to *politics, social justice, and structural inequalities.* And they rarely connect issues of cleanliness to a caste-based Hindu social order that has historically governed notions of cleanliness and purity in India. The narrativization of SBA assumes some normative logic of cleanliness, articulated through Hindu filters, referents, and symbolism that intersect with neoliberal logics of individualism and privatization (for example of filth/shit and thus the body itself) that function as authority devoid of context and social hierarchies.

In the context of SBA, especially woeful is the lack of any attention to environmental justice, an issue that I discuss more comprehensively in the final chapter. For instance, there is nothing in the SBA campaign that addresses the tragedy of Bhopal, when around forty tons of methyl isocyanate gas accidentally leaked from a Union Carbide factory and was carried by the wind into the surrounding slums in the outskirts of Bhopal on December 2, 1984. An estimated 5,300 people were killed and more than 570,000 were injured and poisoned (Withnall 2019). In 1989, Union Carbide paid $470 million (roughly 750 crores rupees) to India as a settlement for the disaster, but that was woefully inadequate, and the government had asked for ten times as much (BBC 2023). The US Supreme Court would not allow victims of the Bhopal disaster to seek damages in a US court, and the Indian government has actively tried to suppress "any research which proves the long term systemic or genetic damage caused by the gas explosion" and "protect the corporations involved" (Ellis-Petersen 2019). Many people in the Bhopal area still suffer from cancer, blindness, respiratory problems, and immune and neurological disorders. Additionally, there is very little infrastructural support for health, or even for attempts to clean up the water in the area. Many still have not received any significant compensation. A few years back, Greenpeace found significant amounts of continued water contamination and disabled babies still born today (Greenpeace 2010). Yet there is nothing on this kind of filth and dirt in the Clean India movement.

Nor is there any critically oriented mention of global warming, of the frequent and increasing floods and cyclones that affect so many cities in India today, which have profound impacts on human health and even sanitation. While there are voluminous narratives connected to SBA about keeping our seas free of plastic and planting trees to clean the air (for example, Bollywood megastar Amitabh Bachchan's Plant a Tree challenge), these narratives, like so much SBA messaging, take on an individualized and privatized attitude toward cleanliness. Such narratives are also delinked from any acknowledgment (in media and mainstream journalism in India) of the BJP government's heightened neoliberal policies, which allow constant land grabs by corporate entities and accompanying deforestation in the name of development.

If one viewed SBA media narratives, without any understanding of the larger contexts within which cleanliness acquires meaning in these campaigns, one could be seduced (as many are) by the cleanliness initiatives and the facile and individualized linkages made with health and environment. While, on the one hand, the SBA campaign provides a seductive screen for the nation's education about cleanliness and its relation to a healthy environment, on the other hand environmental activists protesting the Modi government's neoliberal policies have been arrested and Greenpeace is not allowed to operate in India now. Nor does the SBA campaign mention the plight of manual scavengers, which is directly linked to the ordering of the Hindu caste system, other than tokenistic nods to Dalits every now and then. For example, there is acknowledgment of manual scavengers in the many televised cleanathons that took place annually in the first phase of SBA on October 2, Gandhi's birthday, and were organized by NDTV-Dettol. But these discussions have not been linked to the Hindu heteropatriarchal caste system and the violence toward Dalits in which manual scavenging is situated. Basnet and Hoque note that SBA publicity campaigns, given their huge budgets, could have been "an effective platform to delink the caste-based relationship between the Dalits and latrines" (2022, 307), but that did not happen at any level of the program. Manual scavenging was addressed simply as a "hardware issue" (2022, 307).

Finally, but shamefully, the absence of any proper sanitation and toilet facilities in Rohingya refugee camps should be mentioned. As the Rohingya are Muslim refugees—and one of the most dispossessed and persecuted ethnic minority populations in the world today—the BJP government has not only tried to dispossess them but also to arrest them. As India is not a signatory to the UN Refugee Convention, Rohingya are not recognized as legal refugees. In a Rohingya camp I visited just outside Delhi in 2018, there were only two makeshift shanty toilets made with tin and tarpaulin sheets. The camp is on the roadside, and snakes and other dangerous creatures creep in. There is no proper water facility. Thus, while the SBA campaign keeps alive the rhetoric of toilet building, cleanliness, and hygiene, its dissociation from any human rights and social justice framework becomes glaringly visible when we look at the Rohingya camps in India. However, if the Rohingya had been persecuted Hindu refugees, then under the Citizenship Amendment Act of 2019 one would have likely seen huge efforts made to build toilets for them that would undoubtedly be praised as a human rights issue by the government and the people at large, who see the Rohingya as a burden on the state. This again attests to the Hindu nationalized logics of SBA initiatives.

GENDER, CLEANLINESS, AND HINDU NATIONALISM

One of the most striking things to note about the SBA campaign is that it is framed by the government and its other sponsors as one of the "biggest women's movement at the moment," a claim made by NDTV on its website in 2017 (Bhattacharya 2017). This sentiment is directly expressed by the prime minister, who frequently lauds *nari shakti* (women's power) as propelling SBA activities. Phrases such as "women power leads the way toward a Swachh Bharat" (Ahuja 2018), "women's needs are key to Swachh Bharat success" (Kidwai 2021), or "Swachh shakti: why more women must come forward to spearhead the sanitation revolution" (Vashisht 2018) are regularly advanced by the BJP to promote the SBA campaign. Media images also regularly highlight women or women's groups engaged in SBA activities such as promoting toilet building in their villages or spreading health awareness. And the government's SBA website and that of NDTV-Dettol frequently showcase stories of "remarkable" women who have fought for a Swachh India (Karelia 2017a).

In functioning as a Hindu nationalist text and in employing the language of "women's empowerment" in ways that are drained of any feminist critique, SBA absorbs the notion of "women's empowerment" into already existing Hindu heteropatriarchal structures.[32] In doing so, SBA narratives keep intact and shore up (as we will see in chapter 3) Hindu anxieties about protecting the nation (symbolized by Hindu women as mothers, daughters, sisters, and wives)—anxieties that are simultaneously situated in the terror of caste and violence toward the Muslim (primarily male) body. Dalit feminist Sivakami has argued that Hindu nationalist projects today offer "no vision for Hindu women except that it intends to prepare and reorient them against their imaginary enemy, i.e., the Muslim man, thus diverting her from her real struggles" (quoted in Sayeed 2021).

In coopting notions of "women's empowerment" into a (Hindu) heteropatriarchal familial protectionist logic, these narratives simultaneously reify gender binaries (sometimes with phrases such as *nari shakti*, which Modi loves to use) at a time when trans and GLBTQ populations are fighting tooth and nail to secure cultural and political recognition in India, despite the existence of a law recognizing (albeit in problematic ways) trans identities as third identities. For example, chapter 3 addresses how campaigns such as No Toilet, No Bride (NTNB), which initially ran in Haryana, encourage potential grooms to build toilets in order to secure a bride in rural areas. Young girls are told not to marry a potential groom whose family does not have an in-home toilet. This refusal to marry into a home without a toilet is seen as women's empowerment. The underlying logic is that the bride/wife will be safe *with* a toilet at home (thus empowered) and will not have to go out to defecate in the fields. The husband in this logic becomes the guardian of his bride's (and the family's) *izzat* (honor), and the woman becomes the bearer of family *izzat*. No such equation between a man going out to defecate and *izzat* is established in SBA narratives. Yet, in equating women's honor/dignity with women's empowerment, the NTNB phenomenon obscures, for instance, how the honor of Dalit women—who are regularly raped by caste Hindu men—has never been a consideration for the nation, and in particular for the current government that positions itself as empowering women. Plus, being compelled to work as manual scavengers in public spaces, Dalit women do not have the luxury to be "indoors" at home. Further, such discourses also obliterate the fact that many trans women or lesbians are not safe at home, where they are often brutalized or harassed by parents and relatives—and sometimes forced into "conversion therapy"—for being nonconforming.

Similarly, such rhetorics also ignore the fact that Muslim women's honor today is not protected just by staying indoors and having access to a toilet. At a time when Muslim families and Muslim men are under constant attack, and Muslim women are targets of rape calls by Hindu men (and even women), staying at home and having access to a toilet does little to "empower" them when messages around them constantly scream that "India is not your home."[33] It is the unmarked (typically middle- or upper-class) Hindu woman who is at the center of the NTNB campaign's essentialist imagination, one that equates (Hindu) women's honor with "women's empowerment," an equation that is pervasive in many spheres of public culture today.

Similarly, as I address in chapter 2, it matters that an unclean nation is symbolized through the abuse of Bharat Mata, and cleaning the nation becomes about cleaning (and thus reempowering) Bharat Mata. This is particularly significant in a climate in which Bharat Mata is being weaponized to suppress any critique of the nation, and to intimidate Muslim populations, often by forcing them to express their allegiance to Bharat Mata as an expression of their allegiance to the (Hindu) nation. The underlying pedagogy of many SBA narratives teaches us to restore the honor of Bharat Mata by cleaning her. So empowering and honoring Bharat Mata becomes equivalent to empowering and honoring the nations' Hindu women, while criticizing or abusing Bharat Mata by dirtying her becomes equivalent to dirtying the nation's Hindu women, and by extension the nation itself as (Hindu) women symbolize the nation. In fact, a problem in much SBA messaging is precisely its *representation of womanhood*—a representation that this book argues reinstates logics of purity, dignity, family, and honor, while subtracting it from interlinked issues of caste, class, heteronormativity, and religion, among other categories—in conceiving the "women's question" as a national question.

Such delinking of women's empowerment, women's power, and women's dignity from feminist concerns echoes what is happening in many authoritarian and right-wing nationalist movements in various parts of the world today. A recent special issue of the journal *Signs* was devoted to this topic, albeit primarily in the context of right-wing Europe. The guest editors, in their opening piece, note how global right-wing nationalisms today foreground gender. However, while the politics of gender is often organized around "pro woman" nationalism, this nationalism is such that "it resists the denaturalizing, deconstructive analysis of gender and sex in critical, feminist, and queer scholarship and directs its efforts toward reinstating dominant essentialized gender and sexual norms. These efforts are often coupled with assertions of racial, ethnic, or religious majoritarianism" (Graff et al. 2019, 548–49). That this is happening in many parts of the world is evidenced in many European nations such as France, Germany, Italy, Sweden, and others. For instance, in France, Marine Le Pen invited more women and gay people to her nationalist and xenophobic National Rally party, and positions the party as a party for women. In Italy, the far right has been very successful in winning over women who ordinarily used to vote for leftist groups. And in Germany and other places in Europe, protection of "women's rights" is often being framed by right-wing nationalist parties as protection of women from the invasion of Muslim cultures in Europe, whose values about women—for example, around veiling—are seen to be incompatible with the rights of European (read: white) women.

In discussing gender and the global right in a recent forum, Cynthia Enloe (2018) posed an important question: In what ways are anxieties about masculinity being vacuumed up by right-wing movements today? I believe this is an important question to also consider in the context of Hindu nationalism's cooptation, resignification, and thus containment of notions such as "women's empowerment." How might such notions really be vacuuming up certain Hindu masculine or broadly Hindu heteropatriarchal anxieties in contemporary India, and how might those anxieties derive from a fear of the "other"—for example, the Muslim body, the Dalit body, the Christian body or the (lower-class/caste) queer/trans body—and a simultaneous desire for a Hindu *punyabhoomi* to which these other bodies constitute a threat or a lack? Sara Farris's important work on *femonationalism*—a term which invokes Jasbir Puar's notion of *homonationalism* (Puar 2007)—has shown how notions of "women's rights" in right-wing nationalist discourses in Europe are today sutured to a xenophobic rhetoric, especially in relation to the seeming "barbarism" of Muslim culture as it "invades" European spaces (Farris 2017). Thus, "women's rights" gets conjoined with a xenophobic liberal modernity and is weaponized against "other" Muslim cultures, especially Muslim men and women whose gender values are seen as incompatible with the seeming progressive values of European, white national spaces. This international trend has manifestations beyond Europe, such as in India today.

In the SBA campaign, femonationalist logics are also visible, and the insights of Farris's arguments and Enloe's query are helpful here, even though the European contexts of which they speak cannot be neatly mapped onto South Asia. As articulations of *women's power, women's dignity/honor,* and *women's safety* constitute a larger rhetoric of contemporary BJP's Hindu nationalism that finds expression in modernizing initiatives such as SBA, such articulations secure a protection narrative of Hindu femininity *as national femininity*, and thus the nation as a Hindu nation. As later chapters will evince, in being organized around the trope of the Hindu woman, such protectionist narratives (overtly or covertly) manifesting as "women's empowerment" reinforce the security logic of the Hindu modern, and its underside: violence. Conversely, such protection narratives pivot on a negligence of the plight of Dalits (for example, there is no real protection of Dalit women against sexual violence from upper-caste Hindu men) and Muslim women (and their increasing harassment in contemporary India). A recent article in *Feminism in India* notes that the "BJP's politics with gender is callously calculated and one that ensures that women remain trapped in the domestic sphere" (Ansari 2021). While "trapped" might be too strong a term here, it is clear when we examine numerous BJP social and development projects that ideologies of domesticity (and purity) constitute the basis against which the body of an "empowered" woman is elaborated, one which continues to be the unmarked yet highly visible Hindu woman.[34]

Numerous feminist scholars of nationalism have noted how the female body—especially of the dominant culture—is often the anchor, symbolic or material, upon which nationalist projects are lodged (e.g., Alarcon et al. 1999; Chatterjee 1992; Enloe 1990; Jayawardena 2016; Kandiyoti 1991; Mankekar 1999; Najmabadi 1997; Yuval-Davis 1993). Yet, these scholars have also reminded us that "women are both of and not of the nation" (Alarcon et al. 1999, 12), meaning that while they often constitute the grounds upon which heteropatriarchal nationalist narratives are staged, and while they are often required to carry the burden of representing the nation as a collectivity (Yuval-Davis 2003), they are frequently excluded from any real access to political agency in national dramas. These points are particularly true of the SBA project.

Whether as a bride or as Bharat Mata, Hindu women who appear in SBA representations signify national space and the national family, while non-Hindu women are more or less absent from this representational regime of cleanliness. Thomas Blom Hansen argues that contemporary Hindu nationalism attempts to resolve the "women's question" through a strategy of "controlled emancipation" where women's desire for autonomy and visibility in the public sphere are "suture[d]" to a "protective canopy" (Hansen 1994, 82) of Hindu nationalism. While Hansen's point is an important one, what needs to be also underscored is that this logic of "controlled emancipation" really refers to *Hindu women*. Where Dalit, Muslim, Adivasi, lesbian, or even transgender women are concerned, there is no "emancipation"—controlled or not—from a Hindu heteropatriarchal national order. (For instance, at the time of writing, trans women in India are not covered by rape laws, and even as the BJP attempts to recruit some trans women to their Hindutva cause, sexual assault against trans women abounds.) In fact, as many others have also noted, the very few times in contemporary contexts that Muslim women have been positioned as being "saved" by the nation, that "saving" really has functioned to demonize Muslim men. In Modi's India, this is evident in the Triple Talaq legislation. However, this supposed rescue of Muslim women from seemingly barbaric Muslim practices evoke Muslim men as a barbaric threat, and the legislation functions to shore up the security politics of the Hindu majoritarian state.

Cynthia Enloe famously argued that nationalist projects rarely begin with women's issues as a starting point; rather, they emerge from "masculinized memory, masculinized humiliation and masculinized hope" (Enloe 1990, 44) often materializing from a sense of being emasculated. Contemporary Hindu nationalism in India gains its power and strength by precisely constructing and mobilizing a false sense of Hindu men being disempowered, specifically, but not only, by Muslims and especially by Muslim men through centuries, since the establishment of the Mughal Empire in India in the sixteenth century. This then leads to a simultaneous mobilization and construction of certain forms of Hindu masculinity that will and can protect the (Hindu) nation today. Anand notes that "the politics of Hindutva is one where the construction of a desired masculinity (ideal Hindu male, virile yet with controlled sexuality) requires the destruction of competing masculinities and men" (2005, 207). This competing masculinity is not just Muslim men or any "othered" men, but also seemingly "effeminized" (that is, unable, or unwilling to protect Bharat Mata) Hindu men. This, of course, is not a new rhetoric—it is this sense that led to the assassination of Mahatma Gandhi after independence by Nathuram Godse, an RSS product and close associate of Savarkar, who felt that Gandhi's support of Muslim populations and the division of India was creating a culture of effeminate Hindu men. Assassinating the man (Gandhi) who was feminizing Hindu men was a way of asserting a militant Hindu masculinity. The sense of Hindu men being disenfranchised in relation to Muslim men and Muslim culture has in recent times seen continued and violent expressions in "love jihad" attacks on Muslim men.

Gökarıksel, Neubert, and Smith discuss such anxieties among majoritarian groups through the concept of "demographic fever dreams" that highlight "the role of demography in driving politically pertinent anxieties" (Gökarıksel et al. 2019, 562). Demographic fever dreams are intimately tied to anxieties of dominant masculinities in different nations where authoritarianism is emerging or solidifying, for the fear is that changing demographics—the presence and perceived dominance of the "other"—will wipe out men's power and hold on the nation. Yet these are dreams in the sense that they are illusions or delusions, but nonetheless they constitute a real material force and even violence in political culture.

Hindu hetero-masculine anxieties frequently underlie the development initiatives of the BJP such as SBA. As we will see in chapter 2, it is more often than not men—Hindu men—who are chastised in SBA rhetoric for being undisciplined and for littering the nation; they are the ones who have seemingly forgotten what it means to protect the nation (imagined as a Hindu female body) from filth and dirt. This leads to a call for awakening these men, a call which links to the security feature of Hindu modern governmentality, as well as to specific practices of social media mobilization at which the BJP has become strikingly adept.

Discipline is a central tenet of ideal Hindu masculinity and the Hindu body in general, especially as articulated by the RSS and its associated affiliates. Bodily discipline is constantly showcased by Modi himself. We hear stories about how he wakes up early and does yoga; how he is health conscious and believes in physical discipline. Images of Modi doing yoga with thousands on International Day of Yoga served to cement in the nation's imagination the connection between physical discipline and good governance. Schemes such as Fit India, launched by the government, highlight the importance of bodily discipline and can be understood in conjunction with aspects of the SBA program. Banu Subramaniam (2019) has recently used the notion bio-nationalism to highlight the centrality— the discipline—of the body to (contemporary) Hindu nationalism, which continues the RSS project although not directly. Bio-nationalism is prominently at work in SBA as disciplining the body and its primitive impulses is central to imaginations of national cleanliness. In media platforms, including social media such as Facebook or X, images of schoolchildren in uniform taking a pledge to clean the nation have been frequently displayed (figure 1.5). The framing of these images echo, perhaps intentionally, RSS images of volunteers in uniform taking various pledges

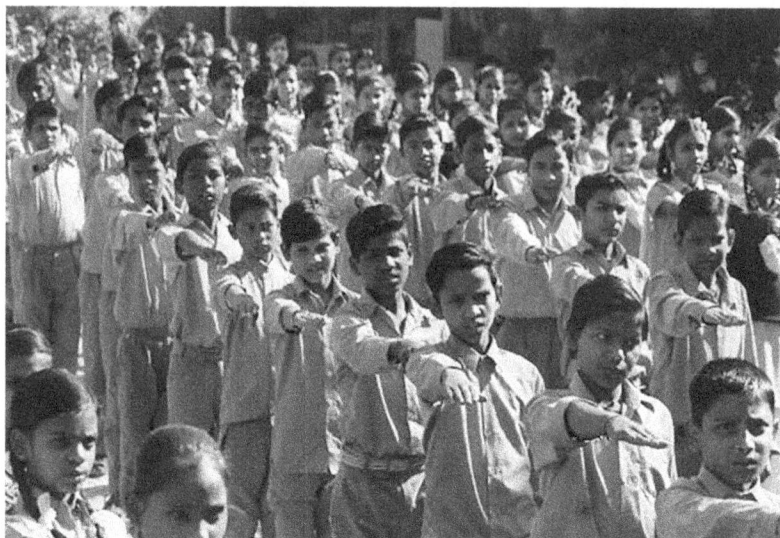

FIGURE 1.5 Children in school uniforms pledging to serve the nation by cleaning it. This image is featured on the government's SBA website, https://swachhbharat .mygov.in/timeline/activities?page=368.

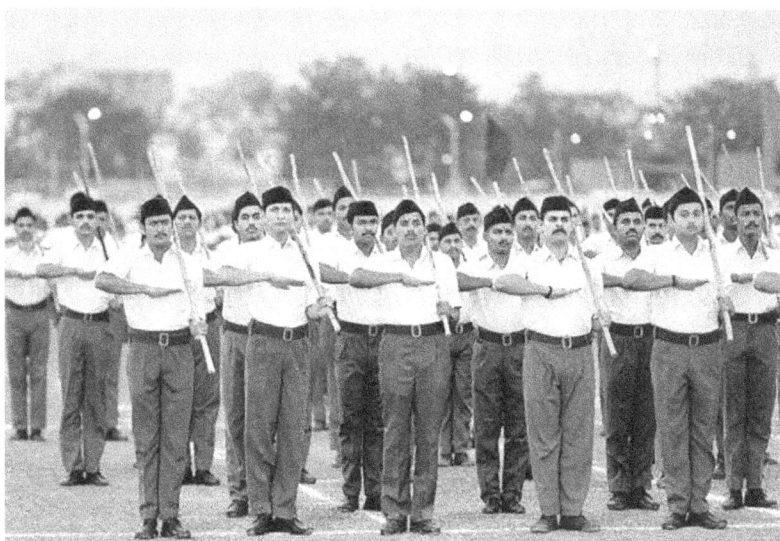

FIGURE 1.6 RSS volunteers taking a pledge at headquarters in Nagpur, India, 2018. *Religion News Service*, June 7, 2018.

(figure 1.6), as well as Hitler Youth in Nazi Germany pledging to subscribe to Nazi principles.

What I find especially striking about these images is that if one did not know that they were related to SBA, one could easily see them in continuity with images of the RSS and others from Nazi Germany. The very visual framing of such images betrays the fascist strains of the current Hindutva project, just as these strains also manifest themselves subtly in various projects of the current government such as SBA.

The materials upon which this book and my knowledge of the SBA campaign are based include a broad mediascape of both official and unofficial materials promoting the program. This mediascape also includes numerous videos about SBA that were/are available on YouTube, Facebook, Instagram, and X. In the fall of 2019, I viewed over three hundred videos to get a sense of the kind of messaging promoted in the SBA mediascape, paying attention also to the comments that accompanied these videos and the ways in which they circulated. Additionally, I viewed around fifty short films on cleanliness created by everyday citizens that were submitted for the 2016 SBA short film contest that was sponsored by the government in its tie with the prestigious National Film Development Corporation (NFDC). I studied the 2016 contest as this was the first time that the NFDC partnered with the government to inspire citizens to engage with the SBA campaign in a creative manner. These films, especially those that won awards or were officially recognized by the NFDC and the government, now have a dominant social media presence and hence are easily accessible. Some of these NFDC films are also showcased on the government's SBA website (at the time of this writing), which is an important means through which India represents SBA to national and international communities. What these NFDC films evince is how the SBA mediascape encourages citizens to use their creativity to visualize—whether through drawing contests in schools or through self-created films and videos—a clean nation. There are in fact even Swachh Bharat drawing tutorials floating around on social media platforms whose aim is to teach youngsters how to draw a Clean India map or image. These, and other social media videos, represent the blurred lines between contents produced by public entities and private citizens, demonstrating how content generation that is allied with the state's vision of a Clean India is being incentivized and encouraged. A similar dynamic plays out in SBA-related content produced by the entertainment industries, which is not always directly produced by the state, but is not untethered to it either.

My analysis also extended to images related to SBA appearing on social media such as X and Facebook, and sometimes also on Instagram. These images are typically posted by everyday citizens, SBA officials, and media networks, as well as government organizations and sometimes the prime minister himself. They include anything from visuals of Bharat Mata represented through cleanliness, cleanliness activities in neighborhoods, paintings and posters of Clean India created by schoolchildren or everyday citizens, to stills of media clips celebrating Swachh Bharat, or ads promoting SBA.

Taken together, all this provided data about the national discourse around SBA as well as more localized campaigns and representations on the ground. Further, I consulted hundreds of mainstream newspaper reports on SBA, many of which highlighted important campaigns that were mobilized around cleanliness in the first phase. Such reports provided insights into not only national SBA discourse, but also local manifestations of SBA as well as international coverage of it. Additionally, I examined speeches by politicians, especially the prime minister, as well as the government's SBA websites. All of this enabled me to derive a broader sense of how cleansing (and the nation) was being rhetorically constructed, and who (and what) was being included and excluded in this rhetoric. This initial research also enabled me to pay particular attention to those campaigns that were seen as important to this cleanliness program such as No Toilet, No Bride and the campaigns mobilized to surveil (and even enforce) cleanliness activities in small towns and villages that I analyze in this book. My attention to the interlinkages between the official SBA mediascape and unofficial realm of SBA media (such as videos created by BJP supporters, everyday citizens, the entertainment industry, celebrities, and so on) also helped me to theorize how the mediation of SBA links with broader formations of digital Hindutva governmentality, as well as to locate occasional critiques of SBA that have circulated in alternative or counter-establishment media spaces.

CHAPTER OVERVIEWS

In order to advance this book's primary thesis that the governance of cleanliness invited through the SBA campaign reveals a Hindu nationalist agenda and illustrates the workings of a Hindu modern governmentality that mobilizes gender, caste, class, and sexuality in order to secure a project of Hindu (nationalist) modernity, of which SBA is a part, chapter 2 explores how the image of Bharat Mata (or Mother India) functions in the SBA mediascape. To highlight the specific type of political work that occurs through the representations and circulation of Bharat Mata in this mediascape, I first offer a discussion of the current political climate in India, where the figure of Bharat Mata is being weaponized by right-wing Hindus and the BJP government to represent any critique of the nation as a betrayal of the purity and divinity of Bharat Mata. I demonstrate how this logic of betrayal also plays out in the SBA mediascape by analyzing videos circulating on social media, many created and uploaded by everyday citizens, in which national space that has to be cleaned up is represented through the appearance of a Bharat Mata that has been sullied by the dirt and filth of its citizens (and thus betrayed), and whose divinity and purity now needs to be recovered by excising filthy elements. I specifically discuss how it is often men (more than women), and particularly Hindu men, who are seen as dirtying public space that suggests how Bharat Mata, instead of being protected by her sons—which is their "duty"—is being abused by them; how Bharat Mata gives *darshan* (a Hindu religious act of seeing the divine) to some of her citizens who are awakened to a new consciousness about purifying and protecting national space; and how issues of cleanliness, being embodied by a divine Hindu female figure such as Bharat Mata, delinks cleanliness from social justice concerns around caste, environment, class, and even sexuality.

Chapter 3 analyzes the No Toilet, No Bride (NTNB) campaign, which initially began in Haryana but has become more pervasive, particularly in the first phase of SBA, in which SBA messaging advises potential brides in rural towns not to marry a groom whose house does not have a toilet. The groom's house not having a toilet is presented as a threat to the woman's safety, dignity, and honor for it forces her to go out to the fields to relieve herself, thus inviting sexual assault. As this chapter demonstrates, the attention of the SBA campaign on women's empowerment and women's honor—as expressions of the seeming modernity of the campaign—is, however, organized around the body of a heterosexual Hindu woman and Hindu hetero-familial protectionist structures. Consequently, it obscures any discussion of the constant violation of the dignity and honor of Muslim women (who are subject to open calls by Hindu nationalists to rape them) as well as Dalit women (who are subject to regular rapes by upper-caste Hindu men that are overlooked in the nation). Furthermore, the NTNB campaign neglects the issue of gendered labor and its entanglement with class and caste, for it is usually women (and in middle- and upper-class households, Dalit or poor women, or men), who typically clean latrines.

Chapter 4 addresses the coercive nature of the SBA campaign, where punitive actions are employed by *swachhagrahis* (often self-appointed "volunteers" or anonymous city groups), or local officers, to enforce cleanliness in ways that often adversely affect the poor, Adivasis, Dalits, and Muslims. I situate this coercive culture in a larger context of punitive populism and a "will to punish" (Fassin 2018) that has gripped authoritarian-leaning states like India today. In revealing the numerous coercive practices through which *clean citizenship* is being enforced, this chapter highlights the mediated surveillance mechanisms that are at the heart of SBA's coercive culture, which I tie to the rise of toxic and punitive hetero-Hindu masculinity in India today. I address how this is symptomatic of the normalization of majoritarian (and often vigilante) violence against minorities and the poor, and which illustrates how state violence today has moved from a state of exception (Agamben 2004) to the state of being normal.

The final chapter discusses what a desirable national cleanliness program might look like. Contrary to how cleanliness in the SBA campaign has been linked to Hindu nationalist neoliberal logics, this theoretical chapter argues that national programs of cleanliness must be intrinsically linked to social justice frameworks and structural inequalities. The chapter offers some conceptual anchors through which to rethink national cleanliness, and advances some ideas about how a national program of cleanliness—rather than national cleansing—might be executed (in India). For example, I invite people to rethink cleanliness as an assemblage. I also contend that a national cleanliness program must be delinked from neoliberal policies that result in landgrabs, deforestation, and thus population displacement and homelessness. Further, this chapter invites a turn toward the planetary in rethinking cleanliness. Overall, the chapter offers insights into possible alternatives to a Hindu national*ist* cleansing program such as SBA that has been wedded to Hindu modern governance and its neoliberal and authoritarian structures.

GLOBAL RELEVANCE OF THIS PROJECT

The SBA campaign can be seen as part of a larger trend that seems to be emerging in many parts of the world, where the language of cleanliness appears in many authoritarian nationalist projects and their fusion with neoliberal logics. In China, a toilet revolution has been underway since 2015 under President Xi Jinping and his authoritarian regime. Aware that

China looks unattractive to tourists due to its poor toilet facilities, the state has been conducting an awareness campaign on cleanliness, sanitation, and toilet building. The goal is to produce a gleaming image of China that fits with China's assertion of its national pride and might on the global stage. According to NPR, as of 2018, three years since the launch of the program, China "has spent 21-billion-yuan ($3 billion) building or renovating 68,000 public bathrooms at tourist sites in major cities and in rural areas" and is also "attempting to clean up users' behavior" (Xu 2018).

Singapore, on the other hand, has always branded itself as a clean nation, intolerant of dirt, filth, and unclean public practices. This has been linked, in its self-narrative, not only to its economic prosperity but also to its vision of clean government (that is, a clean nation serves as a metaphor for a clean administration). Many news reports have suggested that the BJP government's Clean India initiative has been influenced by Singapore's 1986 Keep Singapore Clean campaign that was instituted by Lee Kuan Yew, the erstwhile founding father of Singapore whom Modi personally admires. When the current prime minister of Singapore visited India in 2018, he noted "parallels in Singapore's and India's sanitation journeys" (*Times of India* 2018b).

And then there is Rwanda. Seen by many as becoming one of the cleanest nations in the world, the capital Kigali shines and sparkles. This cleanliness infrastructure, however, has been built at a price—of human rights violations—under the authoritarian President Paul Kagame, who has instituted national cleaning days and whose model of governance is one of "developmental authoritarianism" (Matfess 2015, 181). Human Rights Watch has noted brutal tactics to make streets clean, and documented police and security forces killing people for stealing bananas, a cow, or a motorcycle (cited in Peralta 2018). Police sweep the capital for street vendors, street children, beggars, and sex workers in order to "clean" streets of unwanted elements, who are then sent to rehab centers in unsanitary and unhealthy conditions and are even beaten by other detainees (Peralta 2018).

If China, Singapore, and Rwanda evidence the connection between national cleanliness projects and authoritarianism, there are other nations that have mobilized the language and metaphor of cleanliness to promote a near fascist national vision. In Brazil, former President Jair Bolsonaro came to power promising a "cleansing" never before seen in the history of the country—a cleansing of left-wing "criminals" (Cowie 2018). Similarly, President Rodrigo Duterte of the Philippines engaged in his famous drug wars, which many describe as a police-backed "social cleansing" project

(Tan 2018). More recently, Duterte's social cleansing project targeted *tambays*—loiterers hanging out on streets—for potential unruly behavior that can cause a nuisance to the public. General Joselito Esquivel, a police chief from Manila's largest suburban district, stated: "What we want to deliver is an atmosphere of safety. . . . We're trying to enforce against crimes like [being] half-naked or urinating in public" (Gotinga 2018). Others such as Donald Trump have used cleanliness metaphors especially in relation to immigrants when, for instance, he referred to Haiti, El Salvador, and some nations in Africa as "shithole countries" whose people need to be barred from entering the United States. In his 2024 campaign speeches, Trump also referred to the United States as a "garbage can" because of immigrants coming from all over the world; that is, the immigrants are the garbage making the United States dirty. Similarly, dictators like Syria's former President Bashar al-Assad have used the language of cleanliness to refer to Aleppo and the elimination of terrorists in that region.

One can find more instances of various deployments of cleanliness, especially in emerging authoritarian nationalist projects. However, I make no claim that all nationalist deployments of cleanliness are necessarily and always tied to authoritarianism. What I am simply suggesting—observing—is how the logic of cleanliness has emerged in recent times in regimes heading toward, or already engaged in, authoritarianism, even ostensibly democratic ones. And this cleanliness logic is often mobilized to assert or recover a sense of national order, power, or, in many cases, national purity, that is seen as being eroded by immigrants, cultural others, internal conflicts, and all those who threaten "our" way of life—whatever that "our" is in different national situations.

Such interrogations, as offered in this book, may reveal more insights into the growing rise of authoritarianism in the current moment and what practices and modes of governmentality they employ to institute a homogeneous national order. This book, situated in the authoritarian climes of contemporary Hindu nationalism in India, is one small effort toward such interrogation.

TWO

PURIFYING BHARAT MATA

It is the duty of all 125 crore citizens that the blot on Mother India about lack of cleanliness . . . we have to remove it as her son, her daughter, her child. We have to do it together.

—NARENDRA MODI

This image of Mother India is never that of a Dalit Bahujan or Adivasi or Muslim or tribal woman or that of any other minority community. She must belong to not only the upper caste but upper class too.

—POONAM SINGH

This chapter focuses on how the Swachh Bharat Abhiyan (SBA) campaign is organized around the trope of the nation as a Hindu mother—what in India is deified and sacralized as Bharat Mata (Mother India). This trope, as Dalit scholar Kancha Ilaiah notes, is ultimately "a 'Brahminic Mata,' an embodiment of the cultural code of Manudharma" (Ilaiah 2018). The mediation of cleanliness through the hetero-gendered Brahmanical figure of Bharat Mata in the SBA campaign, I demonstrate, intersects with and contributes to a larger Hindu nationalist climate today where the figure of the Bharat Mata has become the metaphoric ground upon which struggles over who belongs and does not belong to the nation are violently unfolding, both at an everyday populist level as well as in official state narratives of the Bhartiya Janata Party (BJP).

In their representation of cleanliness through the trope of Bharat Mata, SBA mediascapes—including official media campaigns, news accounts, and posts originating from the private social media accounts of supporters of SBA—articulate particular features of the Hindu modern.[1] Specifically, analyzing Bharat Mata's centrality to SBA provides key insights into how land is becoming homogenized and sacralized as Hindu (thus invoking a *punyabhoomi,* a "sacred land"); how particular development aspirations, too, are becoming sacralized—in this case cleanliness through its association with a Hindu goddess figure; how protecting Bharat Mata is being equated with programs of protecting the nation through cleansing it; and how imperatives to cleanse the nation implicitly evoke security features of the Hindu modern that include but also go beyond the security apparatuses of the state to often produce violent results in everyday spheres. Furthermore, understanding how SBA social media campaigns endlessly mediate Bharat Mata as needing cleansing elucidates the viral spread of a Hindutva informational assemblage that sutures cleaning up India—of litter, of filth—with cleansing it of all impure elements. This informational assemblage both draws on and feeds into larger Hindu nationalist anxieties in contemporary India, where political dissidents are being attacked, Muslims are being lynched, terrorized, and threatened with rape, and Dalits (especially Dalit women) are facing increasingly violent working conditions and bodily (including sexual) danger, all in the name of protecting Bharat Mata.

The rhetoric of the nation as an unclean mother burdened by her people's filth dominates many media narrativizations of SBA. Such rhetoric sets up an equivalence between the freedom struggle in India against British colonizers—when the trope of Bharat Mata was charged up to mobilize the nation against the British occupation—and liberation from current filth and dirt located within the nation. This equivalence becomes explicit in SBA media campaigns that have taglines such as "Satyagraha to Swachhagraha: Chalo Champaran," which evokes the launch of Mahatma Gandhi's satyagraha (that is, nonviolent) movement in Champaran. Yet unlike in Gandhi's time, SBA narratives come from an overtly majoritarian state that exerts expansive authority over Indian national subjects and civil society and space, including through military might and censorship powers.

The articulation of Bharat Mata to SBA via viral mediatization produces a hetero-gendered patriotic logic mobilized around a Hindu frame of cleanliness. In this frame, cleanliness becomes ensconced in logics of religious, ethnic, and caste purity, since Bharat Mata, in her various incarnations as idealized female figures or goddesses, has *always* been a Hindu figure. The use of a national Hindu mother figure in SBA discourse to narrativize the nation not only renders India as a natural familial space connected by bloodlines (that is, by the womb); it also reveals how "nationalism negotiates with the most private in the interest of controlling the public sphere"

(Spivak 2009, 90; see also McClintock 1995). But this negotiation is never homogeneous, as the private or the domestic that contemporary Hindu nationalism negotiates with is already riven by inequalities of caste, class, gender, religion, and sexuality.

The engendering of the nation through a mother figure has been a constant in nationalist narratives of many nations (e.g., Abu-Lughod 1998; Mankekar 1999; Najmabadi 1997; Shome 2014; Yuval-Davis 1993, 1997). Thus, while Elleke Boehmer argues that "the image of the mother invites connotations of origins—birth, hearth, home, roots, the umbilical cord—and rests upon the frequent, and some might say 'natural,' identification of the mother with the beloved earth, [and] the national territory" (2009, 27), what needs underlining is that it is the (seeming) natural identification with a mother figure from a *majoritarian culture* that results in the naturalization of national territory and the imaginary of the nation-state. In metaphorizing the Indian nation that must be cleansed via the idealized Hindu goddess figure of Bharat Mata, SBA reinforces a logic of Hindu origins and a "natural" Hindu family—connected by the (Hindu) mother's womb—into which Dalit, Muslim, Adivasi, and Christians cannot "naturally" fit. All this makes the (Hindu) national family imagined via Bharat Mata as sacred, and the land on which this national family resides (and that now requires cleansing) a *punyabhoomi*, an idea which centrally informs the governmentality of the Hindu modern and its obsessions with pure origins.

This evokes other questions that further call attention to the caste/class/gender/religion/sexuality nexus on which the trope of Bharat Mata pivots: Who can the Bharat Mata *not* birth and who thus *cannot* be clean/ed and made pure because they cannot be birthed by the Hindu figure of Bharat Mata or because their "origins" (seemingly) lie elsewhere—outside the Hindu reproductive matrix. Thus, SBA mediascapes evince how contemporary Hindu nationalism mobilizes and *viralizes* a hetero-gendered and casteist national form—the Bharat Mata—to advance Hindu modern logics of naturalizing and consolidating the nation as Hindu through governmentalities of national cleansing that promise national development.

BHARAT MATA IN INDIAN NATIONALISM

India nationalism has always been informed by what historian Sugata Bose calls a "mother complex" (2017, 16), a term he uses not to suggest a psychic disorder in the Freudian sense but a phenomenon in which imagining the nation has always involved imagining a Hindu national mother: Bharat Mata. Indian nationalism's mother complex has historically manifested itself through the image of a divine Hindu figure who is often a goddess but is frequently also an ideal Hindu mother or woman framed in the tradition of mother goddess (Ganesh 2010, 74). Her Hindu-ness is sometimes marked overtly—when she is imagined as a Hindu goddess for instance—and sometimes less overtly, as when a Hindu woman is represented as a national mother.

Initially appearing as a rallying cry, *Vandemataram*—"Hail to the mother," or "Victory to the mother"—in the Bengali novelist Bankim Chandra Chattopadhyay's famous late nineteenth-century novel *Anandamath*, the trope of Bharat Mata made its first *visual* appearance in a painting by Bengal School of Art founder Abanindranath Tagore. Considered to be the father of modern Indian art, Tagore's works often expressed *swadeshi* values—that is, preference for Indian goods and aesthetics over European/British ones. Since then, this trope has had a long history in anticolonial Indian nationalism, as well as postcolonial India (Chatterjee et al. 2014; Davis 2018; Guha-Thakurta 2016; Jain 2007, 2021; Pinney 2004; Ramaswamy 2010). For example, it appears visually in bazaar art, posters, calendars, and prints (Jain 2007).

Scholars have emphasized the importance of the visual—and particularly religiously charged visuals such as Bharat Mata—in various constitutions of Indian public culture. This religiously charged visuality, which has consistently informed Indian nationalism, makes "the visible" a cultural logic that Pinney (2004) identifies as an important difference from Benedict Anderson's famous (and sometimes universalized) theorization of nationalism, which (for Anderson) arose as the religious order and messianic time was waning in Europe (Anderson 2016). In contrast, in India, since the struggle for independence, the circulation of religious images such as Hindu gods and goddesses has revealed a significant *affective modality* in imagining the nation. Pinney (2004) and other scholars have contended that, unlike in Europe, in India the affective field of nationalism has expressed itself frequently through Hindu divine embodiments, or what Ramaswamy terms the "anthropomorphic-sacred" (2010, loc. 1638 of 4238), in which Bharat Mata has been central. As Sarkar has further posited, over the years "through long and continuous usage" this Hindu mother/goddess figure has acquired a "seeming naturalness about it" in national history (1987, 1). Indian nationalism thus has always been situated visually in a uterine economy, which is by definition a religious and casteist one. That is, it has been shored up by exchanges and circulations of the body of an ideal Hindu mother who is often sublimated as a goddess.

Notably, Muslim populations, even in the early twentieth-century anticolonial nationalist movements in India, were never fully at ease with the Bharat Mata trope serving as a symbol for the nation. For instance, Muhammed Jinnah, the Muslim national leader of the Indian Congress Party in pre-Partition India—and who went on to become the first prime minister of Pakistan after Partition—saw the trope as "not only idolatrous . . . in its origins . . . but also a hymn to spread hatred for the Musalmans" (Bhattacharya 2003, 12). Similarly, Neha Singh notes that the social reformer and Dalit leader B. R. Ambedkar too had been uncomfortable with the idea of Bharat Mata, finding it to be anti-woman and Brahmanical. Rather, he coined the notion *Bahishkrit Bharat* "to convey the notion of a fractured nation" (N. Singh 2017). Despite these rumblings, Bharat Mata nonetheless served a unifying function in pre-independence struggles through which a nationalist anticolonial bond was forged across communities in the name of liberating the national mother who was seen as having been humiliated by foreign takeover (and which had seemingly emasculated the nation's sons). Some Muslims, such as legendary bard Kazi Nazrul Islam, even composed songs devoted to Bharat Mata during the struggle for independence.

If the nation is an invention (Hobsbawm 1983) whose constructedness or inventions of traditions occur through repetitions, then Bharat Mata has been one of the most repetitive constructs through which the nation has been naturalized as sacred (a Hindu sacred) over time. Yet, a paradox is that the very naturalization of the nation as a sacred space through figures such as Bharat Mata or other Hindu goddesses is betrayed as a *construction* when we accept that this national sacrality has always been *partial* for it cannot, by its very embodiment in a Hindu goddess/figure, bring into the folds of its sacrality those bodies to which the Bharat Mata typically cannot be a mother; although, as indicated earlier, recent moves by the BJP and the Rashtriya Swayamsevak Sangh (RSS), a Hindu nationalist organization, have attempted to integrate some minorities into the Hindutva project, primarily to secure votes—but without upsetting the caste/religion hierarchy (Gupta 2021).

While the Bharat Mata figure was charged up for anticolonial purposes in the Indian nationalist movement against the British, it was not always at the forefront of state discourse following India's independence. During the Nehru years, a conscious attempt was made to not imagine the nation in terms of Hindu goddesses, consistent with Nehru's secularist agenda. Nehru was careful in immediate post-independence India not to irritate minority Muslim populations, given the Hindu-Muslim tensions that had informed the birth of the new nation. While organizations such as the RSS and more broadly the Sangh Parivar (a collection of Hindu nationalist organizations) have always articulated their right-wing Hindu agenda through an invocation to Bharat Mata in post-independence India, the Sangh's agenda was not as mainstream in post-independence India as it is today. It is only with the gradual rise to prominence of Sangh ideologies in the later years of the 1980s, when the BJP party was also gradually coming into power, and then continuing in the 1990s and early 2000s, that the BJP's stronghold was asserted in various parts of the nation. It is around this time that various Hindu figures and myths slowly but surely began to creep into and dominate the mainstream of late twentieth-century postcolonial India. Mass media played an important role in this development. Rajagopal (2001) has demonstrated how the rise of Hindu religious epics in the late 1980s and early 1990s such as the Ramayana and Mahabharata, televised by the state-owned broadcaster Doordarshan, coincided with the gradual rise of Hindutva.[2] The final thrust of the mainstreaming of Hindutva (soft and hard) has become evident only now since the ascendancy of the Modi-led BJP government and its agenda to create a Hindu Rashtra, or nation.

Even as the trope of Bharat Mata existed in Indian national consciousness ever since the struggle for independence—conferring a divine legitimacy to the nation despite claims to secularism in the post-independence Nehruvian years—the ideologies associated with figure of the Bharat Mata, as scholars have noted, have never been fixed. As Geeti Sen notes, Bharat Mata "has continued to transform, adapting to differing political agendas" (2002, 173). In other words, *what* nationalist work the trope has performed in different times has to be understood through attention to the context of the times. We cannot understand the politics of Bharat Mata outside the context within which it is performing ideological labor and being articulated to a particular national order. Thus, to explore *what* work the presence of Bharat Mata in SBA campaigns performs, it is necessary to first understand how the figure of Bharat Mata functions *today* in the larger political and social climate of India.

BHARAT MATA'S FUNCTIONING TODAY

There are three main differences that distinguish Bharat Mata in the contemporary landscape of India from earlier independence struggles. These differences are important to note to better understand how the figure of Bharat Mata works in and through SBA mediascapes. These differences also embody specific features of the Hindu modern that pervade the contemporary Indian polity that has produced the SBA program, and that is being frequently cleansed, covertly or overtly, by its methods of governmentality.

One difference from the earlier anticolonial era is Bharat Mata's heightened presence in social media today, where everyday citizens can create images of Bharat Mata and attach them to patriotic or Hindutva messages and handles. That is, the deployment of Bharat Mata today does not just occur in official state narratives or in media industries such as Bollywood and commercial art. Social media has enabled Bharat Mata's presence to become more pervasively quotidian and mundane given the scale of social media and the speed with which it moves. Mankekar and Carlan (2019) argue that today's digital media, in conjunction with other forms of media, plays a big role in remediating nationalism as visceral and viral. That is, digital media not only propagates virality, but this virality can be productive of deep affective responses, including nationalist ones. As Hindu figures such as Bharat Mata move speedily through digital platforms, the intensity of the affective field secured by such figures becomes much stronger than previously when Bharat Mata resided in fixed pictorial forms. Thus, today through social media the trope of Bharat Mata more easily—and with greater immediacy—solicits and invites charged national affects.

Social media and its digital platforms enable a speedier "distribution of the [Hindu] sensible" (Rancière 2004, 13) through enabling the creation, sharing, liking, and commenting on the figure Bharat Mata via networks that participatory social media practices help organize. Facebook alone has public groups devoted to Bharat Mata with names such as Bharat Mata Ki Jai, Jai Bharat Mata, Jai Hind Bharat Mata, and Hamari Bharat Mata (Our Bharat Mata), among others. Users of X regularly communicate (sometimes with the prime minister himself) by invoking Bharat Mata to express pride about the nation. For instance, while celebrating India's various achievements in the recent 2021 Olympics, congratulatory messages were frequently framed by Bharat Mata Ki Jai. So, Bharat Mata has a solid online presence that is now also user-generated (and not just state-generated) and has become "viral and visceral" (Mankekar and Carlan 2019, 203).

Recent scholarship on social media argues that the speedy transmission of messages via social media is not simply a matter of the technical infrastructure of digital platforms (Gray 2015; Jenkins et al. 2013; Mankekar and Carlan 2019). There is much more going on. Bishnupriya Ghosh writes that "social media platforms are affect-machines. They amplify political affects" (2020, 11). Herman Gray further argues that the spreadability of social media evokes feelings that "exceed the legibility of [the] semiotic meaning" of an image or video (2015, 1108). Because of the level of direct participation enabled by everyday citizens (for instance, the act of creating and uploading nationalist messages, and the act of liking and sharing them), social media allows a greater production of fandom or attachment toward devotional objects such as Bharat Mata because there is an immediate intimacy with the content (Jenkins et al. 2013). It is much easier to become a fan or lover of an object (in this case Bharat Mata, or more largely, the nation as embodied by her) when one has direct ability to create, share, or spread media content about that devotional or loved object. Indeed, social media today enables all types of mediated activism, and in this context, the marrying of cleanliness to Hindu referents, values, and logics in SBA imbues the campaign with potential virality. However, "Hindutva online" (Udupa 2019, 3148) is not a monolith, as people from diverse backgrounds (often anonymously) engage in it; this means that supporters of Hindutva are not just from hardened Hindu heartlands as our stereotypes might have it. They can be urban, highly educated, modern, English-speaking, and in white-collar jobs, just as they can be in semirural areas, without much education (especially Western), traditional, and employed in low-level (or nonurban but well paying) work. Yet the majority of them typically have various degrees of access to social media. The point is that Hindutva online (and offline) crosses various demographic borders in securing an otherwise heterogeneous internet space as a homogeneous Hindu "affect machine" that is also a political machine.

The second difference—and an important political one—is that today Bharat Mata is often portrayed in dominant public discourse as being attacked *not* by an external enemy but frequently by her own citizens (her "children") who (seemingly) disrespect her and thus fail to protect her honor. Thus, she must be protected from within. How this message connects to specific security logics of the Hindu modern governmentality, where securitization has turned inward, will be further discussed in later chapters, but here it is important to note how this difference encapsulates what Tapati Guha-Thakurta terms an "epistemic transference" of the Bharat Mata trope from earlier anticolonial nationalist movements against the British to present times: "The nation is now an object of *enforced loyalty*, calling for a new pedagogy of patriotism and citizenship. Perhaps the greatest irony lies in the way the charge of 'sedition' has passed from the colonial state which used it against these mythic pictorial allegories of the motherland to the nation-state which is now turning it against all who refuse to offer their homage to this icon" (2016, emphasis added). Similarly, Geeti Sen contends that in anticolonial struggles against the British, Bharat Mata was "invented to effect national unity" against British colonizers (2002, 173). But today, with the hardening of Hindu nationalism, she is used to "effect *religious unity*" (2002, 173, original emphasis), particularly against internal threats.

The third difference is that in contemporary India under the BJP, Bharat Mata has acquired a new currency whereby it is used to discipline dissidents and those who are not seen as being a part of the Hindu national space (Muslims, Dalits, Adivasis, and more). This is another example of the security feature of the Hindu modern whose underside is increasingly violence—toward anyone seen as antinational. Today, under the BJP and an increasingly violent Hindutva, Bharat Mata terrorizes the nation's "others." In contemporary India, if you do not cry or hail Bharat Mata when there is a demand for it (at national or public events, or when you are bullied by Hindutva goons, as many Muslims and Dalits, and increasingly Christians, are), or if you critique its growing pervasiveness in the polity, you risk being branded a traitor. Thus, you need to be taught a lesson in the name of Bharat Mata. It is this teaching of a lesson in the name of Bharat Mata today that is different from the way in which the trope functioned in anticolonial independence struggles. Anticolonial nationalists during independence struggle against the British did not use the trope of Bharat Mata to attack fellow citizens. Nor did they use it explicitly to institute a religious Hindu order, although clearly as suggested earlier, Hindu-ness has always informed Indian nationalism. Today, Bharat Mata has acquired a necropolitical potential that is a significant departure from earlier times. And this necropolitical potential is amplified especially at intersections of gender, religion, and caste, for it is often in the name of protecting national honor personified through an ideal Hindu mother figure such as Bharat Mata or a Hindu woman (and never a Dalit or Muslim woman) that violence is used to target "others" who seemingly threaten this honor. Thus, violence is conceptualized and justified as a form of filial protection of (Hindu) womanly (thus national familial) honor.

For instance, in October 2021 Arbaz Mullah, a Muslim in Karnataka, was found dismembered and killed for being in a relationship with a Hindu girl. Allegedly, he was killed by the Ram Sene, a right-wing Hindutva outfit (*Hindu* 2021b). In 2019, in Barpeta in the state of Assam, some Muslim youths were thrashed by a little-known Hindu right-wing organization that forced them to utter "Bharat Mata ki Jai," "Pakistan Murdabad" and "Jai Shri Ram" (PTI 2021b). In 2018, in Muzzafarnagar in Uttar Pradesh, a Dalit youth was violently beaten by three men and forced to chant "Jai Mata Di," another variant of Bharat Mata (Firstpost 2018). Dalits are regularly targeted by cow protectionists today as some Dalit work involves skinning dead cows and cows are seen as a mother figure in the Hindu social order. And then there is the horrific Kathua case: an eight-year-old nomadic Muslim girl from Kashmir was gang-raped and then killed by Hindu goons. Many Hindu nationalists—including some officials from the BJP—rallied in support of the accused with the national flag in their hands, chanting "Jai Shri Ram," "Bharat Mata Ki Jai" (glory to the mother) and "Vandemataram" (Hail Mother).

That any perceived betrayal to the Hindu order is seen as a betrayal to Bharat Mata was most visibly evidenced in a case involving Jawaharlal Nehru University, a premier research university. Students' (as well as some professors') protests of various state and Hindutva practices met with arrests. Defending the government crackdown on the university, Union Minister Smriti Irani stated that the nation will never tolerate any insult to Bharat Mata (PTI 2016a). Expressing loyalty to Bharat Mata is tantamount to saying that that you are a faithful son or daughter of the nation—that you belong to the national family that coheres around Bharat Mata. In the rhetoric of BJP and RSS leaders, the nation embodied in Bharat Mata thus precedes the social. As Nivedita Menon writes:

> If the Nation is a body—the body of one's own mother—then it precedes its children; or is constituted by its children. . . . From this . . . follow[s] the implied hierarchies of birth and origin among the children. . . . From this follows the idea that the children cannot leave the mother, for that implies amputation, the dismembering of the maternal body, an act that none can survive—neither the mother nor the children. (2017)

Given this charged political climate, in which Bharat Mata as a Hindu mother figure is weaponized to demand loyalty to an increasingly authoritarian Hindu national order and state, the voluminous presence of the Bharat Mata trope in SBA narratives today demands deeper investigation.

BHARAT MATA IN THE SBA MEDIASCAPE

I now return to the SBA mediascape to examine how the trope of Bharat Mata is being organized, how it is circulating, and how the SBA social media space—in linking Bharat Mata to a pedagogy of national cleanliness—puts forth a larger narrative about the nation. This narrative is that the nation is being betrayed by its own citizens, especially Hindu sons, who have seemingly forgotten their duty of protecting Bharat Mata, specifically from dirt and impurity. Citizens, therefore, must now redeem themselves through cleansing and purifying the nation.

In my research on the utilization of the trope of Bharat Mata in the SBA mediascape, I analyzed campaigns in multiple media, but in keeping with the importance of the visual realm and the phenomenon of virality to contemporary Hindu modern governance, I focused primarily on videos that were uploaded on and shared across non-encrypted social media platforms such as YouTube, Facebook, and X.[3] Some of the videos on social media are the creations of everyday citizens. Others are advertising campaigns produced by corporate advertising companies, some of which were selected by the government to produce professional quality ads for the SBA program, including some first released on television, that became widely shared via social media. Some videos fall in an in-between category (between private and government), such as in the case of private citizen videos produced for government-sponsored contests managed by the National Film Development Corporation.

Because my initial research and readings on SBA (including many of Modi's speeches at and around the time of the launch of the campaign) had already helped me realize that the entire SBA program was being anchored by the figure of Bharat Mata, I then narrowed my search by juxtaposing the phrase Swachh Bharat (or at times Clean India) with the terms Bharat Mata, Mother India, Goddess, and Mother. Unsurprisingly there were overlaps across platforms. While there are many videos that frequently use a female figure to represent the nation or cleanliness, I particularly scanned available videos (over thirty) that *overtly* employed Bharat Mata or a mother (or at times a goddess) figure to connect to cleanliness and hygiene. For inclusion in this chapter, I selected four representative video campaigns that have a strong social media presence (at the time of writing) and best capture the larger rhetorical logics through which Bharat Mata is equated with the national body that has to be cleansed.

Papacharissi argues that stories on social media "collaboratively networked together" through different platforms produce "soft structures of feeling" (2014, 32). As she states, "technologies may network us, but it is our stories, emergent in these structures of feeling that connect us (or disconnect us, for that matter)" (quoted in Jenkins 2015). Having said this, it is important to note that, in the case of Bharat Mata and cleanliness, the ability to share and circulate content and stories in social media is not that open. The networked production and distribution of Bharat Mata in SBA social media space produce soft structures of nationalist feelings that secure a Hindu sensibility toward cleanliness that is dangerous in its exclusions. My research on the presence of Bharat Mata in SBA-networked culture reveals that it is primarily Hindu people (as signaled by subscriber names or X handles) who create, upload, and circulate images of Bharat Mata in order to participate in, and thus secure, a networked consciousness around national cleanliness. Further, the very poor, especially from rural villages, for the most part do not have this kind of ability, due to lack of easy uninterrupted access to the internet or the kind of media literacy that is required to design such video content. Thus, one can surmise that it is primarily middle- and upper-class urban or semirural Hindus who create cleanliness messages on social media organized around the trope of Bharat Mata.

Additionally, there are hardly any critical videos, images, or comments uploaded and shared about Bharat Mata in SBA social space that *critique* the use of Bharat Mata in cleanliness narratives or that mark the Hindu-ness, and presence, of Bharat Mata in a national development project. There is also hardly any critique of SBA social media that brings up issues related to Dalits, Muslims, Adivasis, and the poor, who may have a disjunctive relationship with the Hindu goddess-like figure of Bharat Mata that organizes so many SBA logics, as well as alternative conceptualizations of (or differential access to resources related to) cleanliness compared to those of the middle and upper class. When critiques have been offered, they have primarily come from left-wing online magazines such as *Scroll* or the *Wire* and do not typically find their way into the various SBA social media platforms that mobilize a national Hindu pedagogy around cleanliness. Overall—and this is alarming—one does not witness much contestation of the figure of Bharat Mata in social media videos, posts, and campaigns advocating national cleanliness. The equation between cleaning Bharat Mata and cleaning national space—and the divinity that it evokes—is simply uncritically naturalized and even celebrated in the vast majority of circulating social media content. Consequently, the videos, images, comments, and stories that are created about national cleanliness and anchored in the body of Bharat Mata reflect Hindu (middle- and upper-class/caste) values about cleanliness and national purification, values that such content also helps to spread and amplify.[4]

This moves us to an important point. The SBA social media space is remarkably homogeneous, reflecting a trend that often informs social media platforms in which a group form or collectivity "harvests the strengthening of already existing ties" (Ghosh 2020, 15). This encapsulates Wendy Chun's discussion of homophily—that is, how social media, instead of really being open, functions as gated communities that re-entrench social inequalities (Chun 2016). This homogeneity of SBA social media space is reflective of how social media, under the Modi administration, is increasingly being policed and consequently self-policed.[5] Anything that is perceived to be an insult to Mother India or hurts Hindu sentiments will usually be shot down by users. And now social media platforms are being legally obliged to do so under the laws passed in the Modi government's second term, whereby any post the government deems unlawful, hateful, objectionable, or antinational has to be taken down by the platform owners and the identity of the original poster has to be revealed if the government requests it. This demonstrates how social media space itself functions as another realm of national space that is seen as requiring cleansing through the *sanitization* of dissent. Yet it is ironic that the same social media also operates as a space where vile and hateful comments are regularly expressed by Hindu nationalists against perceived anti-Hindus or antinationals. There is no sanitization there. Indeed, the social media space through which SBA has been primarily promoted and through which it has performed its mass pedagogical function in which cleanliness and Bharat Mata have been linked in Hindu patriotic ways demonstrates the powerful workings of informational Hindu modern governmentality in constructing the nation as a Bharat Mata needing cleansing and purification.

The remarkable ideological homogeneity of SBA social media space that links cleanliness to (Hindu) nationalism—overtly or covertly— is further enhanced by the fact that many of the stories and videos of cleanliness are repetitive, evincing the collaborative and habitual (Chun 2016) nature of networked content. Chun characterizes repetitive activities such as liking, updating, sharing, and so on as constantly producing connections as "habits" that remain invisible or become naturalized so that we are not even fully conscious of engaging in such activities. Thus, "individual tics become indications of collective inclinations" (2016, loc 210 of 5754). In the case of SBA, such habits—for instance, the liking or sharing of a Bharat Mata image to celebrate cleanliness—also reveal the presence of the *religious in the mechanical* since ideologies of Hindu nationalism today circulate primarily through the digital sphere. In SBA social media spaces, someone may have viewed a video of Bharat Mata symbolizing national cleanliness on YouTube, and then created another video with a similar theme and uploaded it on YouTube or some other social media platform. We will see such repetition of themes and storylines when I analyze some of the videos circulating in SBA social media space and demonstrate how certain "habits" (in Chun's sense) about national cleanliness get secured through repetitive deployments of storylines organized around Bharat Mata. The constant updating and liking of Bharat Mata that function as "habit" in the SBA social media space are acts of embodiment, for they create a "grouping of bodies" (Chun 2016, loc. 247 of 5754) just as they penetrate those bodies affectively.

In what follows, I first discuss several themes or storylines through which Bharat Mata is made to stand in for the nation that must be cleaned and that surfaced in much social media content, particularly videos, focused on SBA. Specifically, I explore the following themes: first, the abused and suffering Bharat Mata; second, the subjugation of Bharat Mata through filth as being worse than her pre-independence colonial subjugation; third, the receiving of *darshan* (or divine vision) by select citizens, particularly those who have "woken up" to see the state of filth covering Bharat Mata (and thus the nation); and fourth, the production of fear in citizens who dirty streets or let others dirty streets—fear that goddesses will abandon them. In my analysis, I address how these themes evident across official and popular SBA mediascapes variously link up with or reflect logics of the Hindu modern.

Following this, I offer a discussion of how the story of imperiled Bharat Mata's purity that organizes the cleanliness narratives of the SBA campaign ruptures when we address the issue of Dalits, Muslims, and environmental justice concerns, which are conspicuously absent in SBA mediascapes.

Any Indian student who went to school in postcolonial India during the 1950s through the 1980s will remember being exposed to some vernacular literary text that had a story of anticolonial nationalists liberating Mother India or Bharat Mata from the British. One pattern in such stories remains vivid in my mind. It is about how the sons of the nation made it their goal to liberate the national mother from bondage and suffering brought about by the European colonizers. Such stories, beyond attempting to activate our patriotism for the nation, aimed to instill in us—but especially young Hindu boys as future protectors of the nation—the importance of respecting your mother and never letting her suffer or be humiliated. To be able to protect and serve one's mother was/is to be a dutiful citizen/son, and as sons in particular who took care of their mothers garnered praise from neighbors and relatives, this patriotic message was patriarchal.

In this common discourse, the religion of the sons generally went unmarked; yet looking back now, I realize that the appellations—whether in Bankim Chandra Chattopadhyay's *Anandamath,* Tagore's texts, or other pre-independence nationalist texts—were almost always imagined as Hindu sons. Muslim sons had a tense relation with the Brahmanical trope of Bharat Mata. As Dalit sons and their plight were not even acknowledged by upper-caste nationalists, they rightfully harbored suspicions that the Brahminical structures of Indian nationalism could not secure their freedom. Hence Dalit sons such as Ambedkar and Phule, due to their critique of Bharat Mata's Brahmanism (and the casteism of the Indian National Congress), came to be framed as *desh drohis* (antinationals) by many in the Congress-led nationalist movement.[6] Today's patriotic messaging centered around calls for citizens and especially sons to protect Bharat Mata draws on this particular lineage of anticolonial nationalist discourse that Muslim and Dalit citizens have long critiqued as exclusionary to them. In the ways that it also constructs a version of Bharat Mata's well-being predicated on male protection, it also substitutes a limited notion of women's protection for more expansive and inclusive notions of women's empowerment in the nation.

This figure of the suffering mother needing protection is a persistent theme in many of the videos circulating on social media related to SBA, including many created and uploaded by everyday citizens.[7] We learn in these stories that citizens abuse Bharat Mata by sullying her and throwing filth on her. Consequently, she is no longer recognizable and has been rendered powerless by heaps of filth under which she is submerged. Her purity is tarred by "the people," and she is in danger of drowning. Sometimes Bharat Mata is represented as a youngish woman, sometimes old and frail. In many of the videos, even when she is covered in filth, she retains some visible signifiers of her Hindu-ness and the nation on her body—such as being draped in a sari of saffron, white, and green (the colors of the Indian flag) or wearing a red *bindi* on her forehead (originally in Hindu traditions, this vermillion mark signified a married Hindu woman, although these days it is also worn for fashion). Some of the videos end with a call for an awakening: the characters in the videos who litter national space, often men, are jolted out of their indifference and filled with the realization that they have dirtied Bharat Mata and now must redeem themselves. Bharat Mata, by bringing about such recognition, invites *deshbhakti* (devotion to the nation).

Deshbhakti is a patriotic masculinist notion that was pervasive during the anticolonial nationalist struggle, and it was folded into Hindu nationalism. In recent years, with the aggressive rise of Hindutva, *deshbhakti* has been mobilized to mean service (*sewa*) to and protection of the Hindu nation and its values and culture. It has also been recruited by Modi in many speeches, which socialize young men (read: Hindu men) to become dutiful national subjects by encouraging them to devote themselves to the service of Bharat Mata. One needs little reminder of the fact that Modi constantly crafts his image through this frame of *sewa* to the national mother. The BJP recently marked Modi's seventy-second birthday in 2022 by naming the day *sewa diwas* (day of service).

In the nationalist movement against the British, the call of *sewa—sewa* of Bharat Mata—was an important rhetorical strategy used by nationalist leaders to mobilize young men to fight for the nation. In the hands of the RSS in years following independence, *sewa* was explicitly harnessed to an ideology of masculinist national service through which young Hindu men were recruited to the RSS cause and turned into *deshbhakts*. For the RSS, whose ideologies frequently bleed into the larger BJP culture, *sewa* today is a means to produce *deshbhakti* in order to achieve a Hindu Rashtra (nation). As recently as 2022, Mohan Bhagwat (supreme leader of the RSS) proudly referred to the RSS's work in spreading awareness of *deshbhakti*, noting that those who want to be independent—referring to the nation's (Hindu) people—should also prioritize their security, which can be attained by being a *deshbhakt* (*Outlook* 2022b). It is little wonder then that in a different context he stated that the new generation should be taught to chant "Bharat Mata Ki Jai" as part of the all-round development of youth in India, a ritual that seams together a rhetoric of filial devotion and martial pedagogy to produce a spectacle that can also discipline participants and viewers (*India Today* 2016a).

Such male protectionist appeals around *sewa* and *deshbhakti* reproduce the age-old patriarchal "discourse of protection of women" (especially the mother) where "defense of [her] honor available to nationalism" falls on men (Najmabadi 1997, 445). They also shore up a particular kind of Hindu masculinist heteropatriarchal national protectionist subject position that is linked to the security features (and thus violence) of Hindu modern governmentality. It is a subject position that rests on securitizing the nation, as Bhagwat directly states, as an object of "our" protection and an expression of "our" national independence. As discussed in chapter 1, this securitization exceeds the realms of state militarism and becomes an everyday and even inward-looking logic through which Hindu men in particular are being invited, through discourses designed to appeal to and resonate with them, to *reforge* their relationship with the nation. At a time when the BJP is working to securitize the entire national space of India in various ways, is it is striking to note how the theme of *sewa* dominates many videos that concern SBA.

One video illustrating the agglomeration of themes and visual tropes associated with Hindu nationalist patriarchal discourse is titled "The Real Picture," although in various YouTube and Facebook uploads it is also framed by other titles created by different users (YFI 2017). It was produced by the Yes Foundation, which is a corporate social responsibility arm of Yes Bank. Since 2012, Yes Foundation has emerged, according to its website, as one of the most reputable NGOs in India. The video first appeared on social media in 2016 (it is not possible to determine on which social media platform it first appeared, but that is a moot point). Various users have uploaded it a number of times on Facebook and YouTube. Moreover, the video seems to have been so popular that a similar version was recreated by a regular citizen and uploaded in 2020 on YouTube by a subscriber named Team Divine (Team Divine 2020). In other words, this video is emblematically viral.

On social media pages where it appears, this video is accompanied by comments that offer summaries and reactions to this video. Often official posters uploading the video underline it with comments such as, "Clean India, Green India, Jay [sic] Bharat Mata," "Let's serve Bharat Mata by making India clean," "Wake up India see our Bharat Mata, make it clean," "JAI BHARAT MATA let's come together to make our India neat and clean," "A mind changing video to keep your country clean. If you like we will think that you are patriot toward India." "#Bharat Mata ki jai #Clean India" and "Clean India if you think India is our mother" are other comments that reveal how this video issues its invitation to clean the nation through inviting identification with its titular figure. As one official poster says, "let's serve Bharat Mata by making India clean." Such comments do not simply say "clean your nation if you love your nation"—that would reflect a secular language. Rather, they ask the viewer to love and recognize Bharat Mata. Only then does the argument of "keep your nation clean" emerge, with "your" now a circumscribed construct. What is also noticeable is that every subscriber/user who uploaded this video (or other similar videos) bears a Hindu name or a social media handle containing a Hindu reference, and some can be identified as "internet Hindus," a term the journalist and CNN-IBN deputy editor Sagarika Ghose coined to refer to Hindus who, often anonymously, use social media to proselytize Hindu nationalism and/or attack opponents of their ideology.

This video tells the story of two young urban men and a young urban woman who are enjoying a picnic in a green open park. Their urban and even middle-class status is signaled by the fact that they often speak in English. The main character, a young man named Akash, likes to post selfies on social media, and we see him frequently posting selfies of the group outing. At the end of the picnic, Akash lifts up the picnic mat and throws all the waste items on the ground—plates, bottles, and potato chip packets. He then saunters toward another spot in the park to take a selfie. As he positions his phone in front of his face, he sees on the phone's screen an image of a dirty lady behind him (figure 2.1). The lady is youngish. She has dark hair, a red *bindi*, and dark red lipstick. Her entire body is covered with litter; dark muddy spots smear her face, producing a disconcerting contrast with her calm and serene expression. She wears a white sari with a green border, and a white blouse with an orange border, all adding up to the tricolor of the Indian flag. Seeing this dirty lady, who looks as though she might have stepped out of a horror film, Akash is alarmed.

At this point, the music changes, its new tenor providing sonic cues that something uncanny is about to happen. Akash turns to ask the lady: "What the hell! Who are you?" She replies softly: "Do you not recognize me?"[8] Akash responds fearfully: "I don't know you"—a response that seems to signal (and chastise) a seeming amnesia among citizens, and male citizens in particular, about someone they should know. The lady comments: "Hmm. Well, how will you?" And then with a soft voice and a gentle smile she tells Akash that "Facebook and Twitter contain many of

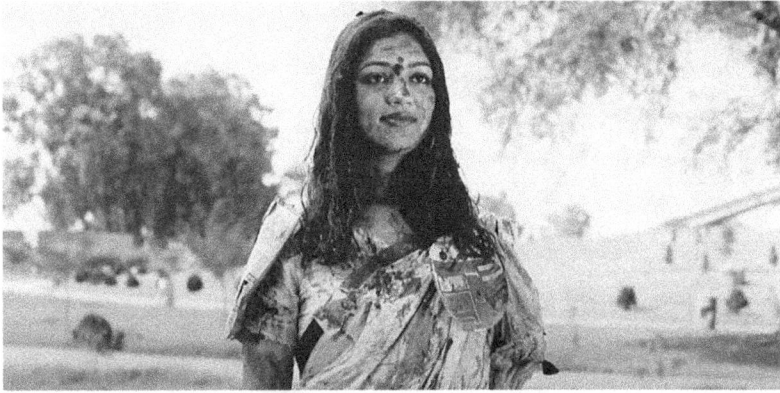

FIGURE 2.1 "Clean India: If you think India is our mother." Still from "The Real Picture."

my earlier photos, which is why people cannot recognize my present dirty state." She then holds up her phone to show Akash an image of her earlier self (figures 2.2 and 2.3). It is an image of Bharat Mata as a goddess wearing a red sari and fine gold jewelry, holding the Indian flag in one hand, leaning against a lion and standing on a big lotus flower. Her entire body covers a map of India.

Both Akash and the audience now recognize that the woman is Bharat Mata, for this image captures a prominent and regal way in which Bharat Mata has been envisioned in Indian visual history. Sumathy Ramaswamy, commenting on this particular image of Bharat Mata, notes how it reproduces the national territory as a "deeply gendered, divinized and affect laden space" (2010, loc. 202 of 4238). By this time Akash is awed by a dawning recognition of who the lady actually is. She asks Akash, pointing the screen of her phone toward his face, "Now you tell me, do I look like this anymore?" She then requests him to upload a photo/selfie of her current filthy appearance on Facebook so that people can see that she is the same person as the earlier goddess image. She hopes that posting a selfie of her current dirty appearance will awaken her children—the nation's citizens—leading to a national consciousness where they realize that she is the same as the iconic bejeweled Bharat Mata, and so that they will no longer abuse her by dirtying her.

The dirty Bharat Mata's request that her current image be uploaded on social media is a rather interesting moment in the video. It captures a trend that marks SBA, a social media trend of citizens (often encouraged by

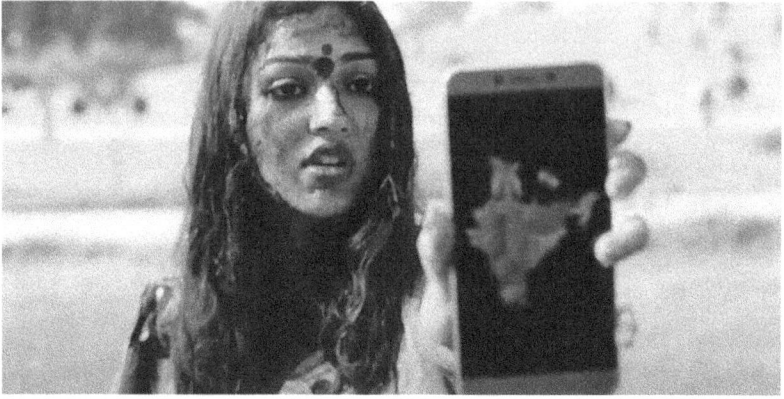

FIGURE 2.2 Still from "The Real Picture."

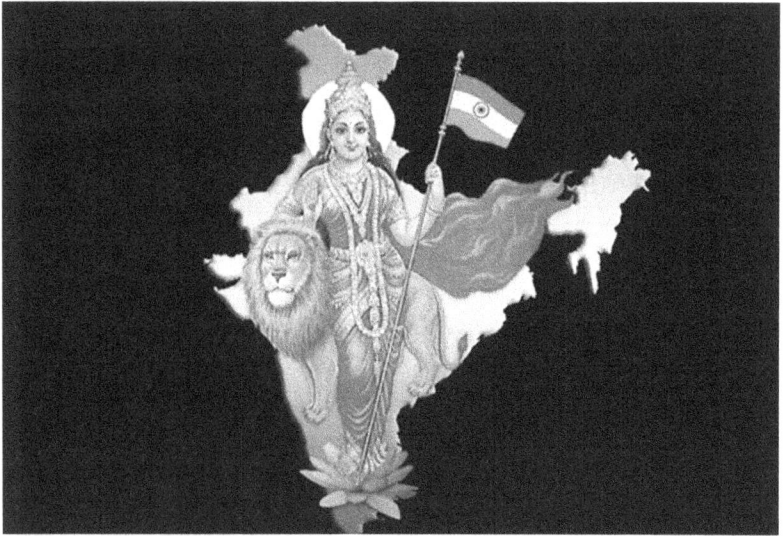

FIGURE 2.3 Still from "The Real Picture."

the government) posting selfies with clean spaces or dirty spaces that they are cleaning up, and sometimes even with celebrities endorsing the SBA campaign. In recent years, scholars have begun exploring the relationship between selfies and nationalism or citizenship (Kuntsman 2017; Kuntsman and Stein 2015; Rao 2018) to explore the "claims made by ordinary citizens via the use of their own networked self-portraits" (Kuntsman 2017, 22). They argue that the selfie, as an aesthetic form, is not simply a continuation of the photographic portrait of earlier times. The very technic is different (Baishya 2015). The selfie secures a sense of liveness—and thus authenticity—that is different from the posed photo taken by a professional photographer. Hence, selfies tend to acquire evidentiary authority about the truth of a person (Baishya 2015). In chapter 3 I return to this matter of the selfie, Hindu nationalism, and SBA more explicitly.

At this moment in the video, even though Bharat Mata is not posting her own selfie but asking Akash to do so, the very fact that a selfie of Bharat Mata can be posted on Facebook for its larger audience to witness creates a sense of authenticity about Bharat Mata—a sense that she is simply not a trope that binds the nation or a spirit that flows through the nation. She is embodied, she *exists*, she is *visible*, she is *real* and *authentic*, and we can *see* her. Her selfie reminds us of this fact. Here, then, is a repeat of what is going in larger Hindu nationalist culture today where Hindu gods and goddesses are brought down to the ground and given a real authority of existence so as to move, mobilize, and awe the citizenry (for example, in the constant erection of statues of Hindu gods and the building of temples). Technology simply enables this earthing of the gods. Divinity and technology fuse in this climate to mobilize Hindu nationalist sentiments. Thus, what we see here is a suturing of Hindu nationalism and its constant invocation of Hindu divinity to a logic of techno-informational modernity that again captures the informational drive of Hindu modern governmentality that is foregrounded in SBA.

This current dirty Bharat Mata is clearly tech savvy—as signified by her use of a cell phone and her awareness of selfies. She is keenly aware that it is in digital space that nationalist mobilization occurs today—a message that is consistent with the way in which digital media is used by the BJP public relations machine, as well as many tech-savvy Hindu volunteers, to distribute Hindu sensibilities in the national sphere. Indeed, in these platform nationalist (Mihelj 2022) times that inform and enable populism today, for the nation to be recognized by the people it must be seen and constantly updated on social media. For Bharat Mata to exist today, to mobilize the people today, she must be seen and constantly updated in various platforms. Bharat Mata in this video is aware that mobilizing her sons to rise up against dirt and filth across the nation requires managing her presence in the online matrix of the nation, which is where she acquires virality for herself and her message. Wendy Chun suggests that "to be is to be updated" (2016, loc. 193), and that things or people no longer updated are things or people no longer cared for. While I would not go so far as to say that "to be" is to be updated (since many people still avoid social media), we can nonetheless import the larger point of Chun's arguments into this discussion and posit that Hindu (populist) nationalism today succeeds in building itself up by constantly "updating" the nation as a Hindu devotional object or body—whether that Hindu-ness is overtly marked in that updating or whether it functions more inferentially.

At the point at which Bharat Mata asks Akash to upload an image of her current state on social media, the video raises the stakes to become more shocking. The background sound rises, and we see urine (from an unseen source) forcefully spraying on Bharat Mata, who endures the abuse with uncanny stoicism. This is the urine of Akash's friend, who is relieving himself on open ground a distance away; we are given a quick shot of this. To make matters worse, a banana peel lands on the already dirty Bharat Mata's shoulders; it has been thrown on the ground by a group of men walking by. Equating the ground with the body of Bharat Mata, these scenes depict the ground, the soil, and the divine yet sullied Bharat Mata as one and the same. We are thus reminded here that national land or territory is a *punyabhoomi*, the rhetorical and material institutionalization of which has emerged as a goal of contemporary Hindu modern governmentality.

Akash, by this point in the video, is filled with shame. He takes a selfie with the current dirty Bharat Mata, uploading it as she requested. He then returns to the spot where he had thrown trash from his picnic earlier. He picks up the trash with the intention of placing it in a bin. The dirty, sullied Bharat Mata looks at him with a proud smile that seems to recognize Akash's inner awakening. The video ends. The final image where credits roll display two hashtags, #Respect_Bharat_Mata and #Swachh_Bharat, prominently on the screen.

In its visual iconography, plot, and paratextual framing, this video illustrates how SBA mediascapes, foregrounding the trope of Bharat Mata, reinforce key logics of Hindu modern governmentality. In particular, it evokes a Hindu divine ethos to frame cleanliness (and development); it sacralizes the land; and it underscores the need for a viral mediation of the nation as a Hindu female body that must be cleansed and rescued—thus reinforcing a Hindu informational matrix.

Many elements of "The Real Picture" reappear in other SBA videos on social media. Foremost among these is the theme of Bharat Mata being abused by her own children (especially men), who dirty her literal body. One popular video entitled "Mother Spitter," produced by Quill Studio in 2016, has been uploaded numerous times on Facebook, YouTube, and X

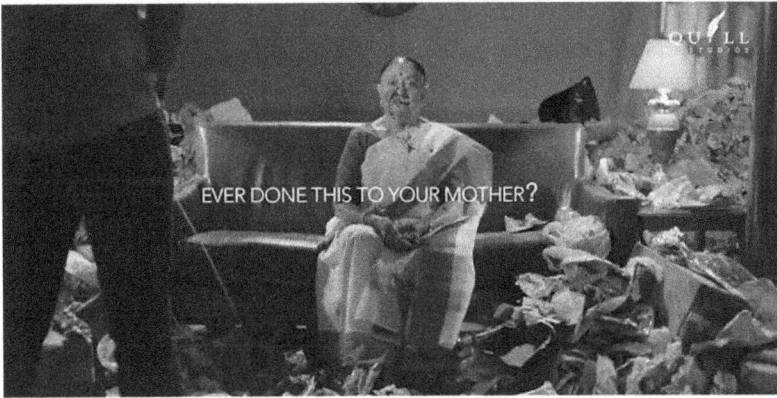

FIGURE 2.4 Still from "Mother Spitter."

(see Anchalia 2018). This ad campaign is significant because it was picked up by the well-known Campaigns of the World, a web portal that selects and displays on its website creative and significant ad campaigns and films from all over the world. At the time of this writing, YouTube registered just over 1.8 million views of this video. It depicts a young man abusing his mother (figure 2.4). In the opening scene, we see the mother sitting in a living room filled with garbage. It is an urban living room, as signified by the modern couch, lamp, and ambiance. It is evening and the room is not well lit. This stylistic visual element—where the room is dark—metaphorizes a crisis of morality, a crisis of light (symbolizing divinity, purity, and so on). The mother is an elderly lady wearing a white sari with a red border—an auspicious Hindu signifier as during religious ceremonies many Hindu women (and especially Bengali Hindu women) wear red-bordered saris. Thus, once again, we see a mother figure, adorned in clothes that visibly mark her Hindu identity, whose presence is being defiled by filth.

We also see a young man sitting on the couch next to the elderly lady. He is her son, and he is on the phone. While talking on the phone, he turns sideways and spits *paan* on his mother's face.[9] The mother looks stoic, not moving, suggesting complete passivity and powerlessness. Seconds later, we see the young man, who has now moved to another part of the room, urinating on his mother's body from afar. We are filled with disgust and anger as this scene shakes us out of any sense of complacency. The screen then fills up with the question: "Ever done this to your mother?" This is followed by another question: "Then why do this to your motherland?"

As this second question flashes on the screen, the colors of the characters in the sentence change to green, white, and saffron—the colors of the Indian flag.

In both these videos, then, we see the continuation of a larger rhetorical theme through which Bharat Mata has been embodied in Indian history, especially during colonial times, when Bharat Mata was depicted as a "suffering mother" (suffering due to European colonial bondage) and it was the duty of her sons to liberate her. In both these videos, the nationalist trope of the "suffering mother" is recentered—*but with an important difference*. The difference is that while during colonial times Bharat Mata suffered due to colonial subjugation now, these videos tell us, the national mother is suffering not because of takeover by a foreign power but by the negligence, abuse, and betrayal of her own children, especially her sons, who are routinely depicted sullying her body (national space). These videos reflect the epistemic transference of Bharat Mata that Guha-Thakurta (2016) discussed from earlier times to today, where attachment to the nation is being enforced by requiring a loyalty to Bharat Mata because citizens—her own children—are seen as abusing her by forgetting their Hindu traditions of cleanliness and purity. Both these videos, while promoting cleanliness, ultimately equate cleanliness with loyalty to a Hindu mother.

THE CURRENT SUBJUGATION OF BHARAT MATA:
WORSE THAN COLONIAL SUBJUGATION

The point discussed above is particularly brought out in a YouTube video (figure 2.5) uploaded in August 2018 and titled "Bharat Mata ke is roop ko dekh kar har Hindustani ki ruh kaap uthegi" (Seeing this sorry appearance of Bharat Mata will make the hearts of every Indian tremble) (Gosavi 2018). The video was uploaded by a Hindu female subscriber who goes by the name Bharat Mata—I say Hindu, again, because a Muslim or Dalit woman in all likelihood would not identify with a Bharat Mata figure. The writer/director of the film is named Akanksha Gosavi. I chose this video because, as in the others discussed earlier, Bharat Mata's body is covered in filth. Thus, it is important for the reader to recognize how pervasive the theme of Bharat Mata being drenched in filth is in SBA social mediascapes.[10] In this video, a prominent moment arises when the teary-eyed dirty lady, whom we do not at first recognize as Bharat Mata, tells a nearby male sweeper:

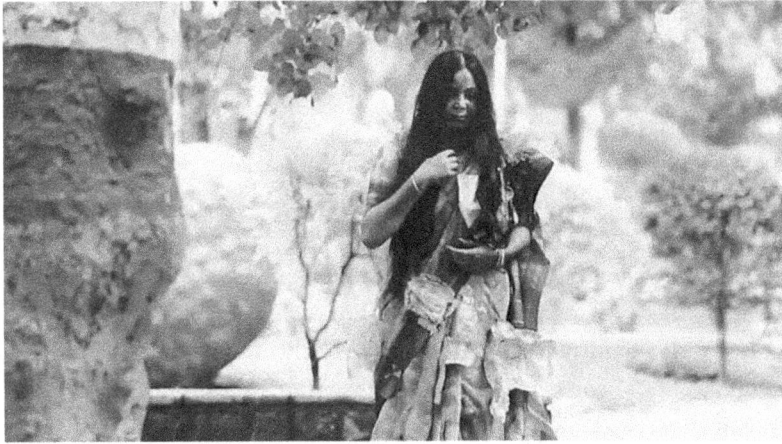

FIGURE 2.5 Still from "Bharat Mata ke is roop ko dekh kar har Hindustani ki ruh kaap uthegi."

I do not understand why people are running away when they see my state. They are the ones who made me like this today. The very children whom I nurtured in my womb are the ones who are abusing me for 365 days. When different foreign invaders looted and exploited me, I did not feel so bad as I do today when my millions of children dishonor and abuse me. I feel as though I have not been liberated yet from the exploitation of the British colonialists.[11]

The video ends with the sweeper waking up. We realize he has been dreaming this entire scene of Bharat Mata. Awakened both literally and figuratively, he takes out the tricolor, the Indian flag, from a box in his room, holds it in his hands, and makes a promise to Bharat Mata befitting of a dutiful Hindu son: "Mata, I will never allow you to be dirty again, until my last breath, irrespective of what others may do."

In this and similar videos, where it is disproportionately men who dirty and abuse the mother, the message is that men (and they mostly seem to be Hindu men) have to be awakened and redeemed—that is, turned into *deshbhakts* by having them realize that the land they dirty is the body of Bharat Mata. It is through such an awakening that they can turn into good citizens—that is, to honor and protect Bharat Mata and be remasculinized as reverent (Hindu) male subjects. This is what happens to Akash in the first video when his realization of Bharat Mata's dirty state leads him back to the spot in the park he had dirtied by throwing away his picnic trash; this is what is also hinted at in the second video, where the young man urinating on his mother's body is chastised with the message, "Ever done this to your mother? Then why do this to your motherland?"—a message that ultimately appeals to men. This is also repeated in the third video, where the male sweeper awakens from his dream and makes a promise to Bharat Mata (and thus the nation) that until his dying day he will keep her clean.

This theme of awakening Hindus (especially Hindu men) has recently emerged as a significant logic in the Hindutva project. I referred earlier to Mohan Bhagwat's comments. But it is now emerging in everyday media sites as well. For instance, a Hindutva website has loudly claimed that "No Hindu politics is possible unless there is Hindu awakening" (quoted in Anand 2005, 204). Similarly, a recent article carried this headline: "From the US to UP, Hindus Are Awakening" (Ratnu 2022). Thus, it is disquieting to see the theme of awakening so prominently at work in what is otherwise being touted by the government as an apolitical project, for the SBA campaign is "beyond politics," or so Modi has claimed.

This theme of awakening Hindus and producing *deshbhakts* through the ethos of *sewa*, while apparently benign, dangerously normalizes the security (and violence) logic of the Hindu modern. For without being *deshbhakts* one cannot feel strongly about protecting Bharat Mata. And at a time in India when Hindu mobs and even everyday Hindu citizens, especially Hindu men, are engaging in all kinds of physical and online attacks on dissenters and "others" of the nation by claiming to be *deshbhakts*, the rhetoric of the SBA campaign and what it has spawned in this vein cannot be disassociated from the larger public culture. In articulating cleanliness through invocations to *deshbhakti* and *sewa*, such SBA rhetoric makes cleanliness a *security* issue through depicting threats to an embodied Bharat Mata whose gendered vulnerability allows for the implicit endorsement of possible violence that may occur in the name of cleanliness. We saw evidence of this in the example offered in chapter 1, where one of the two Hindu men who killed the two Dalit kids in Shivpuri District for open defecation noted that he had been commanded by gods to perform this act. The violence thus becomes a sacred act for the killers. Further, when such potential violence becomes associated with the securitization of the nation as a sacred and divine object, as it does in SBA mediascapes, this violence then can often be protected from critique, for critiquing it becomes the same as critiquing the divine or piety to the divine. It is little wonder, then, that Hindutva mobs who attack others in the name of protecting Bharat Mata are often silently endorsed by the state or the central government that ignores them or frames such violence as a "fringe" issue. In the Shivpuri case, while the Hindu men were arrested, the police stated that they were trying to determine if it was an untouchability issue *or* a superstition issue. Rendering something like this as a superstition issue speaks to how these acts of violence are framed as anomalies, and specifically as non-modern ones, rather than in keeping with the violence of Hindu modern logics. In chapter 4 we will witness many instances of such violence and coercion—especially toward marginalized communities—that have occurred while organizing "cleanliness" in the nation, and which reflect the populist violence of Hindu modern governmentality.

DARSHANIC ENCOUNTERS

The notion of *darshan* is central to Hindu religion, and particularly to Hindu visual culture. Basically it refers to "religious seeing, or the visual perception of the sacred" and it is an "auspicious sight" (Eck 1998, 3). One does not need to be a devotee to receive *darshan*. In Hindu nationalism—in its various phases—the notion of *darshan* was important in articulating the nation through a devotional significance, as when a devotee, or a regular citizen, felt that they witnessed the spirit of the nation in a god/goddess figure (who visited them). There is nothing objective about *darshan*. There is no need to prove if *darshan* happened. The important thing is that an individual believes that they were given *darshan* by a deity or that they were in the presence of divinity or the sacred.

Scholars such as Dipesh Chakrabarty, Lawrence Babb, Arvind Rajagopal, Christopher Pinney, and Diana Eck in particular have addressed the centrality of *darshan* in Indian nationalism and Indian society at large, suggesting that the very act of seeing the sacred makes Indian nationalism a visual nationalism, contrary to Western understandings of India that locate the Indian spirit in an interior landscape (Eck 1998). In his remarkable discussion of imagination in relation to nationalism, Dipesh Chakrabarty takes up the issue of Indian peasants whose sense of being with Bharat Mata "was not based on the training of the mind that print capitalism could administer to the formally educated subject," for "Bharat [India] could indeed be the mother because long before there was newspaper and the novel, there was the age-old practice of darshan" (2000, 177). Arvind Rajagopal (2001), on the other hand, has addressed how the 1980s television adaptation of the Ramayana was able to produce a mediated religious national public sphere at a key moment in the solidification of late twentieth-century Hindu nationalism. He discusses how viewers were transfixed by this media event because many felt that the gods that they had only heard or read about could be now viewed on screen. Many felt the gods were giving them *darshan* (allowing devotees to see them). It is also worth remembering that during his first election campaign, Modi appeared through hologram technology simultaneously to many rural villages in different locations. Some villagers were awed, believing that they were receiving some kind of *darshan* through Modi. This elevated Modi to some kind of an exalted god-like figure.

This centrality of *darshan* in Indian nationalism points to a larger "Hindu scopic regime" (Pinney 2004, 9) that pervades Hindu culture, in which viewing is often endowed with the devotional. This can involve seeing one's own mother in a devotional way, viewing the nation in a devotional way, or even viewing pilgrimage sites (such as the River Ganges at Varanasi) in a devotional way. The concept of *darshan* unsettles the separation between the viewer and the viewed—a binary that has often marked Western notions of vison and viewing—and suggests that in devotional viewing, the viewer (citizen) and the viewed (the devotional object, such as the nation) blend into one. Through *darshan* the viewer experiences themselves as divinely blessed and sees themselves as someone in touch with the sacred. The viewer thus becomes endowed with properties of the divine (but a Hindu divine).

It is remarkable how the theme of *darshan* consistently informs many videos of Swachh Bharat that have been created or uploaded by users. In "The Real Picture" video discussed earlier, Akash receives *darshan* from Bharat Mata—a point that is emphasized when the dirty woman (Bharat Mata) shows Akash an earlier picture of her, and Akash recognizes that she is Bharat Mata. That this *is darshan* is evidenced by the fact that no one else around is able to see this woman but Akash. It is his *darshan* of Bharat Mata (now appearing before him in a dirty state) that awakens him into a new love for the nation/national space that he had littered earlier, a love that is also devotional in nature for it has emerged from a *darshan* of Bharat Mata. It is this awakening that propels him to return to the site he had littered earlier and pick up the trash, symbolic of his new reverence for the nation's grounds (national territory). In the second video, "Bharat Mata ke is roop ko dekh kar har Hindustani ki ruh kaap uthegi," the sweeper dreams the entire video sequence that we as viewers watch. The video ends with him waking up from his dream when he realizes that the dirty woman in his dream is Bharat Mata. So, when he wakes up and makes a promise of cleanliness to Bharat Mata, that promise again ensues from his *darshan* of Bharat Mata.

The framing of many of these narratives through a darshanic encounter with the figure of Bharat Mata situates the nation in divine time (and always a Hindu divine) and thus no time at all—it situates the nation in a timelessness that positions it outside history. The nation appears as a pre-constituted "natural" godlike entity existing a priori, before the social. And the problem with this, of course, is that the nation then cannot be critiqued because it precedes the social.[12] It becomes transcendental, divine. This transcendentalizing of the nation through a Hindu divine timelessness positions the nation, again, as what Savarkar referred to as a *punyabhoomi*, where one can receive sacred visions from deities when one commits to serving the nation (as Akash does in the video). This darshanic logic that invites an attachment to territory through frames of divinity exhibits another way in which the sacralization of land as a feature of the Hindu modern governmentality works in SBA mediations and forecloses the possibility of any critique of Bharat Mata, and of the logics of cleanliness that are anchored by and through her.

The darshanic mode of awakening that informs SBA storylines also makes visible the casteist and anti-Muslim logics underpinning this structure of visuality (that is, awakening) promoted in these videos. If *darshan* produces awakening (as it did, literally, with the sweeper, and figuratively with Akash), the Muslim body—as Muslims do not engage in deity worship—can never receive *darshan* from Bharat Mata or any other goddess form (and thus be a *deshbhakt*). The visual logic of *darshan* already excludes the Muslim body, for *darshan* is a Hindu mode of worship or seeing the divine. The Dalit body is also written out of this holy visual exchange. Kancha Ilaiah (2019) has powerfully written about how in Dalit Bahujan communities, gods and goddesses do not possess an elevated status. Rather, their relationship with the people is egalitarian; there is no distance between gods/goddesses and the people. Ilaiah has noted that, obversely, gods in the Hindu Brahmanical system exist to *create (patriarchal) hierarchy* and fight outcasts.

I bring up this point because the darshanic visual structure that informs many such videos connected to the SBA campaign that attempt to *awaken* citizens to the plight of a dirty nation underscore how structures of visuality in the SBA program are covertly and (sometimes overtly) casteist and anti-Muslim. Not only are there minimal representations of Muslim bodies and no representations of Dalit bodies (other than tokenistic acknowledgment of manual scavenging by celebrities and politicians), but even the visual structures of these media campaigns set up "looking relations" (Mulvey 1975) that are Hinduized. This is because the visual logic of *darshan* can only work when the recipient of *darshan* is Hindu, and the god/goddess offering *darshan* is elevated. As a mode of divine but unequal visual exchange between the god/goddess and the devotee, the practice of *darshan* normalizes hierarchical looking relations that are an intimate signature of Hindu society and its caste/class/gendered system. For instance, domestic servants in many caste-conscious households look down while talking to their master/mistress. Similarly, in very conservative and upper-casteist households, there are wives who may look down while speaking to their husbands (for the husband is supposed to be a god-like figure—*Patiparameswar*), and so on. In structuring many storylines around a visual logic of *darshan*, SBA videos—and even many SBA social media posts—not only reconstitute the citizen as Hindu (and divine, for the recipient of *darshan* is divinized through *darshan*); they also endorse undemocratic-looking relations through which people are being taught to view the nation—and perhaps also its leaders—as being higher and more divine than them.

This relates directly to what is going on in contemporary India. As democracy crumbles, and BJP and Hindutva rhetoric represents the nation as something higher and more sacred than its citizens, we begin to forget that the nation is (and should be) be an expression of the collective will of the people (however fraught that collective may be), protected through secular structures of law and justice rooted in notions of equality. But this kind of a transcendentalizing of the nation, and by extension national governance, is symptomatic of how majoritarian states and parties today, in many parts of the world, are enforcing top-down power structures, often under a shallow guise of democracy. It is within such a model of power, of course, that the ever-pervasive securitization of national space begins to make sense. In the case of contemporary India, this vertical logic of power is being secured by attaching the nation (and national governance) to the sacred, a process that forecloses challenges to this power structure while simultaneously naturalizing it.

This is one of most alarming traits of Hindu modern governmentality as it operates today in India. Whereas in the immediate aftermath of independence, architects of the constitution envisioned national modernity based on liberal ideas of democracy, however fraught that might have been, contemporary attempts to "modernize" the nation through a

Hindu order, and by recruiting ancient gods and goddesses, function to delink modernity from democracy. Hindu modern governmentality and its underlying logics offer promises of citizenly belonging that are increasingly based *not* on political rights and equality but on one's *visible* commitment to serving a *punyabhoomi*—an always already divine land. Images of Modi in sage-like attire is one visual expression of all this, and the mediascape of his signature cleanliness campaign another.

Young Girls and/as Bharat Mata

In some videos on social media, it is sometimes also young children, especially young girls, represented as receiving *darshan* from Bharat Mata such that they become future extensions of Bharat Mata. And like everything discussed earlier, the receiving of *darshan* marks these girls explicitly as Hindu. In one video we see young girls playing outdoors while nearby on a bench sit a couple of young men, chatting (see Omabm Productions 2016). One of the young men drops a banana peel and another a potato-chip packet (again the theme of men dirtying the ground). One girl looks intently at the actions of these young men. And then she looks beyond these men and sees Bharat Mata in the form of a goddess standing a few feet away, looking at her. No one else can see Bharat Mata but her. The little girl walks toward the men and picks up the litter they have dropped. Bharat Mata smiles from afar as though to bless her. Toward the end of the video, we see a statue of Bharat Mata by a traffic circle in the same neighborhood. The same people who had been littering the streets now salute the statue while the children place the litter they have collected at her feet. As they do so, one elderly woman admonishes the children for placing garbage at Bharat Mata's feet while another woman tells them that one should place flowers and not garbage at the feet of Bharat Mata. To this, one young girl replies defiantly that our *dharthi* (earth) is also Bharat Mata, so then why do we— meaning everyone—drop garbage on it? The point is struck home, and everyone is jolted into an awakening.

In another video, a little girl is doing her homework, drawing the map of India in a sketch book (see Mali 2016). However, while trying to adorn the map with the figure of Bharat Mata, the girl becomes frustrated as she cannot sketch Bharat Mata properly. At night in bed, she is still frustrated that she cannot draw the figure of Bharat Mata. After she falls asleep, Bharat Mata, dressed as a young woman holding the flag of India against a dark-blue night sky, visits her in her dream (figure 2.6). She tells the girl, "Dear child, many people are throwing filth all over. If this continues, eventually

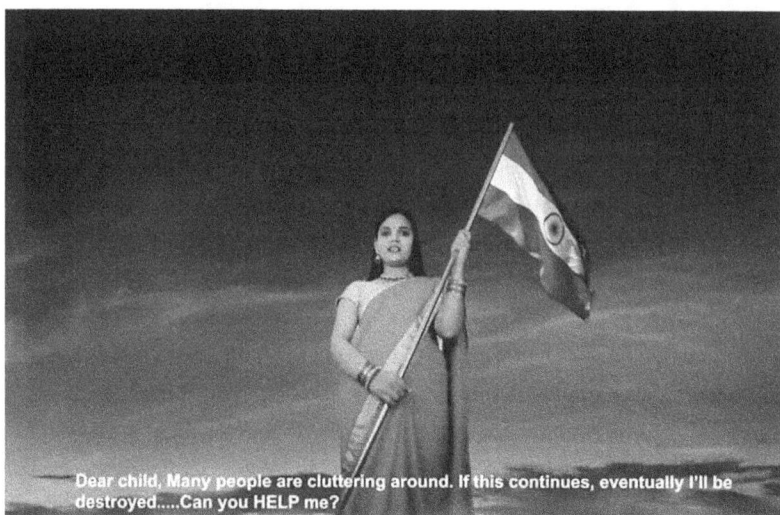

FIGURE 2.6 Still from "Swachh Bharat Abhiyan—Bharat Mata Short Films."

I will be destroyed. . . . Can you HELP me?" This darshanic nocturnal encounter confers a new awareness on the young child. The next morning, she goes around picking up litter in the neighborhood to respond to the divine call of Bharat Mata that appeared in her dream.

In fact, in numerous social media videos, while not all young girls are seen as receiving *darshan* from Bharat Mata—as the two videos discussed above depict—many nonetheless position young girls as the ones who are more aware of the need to clean their surroundings. And there is a frequent theme of young girls cleaning garbage they see on the road or in their spaces. This marks an interesting rhetorical strategy. Children are the future of the nation, and little girls symbolize the nation's future domesticity. They are the future Bharat Matas, and in some films young girls cleaning their surroundings are directly embodied as Bharat Mata (figure 2.7). So, in representing young (Hindu) girls as trying to clean up their surroundings, these girls become the future bearers of a clean, pure nation, and national family. Yet there is a tension in this representational logic. It normalizes the expected role of girls/women in keeping their surroundings and homes clean while also having to represent ideal cleanliness and purity. And this reveals, again, the contradictory ways in which (Hindu) women are positioned by the nation, as addressed in chapter 1 (and non-Hindu women do not necessarily carry the privileging burden

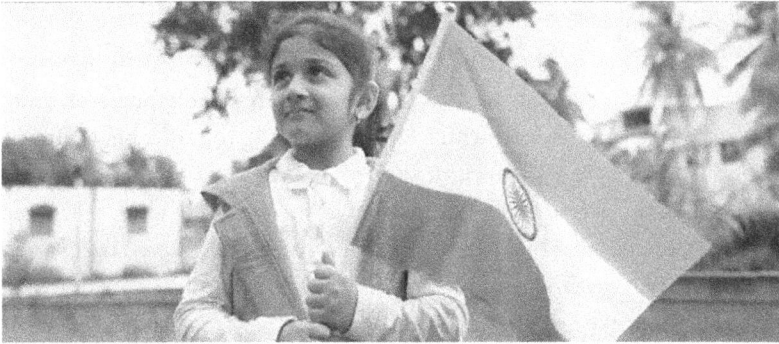

FIGURE 2.7 Still from "Sorry Bharath Mata."

of this contradiction). On the one hand, their labor is associated with the filth of the domestic sphere (garbage in the kitchen, the household, and so on). On the other hand, they are also dichotomously expected to labor to remain pure and clean. We will see this contradiction repeated in another campaign shortly.

The intimate entanglement of the visual logic of *darshan* with the security logic of Hindu modern governmentality takes on particular resonances in the context of Hindu girl figures. It is *darshan* (or the desire to receive it) from a god/goddess that turns one into *deshbhakt*, which is the first step toward turning (Hindu) men into security-citizen-subjects engaging in security and protection of Bharat Mata, an identity they can enact digitally as well as on the streets. If *darshan* from Bharat Mata offers Hindu men a securitized masculinist subject position, *darshan* transforms little girls into future Bharat Matas (goddesses) as they begin to embody national domesticity and cleanliness/purity; they thus also become the objects of security. At a time in the nation where Hindu masculinist violence against alleged "love jihad" campaigns are at an all-time high, this kind of subtextual messaging in a national cleanliness project is especially alarming. In the next chapter, we will see how this messaging plays out where cleanliness logics are organized around the security of (Hindu) women—all possible Bharat Matas. It is also not coincidental that such representations recently led to the naming of a newborn girl in 2018 in the western state of Maharashtra as Swachhata, "purity." And purity, we know, is situated in casteist Brahmanical logics. The last names of the parents indicate they are Hindu. According to several reports, the parents were inspired by SBA campaigns while naming their child (e.g., PTI 2018a, 2018b).

A Rupture That Was Not Allowed to Be: Sanitizing and
Cleansing the Young Kashmiri Muslim Female Body

Most little girls represented in SBA mediascapes are Hindu; however, there is a notable exception, one which ends up proving the rule. Beginning in 2018, a five-year-old Kashmiri Muslim girl named Jannat Tariq seized the attention of the nation and Modi for her two-year effort to clean the iconic Dal Lake, a huge, beautiful lake in Srinagar typically considered by locals to be a heaven on earth, surrounded by the pristine Himalayas and on which many movies have been filmed. Dal Lake, over the years, has accumulated a lot of garbage, but since 1989 and India's occupation of Kashmir, its condition has declined. A video of Jannat cleaning the lake went viral, appearing on numerous news channels and social media platforms that hailed Jannat's cleaning efforts. As her act gained popularity, she was quoted in an interview by Asian News International as saying that "people should not litter Dal Lake and instead use dustbin for throwing waste" (ANI 2018). She received praise on the prime minister's monthly radio address, *Mann Ki Baat,* and his praise was also repeated in his X feed. Her efforts even made it into a textbook used in a school in Hyderabad.

Notably, the nation's hailing of a Kashmiri Muslim girl as an icon of the SBA campaign occurred around the time that the Indian government was stripping Kashmir of autonomy and, as an extension of India's occupation of Kashmir, shutting down its communication networks. With its disproportionate focus on girls and women, the SBA mediascape easily assimilated a Muslim girl in an area that Kashmiris view as colonized by India into the larger Hindu-driven cleanliness narrative. Jannat is simply hailed as one more young girl trying to engage in cleanliness, while her Kashmiri Muslim status and its fraught relation with India remain unmarked. Moreover, Dal Lake is discussed as though it is simply one more dirty site in the nation, when in fact it sits in a region that for the last thirty-five years and more has been one of the most militarized zones in the world, one occupied by Indian paramilitary forces with special powers of arrest and torture. In addition to the contaminants it has absorbed from security-related developments, this militarized zone has been "dirtied" by the blood and bodies of Kashmiri Muslims—many accused of being terrorists by the Indian state and killed by the Indian military. A report in the early 1990s, following the beginning of India's military occupation of Kashmir, noted that Dal Lake is a site "where a number of war-related environmental abuses have converged to threaten the livelihoods of thousands of people and the existence of a treasured ecological gem" (Moore 1994). For example, seasonal tourist hotels have been transformed into military barracks that pump tons of waste into the lake, while the decimation of surrounding forests by the military and its opponents have yielded vast amounts of silt (Moore 1994). Additionally, this highly militarized zone and the Kashmiri insurgency against the occupying Indian state has led to a decline in tourism. Operators of *shikaras* (gondola-like boats) on Dal Lake, a favorite of tourists, do not earn the kind of money that they did earlier. As a result, many *shikara* owners, losing business, have started creating floating vegetable gardens by encroaching on certain sections of the lake, and earning a livelihood this way. This has been at least one reason for garbage accumulating in the lake. Thus, filth in the Dal Lake and its adjoining areas and India's militaristic relations with Kashmir are correlated, and this correlation exacerbates Dal Lake's declining state, whose purification would require infinitely more than the efforts of many small children.

In his powerful study, Suvir Kaul gives a translation of a Kashmiri poet's reflection on an unnamed lake, in which the poet finds not placid beauty but a stranger-like corpse staring at him from the depths of the lake, "steal[ing] [his] musings" (2017, 8). This corpse could be one of the numerous bodies murdered by the Indian state or one of the people who have died by suicide, a phenomenon which has risen during the occupation of Kashmir by the Indian state. The point of this poem, Kaul explains, is to call attention to how the "corpse and the lake, that is unnatural death and natural beauty in Kashmir, inform each other" (2017, 9), and how the lake and natural beauty in Kashmir have been reconfigured by political trauma arising from the structures of violence, including India's occupation of Kashmir, for the last thirty-five-plus years. Yet the celebration (and nationalization/Indianization/Hinduization) of Jannat's image cleaning Dal Lake on many media sites discussing SBA functions to erase the history of India's occupation of the only Muslim-dominant state, which has significantly contributed to Dal Lake's current state. If we had been reminded in mainstream media reports that nationalized this little girl that what she was trying to clean—Dal Lake—cannot be disassociated from India's military occupation of Kashmir, we could perhaps have stepped back and challenged the universalized logic of cleanliness (couched in Hinduist nationalist fervor) in which the cause of filth and garbage in *all regions* of the nation is rendered the same and individualized (that is, the "dirty habits" of people). Thus, although Jannat, a Muslim girl from Kashmir, can never be a future Bharat Mata, her viral image ends up functioning as a visual screen through which India's historical relation with occupied Kashmir and Muslims is cleansed of violence, forced integration, and environmental degradation. Here, the young Muslim (female) Kashmiri subject is rendered an innocent subject, devoid of history and therefore more easily linked to a future that Hindu modern governmentality is attempting to secure in part through campaigns such as SBA.

As I write this, I am haunted by the image of another eight-year-old Kashmiri Muslim girl, Asifa Bano, who belonged to a nomadic tribe. Bano was gang-raped and tortured by a group of Hindu men that reportedly included a policeman and a juvenile—in a Hindu temple in Kashmir—and later beaten to death. This occurred in 2018. Known as the Kathua rape case was, it was, according to several reports, an act of premediated murder, as the Hindu community in the area wanted the nomadic Muslim group, to which Bano belonged, to leave the land (see, e.g., Taneja 2018; *Times of India* 2018a). Bano was racialized as an "other" by Hindu men who used explicitly sexualized forms of violence to sully and kill her in the name of national cleansing.

While Jannat and Asifa experienced markedly different fates, they exemplify how girls' bodies are being instrumentalized as loci of Hindu modern governmentality through cleansing (and "love jihad" campaigns also evince this). Whereas Jannat was deracinated and sanitized, her image seamlessly weaving into the universalized/nationalized (Hindu) logics of cleanliness, her assimilation conceals the tortured ghosts of so many Asifa Banos wandering around in Kashmir, perhaps still hoping for a clean justice—by which I mean a justice that is not simply focused on an individual case but one that emerges from an acknowledgment of the historical and military oppression of Kashmir by the state of India. Only then will future Banos be able to live without fear of the sexual violence that informs the cleansing practices of Hindu nationalists and the military in Kashmir.

All this exemplifies a duality in the SBA campaign. On the one hand, we are constantly reminded that cleanliness is intricately tied to the history of Hinduism and was glorified in ancient Hindu cultures. On the other hand, there is a striking ahistoricity at work. The diverse historical relations of different bodies and regions with cleanliness, shaped by the practices of the Hindu culture that has governed cleanliness through caste and religious-based logics, have resulted in *different and unequal* politics (sexual, gendered, casteist, and religious) around cleanliness, which are being further shaped by the state today. But these unequal relationalities become erased in and through the popularization of SBA and related Hindutva governmentalities of cleanliness. For instance, nothing is made of the fact that

Jannat belongs to the same sphere of young Muslim girls and women in Kashmir who have encountered violent sexual assault including rape by the Indian military and other Hindu mobs since the Indian occupation of Kashmir.[13] Jannat simply becomes "one of us" just as, with the Indian government's 2019 abrogation of Article 370, Kashmir, forcibly integrated into India, becomes "one of us." Yet, like Jannat, Kashmir can never be "one of us." Too many historical wrongs have sullied Kashmir and its bodies. Too much violence and trauma mock the relationship of any Kashmiri Muslim woman or girl with the heteropatriarchal Indian state that is determined to fully "possess" (the feminized) Kashmir against all odds.

Returning more specifically to Bharat Mata, one can argue that the pervasive use of this trope in SBA rhetoric and mediascapes functions to decontextualize how cleanliness is situated in structural/historical inequalities produced by caste, class, religion, sexuality, patriarchy, and even militarism. It delinks the campaign for cleanliness from social justice arenas seeking to mitigate such inequalities. When cleanliness becomes a matter of (Hindu) divinity, as I have argued is happening, it provides the rationale and impetus for exclusionary national imaginings and resulting political violence. One aspect of the rhetoric of SBA, which is enhanced through its embodiment in a divine Bharat Mata, is that the Muslim body—particularly if lower class—is symbolically and materially erased from a clean body politic. The discussion of Jannat exemplifies one instance of such erasure, as her historical specificities (as well as the scale of the cleanup required) are erased. Her visibility, ironically, *is* her erasure, reminding us that it is never visibility per se that grants dignity and recognition but rather *the terms* of that visibility, which SBA shapes through the ways its mediascapes personify defilement and cleansing of the nation. This is also the case with Dalit bodies that will be addressed more fully in following chapters.

Another instance of this erasure of the Muslim body is Modi's Clean Ganga initiative, whose framing intersects with SBA's foregrounding of Bharat Mata. The Ganges is considered the holy river of Hinduism and has historically been symbolized as a divine mother figure—Ma Ganga (Mother Ganges). While the river is quite dirty, due to millions visiting it every year on pilgrimage, its water is nonetheless seen as being pure and containing divine properties. Many use water from the Ganges to cleanse themselves or to heal themselves from diseases, as well as for auspicious occasions. When Modi swept to power in 2014, he pledged to clean "Ma Ganga" (who he said had beckoned him to Varanasi) and committed $3 billion dollars to the Clean Ganga initiative. In Kanpur, which has one of the dirtiest stretches of the Ganges, the Clean Ganga initiative has focused on shutting down Muslim tanneries, seen as polluting the river. Many lower-class Muslims work in the tannery business. The shutting down of the tanneries that are the basis of their livelihood is seen by many of them as a religious vendetta by the government consistent with the larger anti-Muslim climate of the nation. Rahman, president of the Small Tanners Association in Kanpur, stated that "there are many industries in Kanpur, and some of them use harsher chemicals than ours. We have taken steps to treat effluent. Why are we constantly being singled out?" (*Independent* 2010). Reports note that there is no dedicated sewage treatment facility instituted by the government for the tannery industry (Mahaprashasta 2022). Rahman noted that "Since we are Muslim, there is more pressure from the government for us to control pollution" (*Independent* 2010). These examples expose the constant discrepant relationship between SBA and the Muslim body, and how cleaning Bharat Mata often involves (whether intended or not) an assault on, or neglect of, Muslim livelihoods and identities. As with Dalits, the biopolitics of cleaning Bharat Mata is intimately linked with the increasing necropolitics of Muslim existence.

ARTICULATING CLEANLINESS THROUGH FEAR: WHAT IF
BHARAT MATA/GODDESS LAXMI LEAVES YOU?

If the appeal of darshanic encounters with Bharat Mata sutures many narratives of cleanliness, then another affective appeal that frequently powers the SBA mediascape is *fear*: fear that the goddess (Bharat Mata) will abandon "the people" if they cannot keep their surroundings clean. This is the ultimate threat: that people will lose divine protection due to their dirty habits. In a nation such as India, where the divine functions in everyday habits and habitats of people's lives—as when people have altars or temples in their homes, or conduct pujas in their homes every time they embark on an important event—such an appeal to fear can have persuasive effects on people's lives in inviting behavioral change in relation to dirt. It is this fear—the loss of protection from gods/goddesses, instead of a concern with cleanliness per se—that is tapped into by a video campaign that has undoubtedly been one of the most watched videos of the SBA campaign.

The production of fear that (Hindu) gods/goddesses will leave people if they are not clean translates into the idea that people will resultingly stop being Hindu. And the specter of not being Hindu by people refusing or not submitting to Hindu logics, Hindu gods and goddesses, Hindu *sanskar* (traditions), is what invites Hindu nationalist wrath today and the activation of various security mechanisms (statist and nonstatist) to discipline dissidents who challenge or disregard Hindu sacrality as the foundation of the nation. The logic of this video, then, colludes with the security feature of the Hindu modern as well as its sub-logic—the production of fear in order to secure a collective (majoritarian) security state (Inglehart and Norris 2019), which is how authoritarian (populist) governments work today. In the Indian context, however, this fear is being produced and mobilized by invoking a fear of Hindu gods. This ironically also *naturalizes* that fear and consequently naturalizes the security logic of Hindu modern governmentality that mobilizes this fear to govern the nation today.

The video, titled "Don't Let Her Go," was uploaded on social media in 2016. Directed by Bollywood producer Pradeep Sarkar and starring huge Bollywood names such as Kangana Ranaut and Amitabh Bachchan (who provides the voiceover), the video was first uploaded on the Aur Dikhao YouTube channel (Sarkar 2016). With nearly two million views on this channel since its launch, as well as circulating on many other social media platforms such as Facebook and X, "Don't Let Her Go" has become a face of SBA messaging, with its own hashtag, #Don'tLetHerGo. Modi retweeted and endorsed this video on his own X feed, which further amplified its virality.

The basic theme of this video is that if you do not keep your home and surroundings clean, the goddess Laxmi will leave your abode. The goddess Laxmi, along with an amalgamation of other Hindu goddesses— especially Durga, but also Saraswati and Kali—has been represented as Bharat Mata in Indian national history. In Hindu tradition, Laxmi represents wealth, prosperity, and domesticity that come from being a good Hindu. The video depicts three vignettes from a metropolitan city that is unnamed, but which looks like Mumbai. The first vignette depicts a lower-class household in a one-roomed *chawl*, a typical lower-class type of housing in Mumbai that consists of rows of rooms in different levels of a building. In India, many people have small altars in their homes where various deities are set up. In this *chawl*, as the day begins, we see the man of the household praying at a small altar. At the same time, his wife, doing household chores, walks out to the balcony with a bucket full of garbage to dump it outside the building. As this happens, the goddess Laxmi, whose photo was on the altar at which the man was praying, disappears, the photo frame becoming vacant (figure 2.8). As they peer into the now empty photo frame, the man and woman appear puzzled and terrified. We are then given a rapid shot of a rich red *pallu* (the loose end of a sari that is draped over

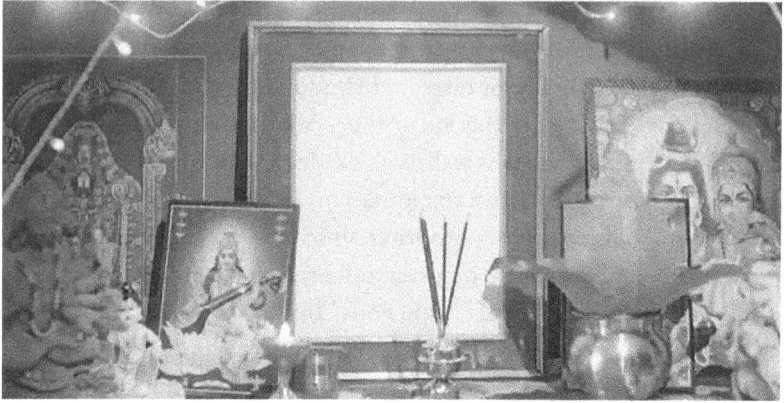

FIGURE 2.8 Still from "#DontLetHerGo."

the shoulder) with gold dots and a green border, which is floating away, signifying the disrobing of a woman's honor that is at the heart of the Hindu epic the Mahabharata and from which followed a war of *dharma* (morality) like none other. This disrobing of a woman's honor and its symbolic implications are etched into the very psyche of Hindu culture, for it represents a crisis of *dharma*. The wife is able to glimpse the floating *pallu* as it leaves her home. She is terrified. As viewers, we are to understand that this is Laxmi's sari, and she has been dishonored (disrobed) and is now abandoning the couple's home. The Hindu goddess of domesticity and wealth will not protect the home anymore.

This same format is repeated over two further vignettes. In one we see a *paan walla* (betel-nut seller) opening his little shack-like shop in the morning. He prays at the tiny altar in his shop, lighting incense sticks in front of a photo of Laxmi. Then he cleans the shop by gathering debris and throwing it on the ground outside. As he does this, the photo of Laxmi disappears from the altar. Once again, we are given a shot of the same red *pallu* floating away. The shopkeeper views this floating *pallu* with a mixture of surprise, fear, and confusion.

The next vignette features a young professional—representing entrepreneurial India—driving to work. He is stuck in a traffic jam, eating a sandwich. The dashboard of the car has a framed picture of Laxmi—a regular feature in many Indian cars. We then see the man throwing the sandwich wrapper out of the window along with a Coke can. As these land on the ground, littering it, we suddenly see the photo frame on the dashboard vacant. As in the other two vignettes, the red *pallu* floats away as the

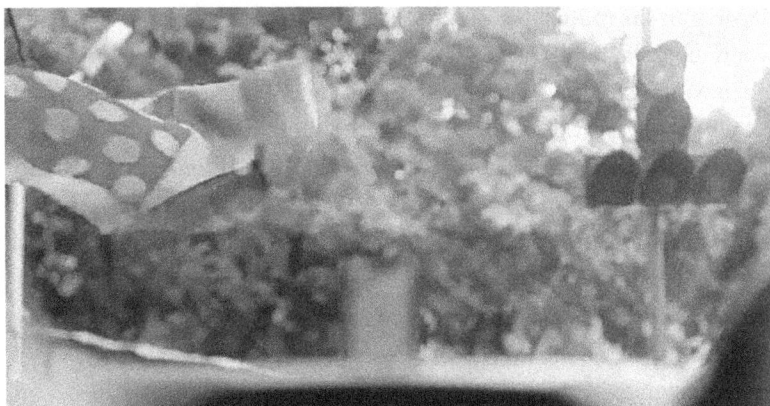

FIGURE 2.9 Still from "#DontLetHerGo."

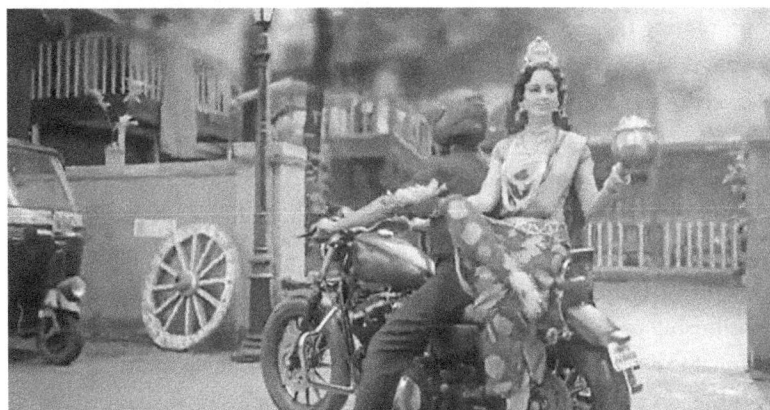

FIGURE 2.10 Still from "#DontLetHerGo."

young man looks out of his car with confusion and fear (figure 2.9). The music changes at this point, and we now see an embodied Laxmi walking away. The camera pans over Laxmi's bejeweled body from the bottom up in a manner that calls attention to her curvy figure. We are given shots of *alta* (red dye) on Laxmi's feet, gold anklets, a gold belt on her waist, a gold necklace, gold bangles, and a gold *taaj* (a kind of crown) on her head. With a pot of gold coins in one hand (signifying her ability to endow people with wealth) and a lotus flower in another (the lotus flower is associated with the goddess Laxmi), she rides away on a trendy looking motorbike driven by an anonymous man in black. A smile lingers on her face as she departs on the motorbike (figure 2.10). The baritone voiceover of Bollywood megastar Amitabh Bachchan takes over at this point. It states that when we are children, we are taught that cleanliness is next to godliness, yet when we grow up, we forget that fact. It continues: "We pray to Laxmi in our homes and yet we dirty the surroundings of that same home."[14] Bachchan's deep voice issues a warning: "make sure that Laxmi does not leave your home" for it is only "in cleanliness that there is *samriddhi* (prosperity)." He further states, "Make India a dream country, a clean country," and asks viewers "to share this video as much as possible." We are then shown a clip of the actress Kangana Ranaut, who plays Laxmi in the video, in her Laxmi attire. Introducing herself by her name, Ranaut states, "I am an Indian and I pledge to keep my country clean." Asking viewers not to litter and congratulating the prime minister for his efforts at making India clean, she reminds viewers that it is time for them to do their bit. She ends by imploring the viewer to share and like the video.

There is a lot going on in this now popular video that is worth noting. First is the erasure of class (which in India is intimately linked with caste), which has been a pattern in so many SBA media spectacles and narratives. This erasure is possible because cleanliness is linked to Hindu divinity. Rendering the situation of the lower-class couple in a *chawl* and the *paan walla* in his shop the same as the well-groomed professional in his car, the video once again constructs a universal Indian body whose access to, and relationship with, cleanliness is seemingly the same. What is erased is the fact that the *chawl* residents and the *paan walla*, belonging to the poor class in India, do not have the same infrastructural access to garbage disposal as middle- or upper-class Indians whose neighborhoods are cleaned regularly by corporation-appointed sweepers, or even private garbage disposal companies.

What is equally important to note are the intersecting gendered dimensions of this erasure. The woman in the *chawl* who drops her household garbage is "unclean" for very different reasons than the lower-class *paan walla* and the prosperous professional young man. Confined to the domestic sphere and having to labor to keep that sphere (and beyond) pure and clean—often without infrastructural support—women's bodies are always in close relation with the dirt and filth generated in a household. This is even more the case for lower-class/caste women who cannot afford domestic help, and who do not live in areas where a garbage collection service is regularly available, as is the case with the woman in the *chawl*. So, when we see Laxmi exiting this woman's household, viewers are invited to chastise her for being dirty and dirtying her surroundings. But the structural barriers and expectations that (still) situate and make women responsible for purity/cleanliness in the domestic sphere (which can be difficult to achieve without help, as is the case with lower-class/caste women) are rendered invisible as Laxmi exits. Instead, dirt and filth are, again, individualized and made to be a matter of "bad habits." As with the case of Jannat, this video, exemplary of many SBA narratives, reveals the consistent erasure of the *historical particularities* of bodies and their *unequal* relation to what is presented in them as filth. In shoring up a universal national body with universal responsibilities toward cleanliness, SBA narratives tell us that history and structural inequalities do not matter.

We see once more in this example the contradictions through which women (Hindu women) are expected to relate to the nation: chastised for being associated with filth (menstruation, domestic garbage, and so on), yet expected to embody cleanliness/purity in the home and the public sphere. The diverse ways in which the female body and ideologies of domesticity (and their intersections with caste, class, sexuality, and religion) are manipulated in SBA narratives will become even more clear in ensuing chapters. Relatedly, by linking domestic honor and prosperity with a female (Hindu goddess) figure, this video, like other Bharat Mata videos, attempts to secure a "clean nationalism" by erasing numerous marginalized women such as Muslim women (who then cannot symbolize national domesticity and honor as these attributes remain imagined through an idealized Hindu female), Dalit women (who are "always already" rendered unclean in the national imaginary), and women who refuse the constraining logic of female purity, domesticity, and its heteropatriarchal associations, such as lesbian women, trans women, and so on (although, as noted earlier, BJP-driven Hindu nationalism makes efforts to coopt some trans women into its religious frames).

Next, we see the articulation of divine cleanliness to a neoliberal economic rationality that demonstrates how in contemporary India logics of the Hindu divine are frequently sutured to a larger neoliberal market culture (Chacko 2019), which, as addressed earlier, is an important feature of the Hindu modern. In "Don't Let Her Go," the well-to-do professional young man symbolizes an entrepreneurial India through metropolitan signifiers such as takeout sandwiches, a can of Coke, and his car, all of which evoke the culture of neoliberal capitalism. The young man is prosperous. Yet instead of prosperity being understood as a symptom of glaring economic inequalities in the nation that are today exacerbated by the embrace of neoliberalism by the BJP government, prosperity is linked to reverence for Hindu culture (its gods and goddesses). So, when Laxmi exits the photo frame in his car—as she does with the other households—the young man's prosperity becomes contingent upon honoring the divine. And we are now to worry that this young man's prosperity will go south because he litters. Interestingly, it is also the young man's littering that is seen as the real problem instead of the automobile-centric hyperdevelopment that powers and pollutes the nation today. The overarching message of the video—that if you keep your homes and other properties clean and do not litter, prosperity (divinity) will not leave you and you will be successful—feeds on the anxieties and dreams (whether achieved or not) of an "aspirational India" (a phrase that was a theme in India's 2020 budget) constantly chasing economic prosperity and upward mobility. The irony, of course, is that the characters in the first two vignettes are not prosperous to begin with, despite possessing photos of Laxmi on their altars, unlike the urban professional young man in his modern car. Laxmi, so far, has done little for them, for if she had, they would have been economically prosperous. Yet the message of the video is to keep cleaning, for then the Hindu divine (goddess/mother) will keep (or make) you prosperous. This individualizes prosperity and poverty. The message also reinforces the inverse logic: those who are not prosperous must be so because they are dirty and inhabit dirty bodies. Economic and structural barriers are delinked from prosperity and linked to the divine (the goddess Laxmi or Bharat Mata) and the divine's desire for cleanliness among her subjects, specifically a type of cleanliness that meshes with neoliberal aspirations.

WHEN BHARAT MATA RUPTURES: OF DALITS AND BHOPAL

This divine script of national cleanliness advanced through Bharat Mata and goddess figures such as Laxmi is brought to a crisis when we foreground the Dalit issue. Dalits have historically been, and continue to be, seen as "untouchables" in Hindu India, and their social positioning is a product of the agelong Brahmanical caste system of Hinduism that is alive and well even today. Dalits are not a monolithic group. There are hierarchies within the Dalit community, where some Dalits have acquired education (and risen to middle-class status), and educated Dalits are mobilizing against upper-caste Hindus. Yet the primary occupation of most Dalits, even today, is cleaning dry latrines in public and private spaces (usually houses belonging to upper-class/caste Hindus), working in sewers, and rag picking. While manual scavenging (the removal of human excreta from dry latrines, sewers, and outdoor spaces used for open defecation in rural villages) is now outlawed, the maintenance of caste-based conditions leading to this practice means that it still continues widely. For example, while Delhi claims zero manual scavengers, in just five weeks between August and September 2017, ten people died trying to enter manholes filled with noxious fumes and human waste (Chatterjee 2017). Census data released in 2011 revealed 794,000 cases of human scavenging in the country (Isalkar 2013). Dalit households that make a living from manual scavenging often face death due to lack of proper personal protective equipment and training to use it. A recent report noted that of "the 1.2 million Indians shackled by this practice, 95% to 98% are women, who are forced to clean dry latrines, carry loads of excrement in leaking cane baskets, clear sewage, discard placenta post-deliveries, work on railway tracks, exhume dead bodies while enduring sexual harassment, social exclusion, dismal wages, and a lifetime's worth of trauma" (Kumar and Preet 2020).

Dalit women in particular work in manual scavenging (while many Dalit men work in public sewers) as the practice is passed down through generations on to young girls, who, post-marriage, tend to work alongside their mothers-in-law. Resistance to taking up this occupation can result in ostracization and alienation from their families (Kumar and Preet 2020). The very nature of Dalit work and the oppressive Brahmanical order in India that demands it continues to restrict the Dalit body to excremental spaces; thus, the Dalit body is always already framed as "unclean"—filth is its survival, its livelihood. For Dalits, to be "unclean" is to survive; to be "clean" is to not survive. Due to the nature of their work, the Dalit body is incrementally situated in what Rob Nixon (2011) calls "slow violence" as their bodies absorb toxins, including those gases emitted from latrines and sewers.[15] Slow violence is "violence that occurs gradually and out of sight, a violence of delayed destruction that is dispersed across time and space, an attritional violence that is typically not viewed as violence at all" (2011, 2). Being situated in an invisible regime of slow violence, as well as regimes of other types of violence, the Dalit body functions as infrastructure for spaces of upper-class/caste cleanliness or, as in the SBA movement, for national spaces that need to be cleaned up to showcase a gleaming India that can invite foreign investment.

In critical infrastructure studies, there is now a growing recognition that infrastructures are not neutral; while often unseen and taken for granted, they are actually political and cultural (Anand 2017; Anand et al. 2018; Berlant 2016; Gitelman 2014; Larkin 2013; Star 1999). While infrastructures have now been studied through a critical lens, what is often less addressed is how (particular) bodies also function as infrastructures that makes possible the life worlds of the privileged and dominant.[16] Simone (2004) reminds us that people's activities constitute infrastructures. If, as Berlant argues, infrastructures are "living mediation[s] of what organizes life" (2016, 393), then we could argue that the Dalit body, while rendered "unclean," is what mediates and makes possible the infrastructures of cleanliness and purity that the upper castes and the upper classes in India—primarily Hindus—inhabit.

Since the impure "untouchability" of Dalits is what makes possible the "self-definition of the upper caste" (Guru 2009, 56) or "the pure untouchable" (2009, 55), as Dalit scholar Gopal Guru terms the upper caste, it follows that the sacrality that Bharat Mata confers on the national text of cleanliness is intimately reliant on the Dalit body as infrastructure, which SBA mediascapes render invisible as such. If Bharat Mata exists as the ultimate sign of (Hindu) national purity, then her "pure" existence is deeply entangled with the Dalit body. Cleaning Bharat Mata (as national space) becomes possible only when we confront the underlying "unclean," "impure" Dalit body that cleans Bharat Mata everyday while being subject to "slow violence." This recognition, if asserted in public and the media culture of SBA, would rupture Bharat Mata as a symbol of a *Hindu* divine, clean, national space and unsettle the Hindu modernistic binary orderings of clean/unclean that are mapped onto upper-caste bodies and lower-caste and outcast Dalit bodies correspondingly.

But such rupturing has not occurred in SBA narratives, even if there was potential for that in a campaign ostensibly committed to national cleanliness. For instance, while sometimes the situation of manual scavengers has been acknowledged in SBA media discussions, these tend to be more tokenistic or uninformed nods to Dalits' work of manual scavenging instead of a deeper examination of the caste problem in India. In 2016 at Kumbh Mela—a major Hindu religious festival that occurs at the banks of the Ganges—Modi washed the feet of the sanitation workers who clean toilets at the Mela in front of the cameras to show respect for their work. But the tokenistic nature of this gesture is revealed by how, in the very few times that discussions occur about manual scavenging in government and nongovernment media campaigns, they tend to focus, as I addressed in chapter 1, on hardware issues like providing safe cleaning equipment, training in the use of this equipment, cash and loans assistance for their families, and removing the stigma that such workers carry.[17] But these do not get to the heart of the issue: the caste system in India that depends on Dalit sanitation workers to keep upper middle-class spaces and homes clean. Ironically, SBA has only heightened Dalit oppression. As more toilets are built under SBA initiatives, Safai Karmachari Andolan, an advocate group for Dalits, argues that Dalits are forced to clean larger numbers of these toilets, often manually, and often without accompanying improvement in sanitation infrastructure or protective gear.

In 2005, the young filmmaker R. P. Amudhan from Tamil Nadu created a short film titled "Vandhe Mataram: A Shit Version" (see Amudhan 2024). *Vandemataram*, "I bow to the mother" or "Hail to the mother," was a rallying crying of anticolonial nationalists in the freedom movement against the British. Thus titled, the film lampoons the celebration of the national mother figure (Bharat Mata) by visually documenting Dalit men and women cleaning shit, working in manholes, and cleaning latrines. While all this is shown, legendary musician A. R. Rahman's song "Vandemataram" plays in the background, highlighting the irony between the song's lyrics, which glorify Bharat Mata, and Dalits working as manual scavengers who have been excluded by Bharat Mata, even as they labor to keep her (national space) clean. At the same time, playing the song against the background of manual scavengers also invites viewers to wonder whether this population—who cleans national space—should be regarded as the *real* children of Bharat Mata, for they are the ones who keep her clean. Not surprisingly, when the film was screened at the VIBGYOR Film Festival in Kerala in 2006, Hindutva supporters tried to stop the screening by filing a police complaint that the festival was showing antinational films. I mention this important detail because the film has been simply erased from the SBA mediascape. Surely, given the outcry that the film caused by highlighting Dalit issues in relation to Bharat Mata, one would have thought that the film and its insights would have been integrated into SBA media campaigns. But I have not found even one reference to the film, and its troubling of Bharat Mata against the background of manual scavenging, in official publicity for SBA or in nonstate SBA media discourses.

Like caste issues that are rendered invisible through employment of divine figures such as Bharat Mata in a national pedagogy of cleanliness, and corresponding erasures of alternative arguments about cleanliness, the SBA mediascape completely neglects issues of environmental degradation.

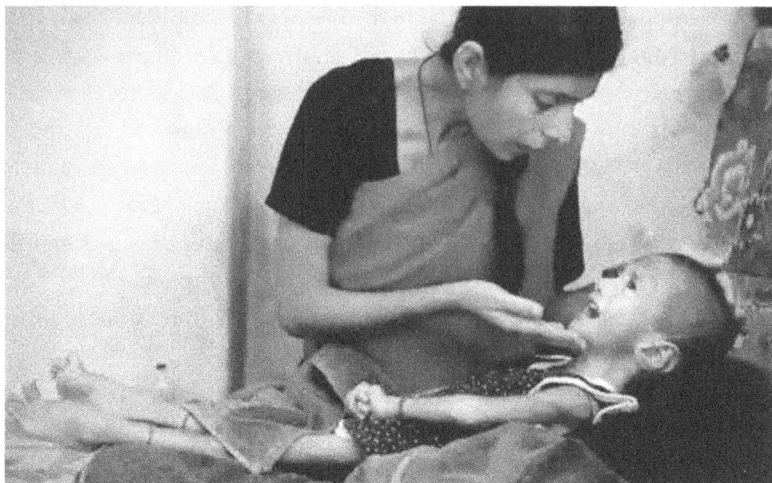

FIGURE 2.11 A Bhopal mother who was poisoned by the gas leak caring for her disabled child. "Bhopal: 25 Years of Poison," *The Guardian*, December 3, 2009.

Environmental crises related to modern, and today Hindu modern, neo-liberal capitalist development are causing death and destruction in India at a scale never seen before. Climate change has impacted several million people in the country. Industrial emissions, pollution, deforestation, and mining in forest lands originally belonging to Adivasis and tribals are resulting in an unclean toxic environment, and this toxicity is only being enhanced by the contemporary neoliberal policies of the BJP and its pro-industry stance. Chapter 5 discusses these issues more comprehensively, but a special mention needs to be made here of the Bhopal case.

In 1984, Union Carbide (now part of Dow Chemical) leaked forty tons of poisonous gas from its factory in Bhopal. It is still the world's largest environmental disaster. There has been no proper cleanup of Bhopal to this date. The water in the surrounding areas of Bhopal is toxic, containing high levels of chlorinated solvents, resulting in widespread cancer among the local population. The toxic air that was created by the gas leak still results in intergenerational disability, with mothers giving birth to children diseased or born with deformities including burned skin or brain fever and dying at ages such as four or five (figure 2.11). There are also women who are unable to be mothers, who suffer multiple miscarriages because their wombs have been injured by the toxic gases still lingering in the air, or who have inherited damaged immune systems from earlier generations who were directly exposed to the tragedy. A recent report noted that Bhopal "still hosts a hundred tons of contaminated waste" (Mandavilli 2018).

Despite the Indian government's negotiations with Union Carbide, the company only paid $470 million in damages in 1989, which is 15 percent of the original settlement money that the government had asked for (ICJB n.d.). This amounted to each gas-exposed person getting 25,000 rupees ($2,200) at the time (Mandavilli 2018). Since Dow Chemical acquired Union Carbide, it has denied any liability, which it pins on Union Carbide's Indian partner. Although the Indian government later asked for $1.2 billion (in comparison to local activists' demand for $8 billion), the money has yet to show up. The state of Madhya Pradesh where Bhopal is situated claims that it is unable to engage in cleanup work and looks to the federal government, which in turn looks to Dow. Forty years after the disaster and despite the song and dance between the federal government and Dow, Bhopal remains a contaminated site causing death and disease.

The diseased wombs of women (potential national mothers), who have inherited toxicity in their bodies from the older generation that was directly exposed to the gas, collide against, and rupture, the national divine text of Bharat Mata that anchors the SBA campaign. When Modi and celebrities keep reminding us that it is the duty of the children of Bharat Mata to clean her up, one has to ask whose duty is it to clean up Bhopal? And to protect the mothers and children of Bhopal? The violent contradiction between the idealization of Bharat Mata and the mothers of Bhopal (or women in other sites, such as Adivasi women displaced from their lands by multinational encroachment and forced into occupations such as sex work in cities) has remained outside of the scope of SBA and its imagining of Bharat Mata.

My concern in this chapter has been to highlight how the central figure of Bharat Mata in SBA campaigns functions as a ruse to depoliticize cleanliness and the idea of an ethnoreligious nation itself while simultaneously enacting the political will of contemporary Hindu nationalism. I have further illustrated how traits of the Hindu modern that are visible in SBA mediascapes reflect larger practices of governmentality in the broader social sphere—practices that in a heightened fashion today exacerbate caste, class, religious, and environmental inequalities. Unless the Dalit body can be structurally "cleaned up," which would entail upending the Hindu caste structure, unless Bhopal (and other toxic sites) can be cleaned up through environmentally conscious social policies, unless cleanliness can be represented as a political issue instead of a Hindu divine issue that leaves almost no room for recognition of Muslim and other minority bodies as clean, SBA will continue to function as a hollow sacred text of contemporary Hindu modern governmentality.

It is embarrassing and alarming that a nation that aims to be a global superpower in the twenty-first century can spectacularize development initiatives such as cleanliness and hygiene management through the invocation of Hindu goddesses and divine figures such as Bharat Mata, but which are divorced from any attention to (the intersections of) caste, class, religious, gender, and environmental inequalities. The hagiographic text of cleanliness performed through Bharat Mata in the SBA campaign and its mediascape is, at the end as at the beginning, a violent text—for what and whom it includes, and for what and whom it excludes.

THREE

"WOMEN'S EMPOWERMENT" THROUGH TOILET MODERNITY

THE NO TOILET, NO BRIDE CAMPAIGN

I am a chowkidar [guardian] of toilets and I'm proud of that. Being the chowkidar of toilets I protect the honour of crores of Hindustani women.
—NARENDRA MODI

You are going to set up 12 crore toilets by 2019. . . . Who will clean the toilets? How many more people will die? . . . [H]ow many more Dalits will die? . . . These are political murders. I have a right to life.
—BEZWADA WILSON

In 2016, a remarkable incident occurred in India. Neha, a young Hindu woman from Kanpur, a city in the state of Uttar Pradesh (a bastion of caste conservatism), rejected the groom to whom her marriage had been arranged on the grounds that his house did not possess an in-home toilet. Apparently, before the wedding, she had made the demand to her future in-laws that they must build a toilet at home. They did not. She broke her wedding and married another young man whose house possessed a toilet. This incident was covered by many print media outlets, and it also went viral as it was picked up by many international news channels. In a widely circulated video, Neha confidently stated to reporters that she was inspired by Narendra Modi's Swachh Bharat Abhiyan (SBA), which called for in-home toilets in rural and semirural towns and villages, but her in-laws had failed to match Modi's vision.[1] Modi's call for building in-home toilets was rhetorically framed in his speeches and in SBA discourse as a way to guard women's honor so as not to compel them to go out to the fields for defecation, wherein they could be exposed to sexual and physical violence.

Neha's story is not unique. Since pronouncements by the SBA campaign that homes in villages and rural towns that do not have a toilet must build one in order to guard women's honor and keep them safe, many young women like Neha have reportedly "refused" marriage without a toilet in their in-laws' home. Some are even being monetarily rewarded by local governments or NGOs for doing so (IANS 2012). The media, fascinated with this "Modi effect," are framing such refusal as a women's revolution and representing it as women's rights activism. Phrases such as "revolution of the runaway brides" (Kumar 2015), "the bride who led a toilet revolution" (Dhillon 2019), and "India's women want a toilet revolution" (Gale and Pradhan 2018) have emerged as typical descriptions of this phenomenon, which has also been referred to as "bathroom justice" (Sachdev 2017). The No Toilet, No Bride (NTNB) phenomenon has played a key role in how the media and the government portray the SBA campaign more broadly as a "women's empowerment" movement.

The No Toilet No Bride campaign was initially launched by the state government of Haryana in 2005 to encourage private toilet usage, primarily among the rural poor. A social marketing campaign, through radio jingles, billboards, and posters, circulated phrases such as "No loo, no I do." Although it preceded Swachh Bharat days, however, NTNB has received a new lease on life with the implementation of the SBA campaign, which has strengthened the narrative that women's safety and honor are linked to the acquisition of in-home toilets (Wells 2017). Especially in the first phase of the campaign, national and local media in India proudly circulated stories of would-be brides in semirural towns or villages refusing marriage or of women already married but now walking out of their marriages because the groom or the husband's household would not build an in-home toilet, thus risking her safety and honor by compelling open defecation. To be noted is that the stories are primarily of Hindu women, although they are never marked as Hindu but as everyday Indian (primarily small town or rural) women. In turn, the heightened national media coverage of the NTNB phenomenon has catapulted it to a global stage, as it was picked up by United Nations Television; the US broadcaster NPR; the British broadcaster BBC; British newspapers such as the *Guardian*, the *Independent*, and the *Daily Mail*; US newspapers such as the *Washington Post*, the *New York Times*, and the *Huffington Post*; the Pakistani newspaper *The Dawn*; and the Singapore edition of Yahoo News, among others.

The pivotal moment of this mass-mediated phenomenon, and one that shows the extent of its popular appeal, was the 2017 release of the Bollywood blockbuster *Toilet: Ek Prem Katha* (Toilet: A love story). The film (S. Singh 2017) is based on the real-life story of an educated Hindu woman in a rural village in the state of Madhya Pradesh named Anita Narre. In 2011 she walked out of her marriage within two days of being wed when she realized her husband's household would not build a toilet, which she viewed as compromising her safety and honor. She only returned to her in-law's home—after filing for divorce—when they constructed one. *Toilet* linked a happy marriage with the possession of a toilet in the groom's house, where the toilet functions as a symbol of women's honor. The A-list Bollywood actor Akshay Kumar—who has emerged as a poster boy for the Bhartiya Janata Party (BJP)—and actress Bhumi Pednekar have since become brand ambassadors of the SBA campaign. They have appeared on shows and in ads advocating for the need for toilets in rural villages and semirural towns in order to ensure women's safety and guard their *izzat* (honor), which in this rhetoric is linked to "women's empowerment." According to many news reports, *Toilet* was an inspiration to many young rural women (Bisht 2018).

The "women's empowerment" logic of the No Toilet, No Bride phenomenon is part of a larger discursive assemblage of developmental nationalism in Modi's India that purports to secure and uplift women. Like other SBA initiatives, the NTNB campaign has garnered praise domestically and on the world stage, and also contributed to Modi's reputation as a modernizer. Yet, even as this initiative has led to the building of some in-home toilets, it has done little to unsettle Hindu casteist heteropatriarchy and broader structural inequalities that unequally affect women's well-being.[2] Indeed, I argue in this chapter that as part of the SBA campaign, the NTNB phenomenon consolidates, in the name of "women's empowerment," a Hindu heteropatriarchal familial imagination in which guarding women's *izzat* (honor) and keeping her safe from assaults in public spaces become the prime rationales offered to men and their families in the Hindi heartlands for building in-home toilets. As the messages and images of the NTNB campaign largely center Hindu women, they implicitly reinforce associations between Hindu modernity (signified by modernizing toilet practices through in-home toilets), national cleanliness, and Hindu women's purity. Moreover, the linkages it makes between modern cleanliness and women's protection portrays the empowerment of women as being most effectively advanced by traditionally male-dominated structures of authority and the Modi-led state.

This chapter particularly explores how the discourse of "safety" and "honor" in the NTNB phenomenon advances a larger Hindu nationalist discourse in the nation today that in the name of (Hindu) women's security, is focused on *regulating women's bodies and sexuality*. Through this exploration, this chapter reveals how this logic of guarding some women's *izzat* via in-home toilet building is intimately situated in the security feature of the Hindu modern that evinces something larger going on in the nation: how the private domain of the family is being securitized at this current juncture of Hindutva in order to "empower" and purify the Hindu national family. Thus, the Hindu woman's body—as an upholder of the Hindu family—becomes a site for securitization. Such securitization of the (Hindu) family that is evident in the NTNB campaign is one of the ways in which cleanliness initiatives visibly connect the traditional Hindu family form with Hindu modern governmentalities of the contemporary Indian nation-state such that the security and stability of the (Hindu) nation-state becomes about the security, integrity, and purity of the (Hindu) family—and thus the Hindu woman. This connection plays an important role in linking rural and urban developmental imaginaries and, relatedly, brings together historical anxieties about the purity and autonomy of post-Partition India with contemporary campaigns to construct a Hindu supremacist polity.

As I have been suggesting throughout, the security characteristic of the Hindu modern is not simply political or militaristic but equally cultural (and they are entangled), where in the name of cultural securitization (that is, preserving Hindu culture) appeals or even demands to protect the (Hindu) nation are made today. Meanwhile, these appeals are increasingly organized around the protection of Hindu women. As Dalit feminist Sivakami (2021) recently observed, there has been a growing discourse in the nation around the "Hindu woman." The proliferation today in India of discourses around women's safety center on (frequently perceived) threats to Hindu women by Muslim men (and other men), all imagined as dangerous, leading to new policies and practices (such anti-conversion laws and the targeting of "love jihad" or setting up Hindu protection helplines) aimed at controlling Hindu women's contact with Muslim and other men.[3] Meanwhile, threats to women from Hindu men are downplayed. This was apparent in the coverage of the case of Shraddha Walkar, a Hindu woman killed in 2022 by her Muslim live-in boyfriend. At the same time as the Walkar case, there were at least two other instances of women being killed by their male partners with Hindu last names, but these did not result in the kind of coverage that the Walkar case received.[4] Fitting into this broader cultural map, the NTNB campaign portrays danger for women as residing outside rather than also inside the (unmarked) Hindu home.

Such discourses about protecting and securitizing Hindu women are not new, to be sure; they have deeper historical roots. What is different today is, first, that they are attached to *national* security frameworks (earlier in the colonial period it was more about communal security); second, they result in the increased normalization and even routinization of Hindu vigilantism, which is also producing authoritarian heteropatriarchal masculinist-protectionist subject positions—embodied by Modi himself—that circulate through various mainstream discourses (including popular culture) today; and third, they are often expressed through a framework of "empowerment" whereby empowering Hindu women is equated with protecting or securitizing them. Again, I should note that typically the Hindu woman is not marked as such in public discourses (unless they are Hindu extremist discourses), but closer analysis of mass media discourses, speeches by ministers and other public discourses (such as development schemes and legal discourses, including anti-conversion laws) reveals the woman who is to be protected (and thus empowered) to be Hindu.

What is continuous from earlier times is the Hindu heteropatriarchal regulation of the Hindu woman's body and sexuality in order to keep pure and stable the Hindu family (and thus the national family; this was evident particularly during the period of Partition violence) and, in the process, to construct imagined threats to that family. What is also common with earlier times (especially around the Partition) is the revival of a Hindu masculinist heteropatriarchal subject position (that thus far has felt weakened by the presence of "others") although the ways in which this plays out today is different.

In this chapter, I show how the NTNB phenomenon feeds into, and draws from, this broader political and cultural climate of majoritarian fear and securitization in the nation today. I argue that the NTNB discourse of protecting (Hindu) women's safety and honor through toilet reform offers a hetero-masculinist and protectionist subject position to Hindu men, specifically by whipping up fears about the potential defilement of (un-stated Hindu) women that can seemingly occur when there is no in-home toilet, and they are compelled to engage in open defecation. As Dibyesh Anand argues, "discourses of insecurity are about 'representations of dan-ger'" (2005, 206). What this chapter illustrates is how something as in-nocuous as toilet building fuses with the Hindu modern security ethos of fear. Through the NTNB campaign, we can see how, in contemporary India, almost everything and anything can be attached to a security logic, which has become overtly intimate, and tends to work particularly on (Hindu) female bodies. For some communities, however, the security ethos of the Hindu dominant state has *always* operated in their intimate spaces (for ex-ample, Dalits, those deemed as "Naxals" or "terrorists," and Kashmiri and northeastern women violated by the military). Today this trend is expand-ing and accelerating, becoming increasingly national in scope, with cleanli-ness logics and vocabularies playing an important role.

THE DISCOURSE OF "WOMEN'S SAFETY" IN THE NTNB PHENOMENON

The predominant rhetoric through which the NTNB discourse constructs gendered logics of securitization is by linking a woman's safety to her per-sonal honor, which is equated with the familial man's (husband/father) honor and by extension the heteropatriarchal nation's honor. Men seeking to marry have a duty to keep their wives safe so that they are not compelled to go to the fields to defecate and risk being sexually assaulted or exposed to prying male eyes. This rhetoric is geared toward rural India, especially the Hindi heartland where most homes do not have an in-home toilet, either because they are poor and cannot afford to build one or they are caught in ancient Hindu traditions where maintaining a toilet inside the home is seen as polluting. As emphasized earlier, although the NTNB discourse fo-cuses on keeping safe an "everywoman" of India, that this woman is norma-tively Hindu ignores the varied and different ways in which "safety" plays out where Dalit (or even Muslim or Adivasi) women are concerned.

Concerns about women's sexual and physical safety undergird the dominant media coverage of NTNB. For example, in 2017, many newspapers reported the case of a twenty-four-year-old woman from Bhilwara who filed for divorce as her husband's household would not build a toilet. The courts granted divorce stating that not having a toilet amounts to "outraging the modesty of a woman" (*News Minute* 2017). Media reports of this incident noted that having to go out to the fields undermined the woman's dignity, for she had to wait until dusk to go to the fields and this exposed her to danger (of sexual or physical assault). The *Guardian* similarly narrated the story of a woman who started a "toilet revolution" that was supported by her mother-in-law and grandmother-in-law. In an interview, the grandmother-in-law stated, "We never knew anything else. This is how it has always been. We had no choice but to go out in the fields. It was hell—getting up so early, the freezing cold in the winters, the fog, *the fear that some man will stumble across you*" (Dhillon 2019, emphasis added). Elaborating on this unsafe situation, the report summarized the grandmother-in-law's comments by noting that during their time in the fields, "men would suddenly appear and start jeering. At other times, a farmer would turn up armed with a stick to run them off his fields. At night, women had to wait for cover of darkness before venturing out" (Dhillon 2019).

The government's SBA media portal has uploaded research reports that constantly assert a link between open defecation and sexual assaults of women. One report states: "open defecation places women and girls in danger, as they often face harassment and assault from men, or are attacked by animals" (SRC n.d.). The title of the report, "Access to Toilets and the Safety: Convenience and Self-Respect of Women in Rural India," explicitly links women's "self-respect" to their safety from violence perpetrated by unknown men, thus justifying the need for a toilet. The government tweet referenced below also echoes this sentiment (figure 3.1). The accompanying image of a lone woman in an open field evokes her lack of safety, reminding us that any harm could come to her in this stark openness. Thus, we are told in the image's accompanying text that we have to ensure the safety of such women by equipping a home with a toilet. This link between open defecation, the need of an in-home toilet, and sexual or physical assault of women has been further emphasized by important NGOs, such as Sulabh International, that focus on sanitation programs. The founder of Sulabh insisted that "rapes can be curtailed if there are more toilets built for women" (PTI 2021a).

Swachh Bharat Urban

@SwachhBharatGov. Jan 9, 2016.

With an absence of a toilet at home, women & girls defecate in the open. This risks their health and safety.

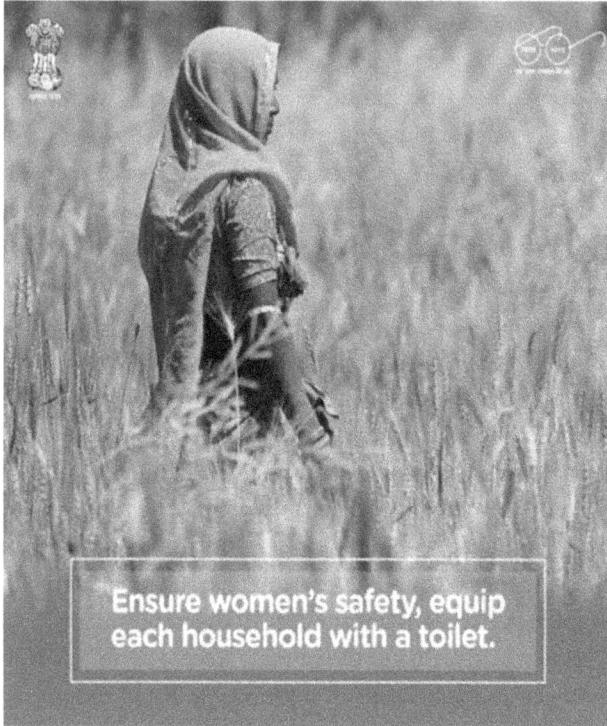

Ensure women's safety, equip each household with a toilet.

FIGURE 3.1

This kind of framing of women's safety is particularly evident in films and advertisements that advance the NTNB phenomenon in the name of women's empowerment. *Toilet: Ek Prem Katha*, the aforementioned Bollywood blockbuster that was released four days before India's Independence Day in August 2017, warrants examination as it was hailed by several media outlets and by Modi himself for representing a "commendable effort to promote cleanliness" (PTI 2017b). Its very launch around Independence Day was meant to stir up nationalist fervor around women's safety. Seen by various state governments as a social-issue film that takes women's safety and empowerment seriously, *Toilet* was essentially promoted by being exempted from taxation in many states, especially those where the BJP is in power.

Women's safety is evoked right from the start of the film. One of the early shots is of a *lota* party where women at dawn are seen defecating in the fields.[5] We see a man on a tractor (presumably a farmer) deliberately aiming the light of his tractor on the women. In this early scene, the fear of sexual assault is evoked as the shining light from a tractor, exposing the defecating women with their saris pulled up to their waist (although the camera does not show us frontal images of this). On the face of it, the attention to women's safety is commendable. In a general manner, I do not deny that open defecation *can* make women vulnerable to all kinds of assault. However, closer analysis of this discourse exposes a monolithic conceptualization of female safety that advances Hindu casteist heteropatriarchal ideologies and makes invisible the relationships between Hindutva and caste- and religious-based sexual violence.

Implicit in this construction of "women's safety" is a unidimensional premise that in-home toilets in rural areas will curtail sexual violence and therefore protect and empower women. Caste blindness is exposed when we confront the sexual and physical atrocities that Dalit women continually experience from upper-caste Hindu men whose proprietary hold over the Dalit female body for centuries—and continuing today—is not necessarily pegged in any way to whether Dalit women have access to toilets in their homes. Dalit women workers in upper-caste Hindu households are often forced to be sexually available to upper-caste men of the household (including households with toilets) or risk their livelihood, for being of the lowest caste, their bodies are not seen as possessing any rights. Dalit families who try to assert their rights against the Hindu upper castes not only have women members (often publicly) raped, but also, as numerous incidents have shown, these raped women are then paraded naked. The frequent public stripping of Dalit women by Savarna (those within the caste system) Hindu men is often geared toward punishing Dalit men, especially those who are found to be in a relationship with upper-caste women or who assert their rights against the abuse of upper-caste Hindus through creating a spectacle of emasculation—that is, "I now take 'your' women, and by doing so, I remind you of your caste position."[6] Anupama Rao argues that this kind of "sexual violence is particularly indecipherable as *caste* violence because it is normalized as upper-caste privilege and experienced as an unspeakable form of intimate humiliation" (2009, 222). At least ten Dalit girls are raped every day in India, but the actual incidences are likely higher than what this statistic conveys.[7]

Such a narrow representation of women's safety in the NTNB discourse reminds us of the urgent critiques of Savarna feminism offered by Dalit feminist writers or writers focused on Dalit feminism and Dalit women's issues such as Uma Chakravarti, Sunaina Arya, Sharmila Rege, Ruth Manorama, Shailaja Paik, Gail Omvedt, and Gopal Guru. Arguing that Savarna feminism has consistently neglected caste, and caste-based sexual violence, in conceiving of women's oppression, and that it has imagined a feminist movement that speaks primarily to concerns of Hindu women from the upper and middle castes and classes, Dalit feminists have argued that, to use Gopal Guru's famous phrase, "Dalit women talk differently" (1995).[8] Their experience of oppression and violence emerges from the intersections of caste, class, and gender; thus, their "talk" about gender oppression is different from that of upper and middle class and caste Hindu women. Ruth Manorama, president of the National Federation of Dalit Women, notes that "certain kinds of violence are traditionally reserved for Dalit women: extreme filthy verbal abuse and sexual epithets, naked parading, dismemberment, being forced to drink urine and eat faeces, branding, pulling out of teeth, tongue and nails, and violence including murder after proclaiming witchcraft, are only experienced by Dalit women. Dalit women are threatened by rape as part of collective violence by the higher castes" (Manorama n.d.). The issue of safety is thus complicated when we factor in caste violence against Dalit women. It is a violence that also invites us to acknowledge that attacks on Dalit women's bodies emerge not just from upper-caste/class Hindu men but also from Savarna women who, having internalized the casteist misogyny of Savarna men, enact or are often complicit in violations of Dalit women in order to reinforce caste hierarchy.[9] This is what one saw in 2006 in the horrific massacre in Khairlanji, a village in the state of Maharashtra. Two Dalit women were publicly attacked and gang-raped by upper-caste men, and their naked bodies publicly paraded before being thrown into a canal. The group of attackers included women as well.

Just as Partha Chatterjee (1989) argued, in a different context, that pre-independence nationalists resolved the "women's question" by confining women to an indoor (*ghar*) domain that was to remain untouched (pure) by the material (Western) influences of the public sphere (*bahir*), in SBA discourses we also see the *ghar/bahir* dichotomy at work. Yet as Dalit feminists have pointed out (e.g., Rege 1998), the classist and casteist assumptions underlying Chatterjee's famous essay ignored how many women in India (such as Dalit women) were involved in Ambedkarite movements. Plus, many lower-class and lower-caste women worked outside the home. Thus, Dalit feminist writers have advocated for an intersectional approach to gender justice, one that, however, has been critiqued by some Savarna feminists (e.g., Menon 2020) as being too Western.[10] Yet, Dalit women's insistence on intersectionality is urgently needed for a nuanced engagement with the "women's question" in India today, especially as "women's empowerment," as one mode of the BJP's developmental nationalism, is being mobilized to signify a logic of Hindu modern governmentality and its alleged production of an ethos of progress.

An important point needs to be underscored here.[11] When Partha Chatterjee (1989) referred to the "women's question" in the nationalism of earlier (pre-independence) times, it was the hygienic upper-caste/class, chaste, pure (Hindu) woman who was the focus (of nationalism). The (perceived) lack of cleanliness, chastity, and purity of women of the lower castes and the lower class, at that time, was not really at the center of (Hindu) nationalist concerns in resolving the "women's question" with the national question. But today, especially with initiatives such as the SBA campaign, the scenario is different. The (seeming) lack of purity and hygiene of the lower-caste/class women, and their habits of defecation, have become the state's concern (in ways that they were not earlier) as the state attempts to "civilize" and "uplift" them into an imaginary status by trying to "cleanse" them through changing their toilet habits (that is, through development). Thus development itself becomes a tool of cultural cleansing and a mode of entry into the bodily intimacies of "stigmatized" women who are to be civilized into a clean (Hindu neoliberal) imaginary of the state. But as indicated earlier, such attempted upgrades (which can also be seen with the Ujjwala Yojana scheme that is aimed at getting poor women to use gas cylinders for cooking, although many cannot afford to refill them as the government subsidy for refills is very low) tend to be individualized. Placing the burden of "cleansing" on the individual woman, such upgrades ignore structural inequalities that result in lower-caste and lower-class women opting for open defecation instead of building private toilets (costly, for a poor family) that are not fully covered by government subsidies, as reports have indicated.[12]

A Dalit feminist standpoint (Rege 2005) that reveals the unequal distribution and recognition of safety in the public and legal spheres of the nation was particularly foregrounded by Dalit activists after the 2012 gang rape and eventual death of Jyoti Singh, who acquired the moniker Nirbhaya (fearless) and "India's daughter." As the nation angrily cohered around the body of this raped Hindu woman, Dalit women noted that the state's recognition of and willingness to investigate a case of rape depends largely on a woman's caste identity, as rapes of Dalit women are often dismissed in police stations in order to protect upper-caste perpetrators (Javaid 2015). The very few times such cases reach, and are recorded in, the courts or police stations, they are framed as "sexual crimes" but rarely as *caste crimes* that are sexually violent in their operation.[13] Gang rapes and other forms of sexual harassment of Dalit women have frequently been met with silence by upper-caste women's groups in India, and this silence, for the most part, continues even today, as was seen in the recent #MeToo movement in India.[14]

The NTNB discourse additionally makes toilet building in villages and semirural towns simply a voluntaristic matter of changing one's mindset and behavior, rendering invisible the political economy of caste. In the film *Toilet*, the father-in-law, a Hindu priest who is reluctant to allow his son to build a toilet at home for his new bride, changes his mind at the end of the film and declares a change from "*soch* (mindset) to *sauchalya* (toilet)." While the SBA mission promises financial assistance to rural homes to build toilets, it does not care to acknowledge that not everyone owns land or property on which a private toilet can be built.[15] Landlessness is one of the biggest structural challenges faced by Dalit populations, especially in rural India. Some 71 percent of Dalits are landless laborers, working on land that they do not own (Yengde 2023). In states that have a greater presence of Dalits, such as Haryana, Punjab, Uttar Pradesh and Bihar, 85 percent are at the mercy of their landlords (Yengde 2023). When Dalits attempt to build toilets, they are routinely prevented from doing so by upper-caste members of the community, just as they are prevented from using communal toilets by the same people. For example, in Mehsana District in Gujarat, a Dalit family had been trying to build a toilet for several years, but their efforts were blocked by upper-caste members of the village. Despite appealing to the authorities, nothing changed for a long time (Bose 2016).

The monolithic construction of women's safety advanced in the NTNB discourse and celebrated by enthusiasts of the SBA program as evidence of the government's commitment to "women's empowerment" additionally reveals its congruence with the Hindutva agenda when we consider the increasing disenfranchisement of Muslim women in India, especially in relation to patterns of sexual and other forms of violence. There is a difference, however, in the way in which Dalit women and Muslim women are articulated by Hindu heteropatriarchal violence that informs the security logic of the Hindu modern. Dalit women (and men) are violated by upper-caste Hindus to keep them under their thumb so that the political (and sexual) economy of caste upon which every Hindu household is directly or indirectly reliant can continue. They are thus imagined as being *within* the Hindu nation-state, even if reviled and grossly oppressed. But they are needed. Where Muslim women are concerned, the subtextual and often direct message is that "you do not belong to the (Hindu) nation"—a message that has a deep historical lineage that informed the birth of independent India—for "you are the source through which the Hindu-ness of the nation can be diluted." It is not that one articulation is less pernicious than the other; rather, it captures the different ways in which Dalits and Muslims (and women in particular) are (dis)articulated by the Hindu state.

For instance, in the Kathua rape case referred to earlier, when Hindu nationalists chanted "Bharat Mata Ki Jai" or "Pakistan Murdabad" (Death to Pakistan) in defense of the accused (Naqash 2019), they positioned the rape as an act of *nationalist labor,* and the raped body of the Muslim girl is thus not seen as belonging to Bharat Mata. In 2021, hundreds of Muslim women were anonymously listed for a live online auction by some Hindu goons in the now famous Bulli Bai case. Bulli Bai is an app that was designed to "sell" Muslim women online without their knowledge.[16] Their photographs were taken from social media sites and doctored (*Outlook* 2022a). Although the auction listing was not about actual selling, it still performed a function of objectifying and denationalizing Muslim women. And one sells that for which one does not have a place in the home. The Modi government has been apathetic toward this unprecedented event while insisting on women's safety on the national stage. One can only imagine what chaos would have been unleashed in the nation if Hindu women had been listed for an online auction. Even more recently, open calls have been issued by some Hindu radicals (including Hindu women) to rape Muslim women. In April 2022, in front of a mosque in Uttar Pradesh, a Hindu priest issued a call for the rape and kidnapping of Muslim women. This was a continuation of Sadhvi Giri's exhortation of Hindu men to "rape and impregnate Muslim women if Muslim men cast even a glance at Hindu girls" in a *dharma sansad,* a Hindu religious meeting (Asthana 2022), to which I referred in chapter 1.

When we consider the larger political climate within which SBA discourses advance rhetoric about women's safety, we see how selective its consideration of safety is. And we are left asking: What kinds of violence (historical and contemporary, casteist and religious) remain unacknowledged and unaddressed as a result of this unequal distribution and recognition of safety that is intimately networked through the larger security logic of the Hindu modern that informs the "intimate" realms of SBA discourse? The partiality of the gendered security logic of the Hindu modern is revealed here, in that it mobilizes fear one way but not the other. This also illustrates how the security logic manipulates ideas (that are seemingly modern) about (Hindu) femininity in order to produce insecurities that contribute to the regulation of the boundaries and intimacies of the (Hindu) family, which in Hindutva discourse often serves as a metonym for the modern nation.

The discourse of women's safety that is part of the NTNB phenomenon likewise remains enmeshed in a Hindu heteropatriarchal framework when it elides issues of domestic violence and marital rape, the second of which still has not been legally criminalized in India on the grounds that a marriage already presumes sexual consent. The NTNB phenomenon idealizes the home (which by default functions as a Hindu home for reasons argued earlier) as a site of women's safety. Senior BJP leaders of the Modi government have opposed criminalizing marital rape, arguing that it will end the institution of marriage (PTI 2022). Disingenuously, Smriti Irani, the minister for women and child development, stated in the Rajya Sabha (the upper house of Parliament) that "to condemn every marriage in this country as a violent marriage, and to condemn every man in this country as a rapist is not advisable in this august house" (*Times of India* 2022a).

Like Modi's Beti Bachao Beti Padhao initiative—which calls for saving girls (in response to female infanticide) and educating them when they reach school age, but looks away when young Dalit girls are raped and even killed by Savarna Hindu men (the Hathras case being a recent example); or, when Muslim girls are listed on an online auction site by Hindu men; or when lesbian or trans women experience violence inside their homes, as for instance through the "corrective rape" phenomenon used by some parents primarily but not only in rural India to "cure" their "homosexual" children by having a male family member rape the lesbian or trans child in order to "fix" her—the idealization of home as a site for female safety in the NTNB discourse makes, by extension, the Hindu nation-state (and the national family) the site for female protection while rendering invisible the casteist and heteropatriarchal logics (and their accompanying violence) through which family ideologies function not only at local levels but also at the level of state policies. As the nation, as the larger family, in discourses such as SBA becomes the site for (Hindu) female protection, we see the solidification, and even celebration, of a Hindu heteropatriar-chal masculinist national protectionist logic that absorbs violence in its performance, and that is also based on patrimony (Grewal 2020). Such a heteropatriarchal, casteist, masculinist, protectionist position of the Hindu nation-state is ultimately misogynist for "protection" invites grati-tude, and thus subordination (in this case of Hindu women) toward the protector (the nation and Hindu or Hinduized men embodying national protection). In connecting the home/family with the nation-state through a logic of female protection/empowerment/safety, such discourses mask how the nation-state, instead of being a site for female protection has—for instance, through the military and security forces—often used sexual and physical violence to discipline unwanted others, especially women, one example being the conflict-ridden areas in India. Northeastern regions such as Nagaland and Manipur, and Kashmir in the north, have numer-ous reported (but also undocumented) instances of women being raped or sexually violated by the military, security forces, or vigilantes, who are given impunity under the Armed Forces Special Powers Act.

It was actually quite possible in SBA discourses to make an argument for toilet building in rural villages without invoking women's security (again, the unstated women being Hindu). One could have offered vari-ous other plausible rationales. But the fact that NTNB discourse makes women's security its prime focus and links it to a happy marriage and family safe under the husband's (or father's) protection causes us to ask a larger question: Within what kinds of political, cultural, and histori-cal frameworks does the safety of a Hindu woman make sense and thus can function as a rationale for toilet building for her protection? In her powerful analysis of the semiotics of violence following the Godhra po-grom in 2002 (in which thousands of Muslims were butchered, raped, and looted by Hindus in Gujarat because of the allegation that a train carrying Hindu pilgrims in the Godhra station was set on fire by some Muslims, even though after two decades the details of the fire are reportedly still not clear) Tanika Sarkar wrote that what made Godhra ultimately possible are legends about "partition time rapes of Hindu women, rapes of Hindu queens under Muslim rule, [and] abductions of Hindu women all through history by Muslims" (2002, 2875). As I discuss in the next section, anxieties about the sexual (im)purity of Hindu women underlined the very birth of (Hindu-dominant) India, following the partition of British India in 1947. In the obsession with women's safety-as-honor in SBA discourses, can one not trace hauntings of similar legends to which Sarkar refers, given the current anxiety-ridden climate about the protection of Hindu women and a (perceived) loss of Hindu power that now must be regained? The next section explores this question through a focus on (Hindu) women's honor as it is represented in the NTNB phenomenon.

LINKING WOMEN'S SAFETY VIA TOILETS TO *IZZAT* (HONOR)

In his speeches on the SBA campaign, Modi has frequently referred to toilets as *izzat ghar* (honor rooms). In India, *izzat* is a highly hetero-gendered idea that typically evokes a woman's honor, and by extension the honor of her family. Modi stated that "if a house will have '*izzat ghar*,' it would upkeep the dignity of the house" (R. Srivastava 2017), a statement that equates women's dignity with the reputational dignity of a home and family as indexed through the perceived sexual behavior(and cleanliness) of its women members. In 2017, the BJP government issued a statement that all toilets constructed with SBA financial assistance should be called *izzat ghar* (*Business Standard* 2017b), although I was unable to find any data about the potential effects of not following this recommendation.

This linking of women's safety to her *izzat* is one of the most troublesome features of the NTNB discourse. In India, the notion of *izzat* is not just gendered but is also enmeshed in casteist logics. It is impossible to think of *izzat* without thinking of caste. Chakravarti and Krishnaraj write, "the honour and respectability of upper caste men are regarded as protected and preserved by women who therefore must be closely guarded and whose sexuality is stringently monitored. Upper caste women are regarded as the gateways—literally points of entrance into the caste system" (2018, 2). Thus, the sexual subordination of Hindu women to Hindu men is preserved in the notion of *izzat*. A caste's or a family's honor rests upon a (Hindu) woman's chastity, respectability, and proper conduct as she becomes the bearer of the family's/community's/nation's values and honor. Nowhere was this more evident than in the immediate aftermath of Partition. Tanika Sarkar notes that a Hindu woman's chastity functioned as the "*condition of the possible Hindu nation. . . .* [It] has a real and stated, not merely, symbolic political value" (2001, 41, emphasis added). Urvashi Butalia further asserts that, "[if] colonialism provided Indian [read Hindu] men the rationale for constructing and reconstructing the identity of the Hindu woman as a 'bhadramahila' [genteel woman]. . . .

Independence and its dark 'other,' Partition, provided the rationale for *making* [*Hindu*] *women into symbols of the nation's honor*" (2000, 152, emphasis added). The issue of the (Hindu) woman's honor (or lack of)—attached to notions of her sexual (im)purity and defilement by an "other" community (particularly Muslims)—informed many state policies of the newly born India. Some historical context is needed for the unfamiliar reader in order to uncover a genealogy that informs current anxiety about the protection of the "Hindu woman" that also manifests itself in SBA discourse.

Sarkar's and Butalia's comments take us right back to the partition of British India into the states of India and Pakistan, where the honor and sexual (im)purity of the Hindu woman and family became linked to narratives of self-legitimation of the newly born India, a Hindu-dominant nation-state. Partition resulted in two directional migrations and displacements. Millions of Muslims and Hindus who respectively chose Pakistan and India migrated to these newly formed states. Many were wrongly displaced in the chaos of this highly disorganized migration. Partition was a bloody affair, resulting in the worst communal violence that history has witnessed. Hindus, Sikhs, and Muslims butchered each other in order to uphold the pride and integrity of their communities and families, and by extension their newly born nations. Women's bodies became the battle ground upon which the war of pride and vengeance was fought.[17] As Ritu Menon and Kamla Bhasin explicate, "the preoccupation with women's sexuality formed part of the contract of war between the three communities" (1998, loc. 547). Scholars have brilliantly documented how Hindu and Sikh women were raped and mutilated by Muslim men; many were abducted to Pakistan, converted and even married to their Muslim-Pakistani abductors (see, e.g., Butalia 2000; Menon and Bhasin 1998). The same was true for Muslim women, as they were abducted or their bodies violated by Hindu men who expressed their rage at Muslims (as the Muslim League had opted for Partition) for the severance and dismemberment of the national body (Bharat Mata). Yet national discourses of the time constructed such Hindu men as exceptions, and abductions by Hindu men were often framed as giving shelter to Muslim women (Butalia 2000, 146). Partition was orchestrated by the British to satisfy Muslim fears (stoked by the British themselves in accordance with their age-old policy of divide and rule) about having to live in a Hindu-dominant nation-state post-independence.

My goal here is not to offer a detailed discussion of the gendered and sexual trauma that haunts the birthing of India and Pakistan. What is relevant for us is how, on the Indian side, the Hindu woman's (sexual) (im)purity became linked to national honor in ways that *it did not* for Muslim women who went to Pakistan from India after Partition (Butalia 2000). Hindu women who had been raped, mutilated, or abducted by Muslim men and taken to Pakistan at this time were largely rejected by their families in India on return, for their sullied state (that is, touched by Muslim men) was seen as a loss of family honor (and thus the nation's honor). Many Hindu and Sikh women committed suicide as a result of being disowned, or they simply disappeared. Hindu and Sikh families, out of fear, also killed their own women—so as not to make them vulnerable to potential sexual assaults by Muslim men—in order to prevent impending dishonor to their families.

Butalia comments on the remarkable efforts made by the Indian state in the aftermath of Partition to "recover" Hindu women who might have been abducted by Muslim men or families and were residing in Pakistan (2000, 151). *What* was at stake in these exceptional efforts, she asks, especially as efforts on the Pakistan side to recover Muslim women from India were not strong? She suggests that at stake was the purification (that is, recovering national honor) of these women and their relocation in their families for only then would the Hindu national family feel whole again and moral order would be restored. This was also about vindicating the "emasculated weakened manhood of the Hindu male" who had allowed this state of affairs "and who would now recover his honor" (2000, 150) through the recovery of these women. *Never once was this about the women themselves.* As the recovered women had to be purified, this involved them submitting to medical examination to ensure that they were not polluting the (national) family by carrying the enemy's children (Menon and Bhasin 1998, 542). Purification also involved forced separation from their illegitimate children in cases where they had been married to, or raped by, a now Pakistani Muslim man (Butalia 2000, 150). When some families refused to take back these "soiled" but now "purified" women, Gandhi and Nehru appealed (largely unsuccessfully) to the families, emphasizing that these recovered women *were* pure (2000, 127). This spectral wound of Partition reveals how the purity of the Hindu woman and its entanglement with the (re)masculinization of the Hindu male (and his honor) that fueled a politics of national honor was the ideological and material ground from which the Hindu-dominant nation that we call India emerged.

It is this genealogy that structures the current moment as the Hindu heteropatriarchal order, gripped again by "demographic fever"—primarily about Muslims (Gökarıksel et al. 2019, 561)—becomes obsessed with the Hindu woman's (that is, Hindu family's) purity and integrity, which is defined as her honor. The logic of the Hindu modern actively shows its workings in myriad legal, social, and cultural campaigns today as the Hindu woman's purity, integrity, and honor become attached to the security frameworks of the nation where it is not about the women themselves but the securitization of their honor, and thus the honor of the Hindu family, and thus the Hindu nation. This securitization of the Hindu woman's honor today has led to the emergence of all kinds of paternalistic, protectionist—and sometimes overtly misogynistic, heteropatriarchal, and violent—masculinist positions that are mobilized by (as well as produced through) various security logics promising to protect and power a Hindu Rashtra (nation) today, including the site of the so-called *izzat ghar*.

In contrast, nowhere in Indian history, even today, has the *izzat* of Dalit women—continually raped and humiliated by the upper castes— been a part of national concern. As Uma Chakravarti's powerful examination of nineteenth-century nationalist discourses demonstrated, when anticolonial nationalist reformist discourses became concerned with the "women's question," it was the Aryan woman's (the progenitor of upper-caste women) honor that became the object of historical concern, while the history of the Vedic *dasi* (the woman in servitude, typically Dalit and lower-caste women) was swept under the rug (Chakravarti 1990). Additionally, *izzat* has rarely been accorded to Muslim women in Indian nationalist discourses. Muslim women were often seen as sexually licentious, courtesans or prostitutes in nineteenth-century nationalist discourses (and were often forced into prostitution in these times). Not much has changed today as evidenced in the Bulli Bai scandal or recent calls for the rape of Muslim women. Bollywood too has a long history of portraying Muslim women as dancers, courtesans, or otherwise sexually "loose."

Additionally, the very logics through which a woman's safety is equated with her honor in SBA discourses excludes lesbian and trans women, a growing population in India that is rightfully demanding that they be recognized as *equal* citizens of the state. The *izzat* that is embodied by a Hindu woman ultimately functions in SBA discourse to shore up the honor of the Hindu casteist heteropatriarchal familial order. To be a lesbian or trans woman is already to violate the family's *izzat*, as seen in the pervasiveness of honor killings that are reserved not just for Hindu heterosexual women crossing caste or religious boundaries but also for lesbian or trans women, who face threats of "corrective rape." The logic of women's *izzat* in the NTNB discourses shores up a caste-ridden, religiously charged, heteronormative private and public binary of the honorable or respectable woman (inside) and dishonorable woman (outside), thus rendering the home/nation as a safe space of belongingness for (Hindu caste) women that must be simultaneously cleansed of queer others, especially those who disrupt Hindu national logics of belonging since there are queer populations who are also being sanitized and appropriated by Hindu nationalism today.

This *izzat* of (Hindu) women in SBA discourses is also being mobilized by corporate power to sell products, thereby strengthening associations between honorableness and neoliberal subject positions the government tends to valorize. The Modi government has reached out to the private sector to participate in SBA toilet-building initiatives. Reports note that this has created new markets in the country.[18] Through such initiatives, and their outgrowths, the discourse of honor is reproduced in many corporate ads that advance the NTNB phenomenon in the name of progress and modernity in order to profit from it. This demonstrates how the ethos of the Hindu modern, as it manifests itself through development, is intimately linked to neoliberalizing initiatives that are remaking India, often by shouldering the financing of national development programs under the guise of public-private partnerships.

One such popular ad, with a pervasive social media presence, was created by the Lowe Lintas ad agency for Astral Pipes (figure 3.2). Its message, aimed at men, is that using Astral Pipes to build a toilet at home for their wives, mothers, or sisters will protect their family honor. In the opening scene of the Astral Pipe ad, we see a group of men getting ready to defecate in the open in the early morning. They soon find themselves surrounded by a group of women from their village who mock and tease them, threaten to take pictures of them defecating, and make them viral in order to shame them. As the men ask these women why they are engaging in such misbehavior when they are the pride of the village, the women angrily retort: "Pride, what pride? Is there pride in being eve-teased when we are defecating in the open?[19] Is their pride in being raped? Forget the pride of the village. First give us pride and dignity by constructing in-home toilets." The women in no uncertain terms tell the men: "Listen carefully, build a toilet at home." As these men acknowledge their mistake—that they have failed to protect the honor of their women—the women threaten that if they go back on their word, they will appear every morning to shame them. The men promise that the work of building toilets will begin immediately. The ad closes with a scene of toilets being built by the men who have purchased Astral Pipes to do so. Having seemingly redeemed themselves, the men of the

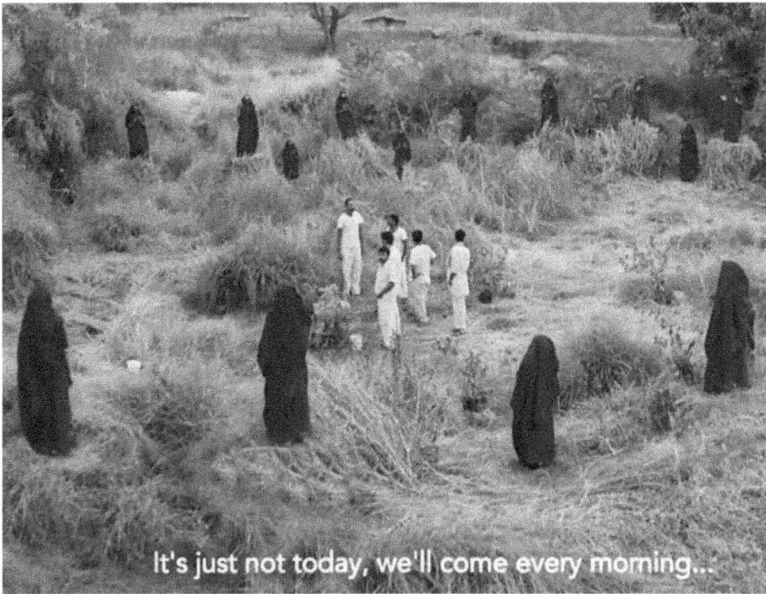

FIGURE 3.2 "Lowe Lintas sends a stern message to the Rural Mensfolk in its latest for Astral Pipes." *Lowe Lintas* (blog), May 23, 2017.

village now guard women's dignity and honor; through Astral Pipes, the empowerment of women harmonizes with the restoration of patriarchal order, which has been made possible with the help of private industry that directly benefits from the NTNB phenomenon. Other companies such as Tata Steel have also run promotions that address how their product has been used to construct many toilets in schools, thus keeping girls and women teachers safe so that they do not drop out (Tata Steel 2019). In this linking of women's honor with corporatism, "market citizens are regulated and disciplined through moral frameworks of Hindu nationalism" (Chacko 2020, 205).

This linkage of women's honor with family honor, and thus national honor, emerges most explicitly in an ad campaign featuring A-list Bollywood actress Vidya Balan that has become an important face of SBA. In a series of ads in 2012 promoting the Congress government's sanitation program, and which have now been revived to promote SBA, the linkage between women's honor (especially a bride's honor) and family honor is underscored. The setting of the ad is a Hindu wedding (there are almost no representations of non-Hindu weddings in the NTNB discourse). Vidya Balan is shown sitting next to the bride as her chaperone, while the

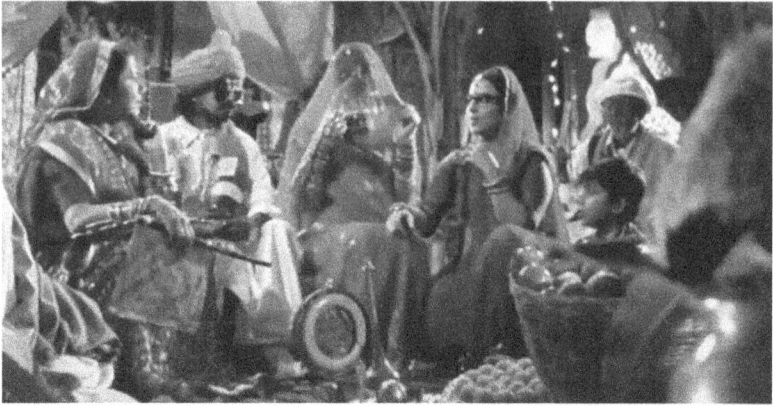

FIGURE 3.3 Still from "Ensure the Dignity of a Dulhan."

groom and his mother sit to the right of the bride (figure 3.3). When the bride drinks from a glass, her *ghunghat* slides down, revealing her face.[20] The sliding down of the *ghunghat* revealing the bride's face is not respectable, especially as it is often a symbol of sexual control, for by covering the bride's or married woman's face, it prevents a potential sexual gaze from a male (other than the husband) falling upon the woman. In the ad, as the bride's *ghunghat* slides off, the mother-in-law hurriedly nudges her son to tell his bride to lengthen her *ghunghat* so as to cover her full face. The bride immediately obeys. Moments later, the bride whispers something to Balan. We learn that the bride needs to relieve herself. Balan, on the bride's behalf, asks the mother-in-law, "Do you have a toilet at home for your daughter-in-law? She needs to go." Because a bride is supposed to be pure and chaste, she herself clearly cannot bring up the "dirty" issue of relieving herself. Mother-in-law replies that there is no toilet at home, and the bride will have to go out in the open. Balan, hearing this, is annoyed. She tells the bride to take off her *ghunghat*. She then chastises the mother-in-law for her hypocrisy, proclaiming "on the one hand, you were concerned that her *ghunghat* was sliding off, and on the other, you are expecting her to go out to relieve herself?"[21] If the bride's honor is violated by open defecation, then the family's honor is also violated. Hence what is the point in covering a woman's face with a *ghunghat* at home if open defecation already violates her and her family's honor?

This theme, where guarding a woman's shame/honor is the responsibility of the husband and his family—for the woman's honor is their honor—is repeated also in the blockbuster film *Toilet: Ek Prem Katha*. There is a moment in the film where Jaya, the female protagonist who ultimately walks out of her marriage due to the lack of a toilet, is seen defecating in the open in the dark, behind shrubs. Her father-in-law—a conservative Hindu priest, ensconced in traditional scriptures, who functions as the prime opponent of in-home toilets—is passing by on a motorcycle. The light of his bike falls on Jaya and he can see his daughter-in-law in that compromised, defecating state. Jaya, ashamed that the father-in-law has seen her defecating, quickly pulls her *ghunghat* over her face, trying to protect her *izzat*. The next morning, in the family courtyard, as Jaya is seen cooking for the family, she refuses to cover her face with a *ghunghat* when her father-in-law arrives. Her husband is extremely uncomfortable with this act of defiance and gestures to her to cover her face. The father-in-law, referring to the previous night's incident, makes light of it, stating, "What is the big deal, she [Jaya] did cover her face [when she saw me]." But Jaya chides him: "If you think that was not a big deal, well from now on, I will not cover my head before you with the *ghunghat*." Jaya's point is that if her father-in-law does not realize how she, as the bearer of family honor, was violated when he saw her defecating, then why should she be expected to maintain her modesty (and thus the family's honor) *in* the house by covering her head with a *ghunghat* in front of him? The *ghunghat* here, as in the Vidya Balan ad, functions as a bordering mechanism between honor and dishonor. The message in both these films is that if the bride's honor is violated by forcing her to defecate in the open, then the (Hindu) family's honor has also been violated. What should be noted here is that an in-home toilet (as a sign of the modern) functions to reinforce traditional and proper gendered expectations and behaviors of the (Hindu) woman. This again reveals how the logic of developmentalism that characterizes Hindu modern governmentality—here, an in-home toilet is a sign of that developmentalism—functions to keep women "in place" in the name of development and empowerment.

Such discourses "inscribe [Hindu] women primarily in terms of sexual honor and shame, fixing their value within the circuits of patriarchal kinship" (Basu 2015, 156). This raises the question: Is a raped woman not worthy of honor, especially as the fear of sexual assault is continually offered as a rationale for in-home toilet building? In her important work on the legal regulation of sexuality in India, Ratna Kapur has noted that while the Indian (read: Hindu) woman's sexuality is constructed as pure, chaste, honorable, monogamous, and confined to the family, once a woman has been raped she loses all protection from the family and community, however much she might conform to dominant norms (2005, loc. 873). For whom then does "honor" function in the NTNB discourse?

Further, such an understanding of a woman's rape or violation in terms of her *izzat* constructs an inner essence of womanhood—such that *izzat* is inherent to being a woman, that it is somehow located *within* her, instead of recognizing that *izzat* (or its perceived absence in the case of "other" women) is itself a heteropatriarchal construction imposed on women. Nivedita Menon provocatively suggests that understanding rape in terms of violation is compatible with patriarchal and sexist notions of a woman's sexuality, and that the struggle is to liberate ourselves from the very meaning of rape (2004, 156). While I am not in full agreement with this position (if I understand it correctly) that rape should not be seen as a violation (for it *is* a violation of the body), I do, however, embrace the larger suggestion in her argument—that to see rape as a violation of a woman's honor and "self" is already to locate that self and honor within a framework of serving, in this case, the Hindu heteropatriarchal (nationalized) family. Rape must be delinked from notions of honor or some seeming essence of a female self. Such framing of rape also makes it impossible to recognize its impact on those deemed to lack honor or appropriate femininity. But the entire semiotic landscape of NTNB frames rape, or other forms of assault, in terms of a woman's honor, and consequently offers a regressive view of female sexuality that is to be understood primarily in terms of a binary: honorable or dishonorable. This discourse also vacates responsibility for rape from its perpetrators—which are not the families who do not have indoor toilets, but rather those who assault and rape.

The honor discourse that informs the NTNB messaging is especially concerning because it feeds into the larger Hindu nationalist climate of today where a respectable woman's place (that is, Hindu women, for other women are not seen as respectable) is imagined through the family. This idea is advanced covertly and often overtly by many Hindu right-wing groups and leaders (who are increasingly asking Hindu women to produce more babies), and it has been especially charged up with the dominant presence of the Bharat Mata trope in public discourse today, as discussed in chapter 2.

However, this familial and domestic discourse, advanced by Hindu nationalist rhetoric, is complex. On the one hand, neoliberal entrepreneurialism—since Modi came to power—through the rhetoric of women's empowerment, provides financial incentives to women to become entrepreneurs (or participate as leaders), thus attaching the notion of women's empowerment to market logics (Chacko 2020) and the public sphere. On the other hand (and these are not contradictory imperatives), women are also increasingly being conceived in traditional familial/ homely terms. Thus, while women may be active in the public sphere when they are serving national development (being entrepreneurs or leaders), when there is no reason for them to be outside, they are attached to familial/homely logics, where they are considered safe and respectable. The NTNB phenomenon does some work toward overcoming the contradiction of these competing visions, encouraging brides to seek personal "empowerment" by leveraging demands for a toilet in the house that will take away their need to go outside frequently. Yet, as Coffey and Spears note, the reality sometimes is also that women *prefer* to go out to defecate because they enjoy "the temporary freedom and sociality that open defecation provides," given that women's movements are severely restricted in many traditional households in rural towns and villages (2017, 151). Recognition of this enables us to complicate the one-dimensional notion of women's empowerment advocated by the NTNB discourses, which offers a very circumscribed version of modernity for women.

There have been recent instances of young women questioning the paternalist narrative of safety within which women's empowerment and respectability have been conceived in recent Hindu nationalist discourses. A famous recent example is the Pinjra Tod (Break the cage) movement. In 2015, young women in Delhi college hostels and paying guest accommodation protested their curfew time, which they pointed out was not extended to men in the same accommodation. The young women formed the Pinjra Tod movement, which grew into a nationwide social media phenomenon that was joined by urban young women from many parts of India. On their Facebook page, Pinjra Tod activists wrote that this "binary of the 'good woman' and the 'bad woman' is the same as 'national' and 'anti-national.' (We) refuse to live by their patriarchal, casteist diktats" (quoted in Borpujari 2016). Important to our current discussion of NTNB, SBA, and gendered nationalism, they created a poster stating: "We won't be Mother India. Nationalism cages women" (quoted in Borpujari 2016). Further, they argued that rhetoric about women's safety actually functions to silence and contain women and deny them freedom in public spaces. All this has occurred at a time when the BJP government has been diluting Sec 498A of the Indian Penal Code, which provides sanctions against domestic violence and dowry harassment, by instituting a requirement that false allegations of domestic violence and harassment will result in a fine of 15,000 rupees. For a middle-class or poor woman in India, this is a big financial amount to risk. Additionally, since 2015 the BJP government has attempted to ease anti-dowry laws in order to prevent their "misuse" by women and their families (BBC 2017). The double standards of the BJP's rhetoric about "women's safety" are further revealed in that the home/family is hardly criminalized when it comes to violence against women, but the (largely Hindu) women's movement concerning public space is surveilled in the name of safety and empowerment. The anti-Romeo squads launched by the chief minister of Uttar Pradesh that I discuss later does exactly this.

The Pinjra Tod movement was targeted by the Home Minister Amit Shah and Hindu right-wing newspapers, that claimed that "under the veil of social reform, [it] shamelessly peddle[s] anti-Hindu, and . . . anti-India narratives" (Ranhotra 2020). Underlying these criticisms is the idealized image of a chaste Hindu woman who must be guarded by heteropatriarchal protectionist structures like the ones supported by Modi's regime if the mores and values of Hindu culture are to be preserved. The Pinjra Tod movement—along with others such as Why Loiter? that started in 2014 in Mumbai by a group of women organizing in response to street violence—resists the idea that women cannot be in public places by themselves without a reason, and that otherwise their place is inside the home, inside the family. As Phadke, one of the pioneers of the Why Loiter? movement, stated, the goal is to critique the "present environment where the discourse of safety has been taken over by the ideas of protectionism" (quoted in Jain 2014) and reassert women's right to public space as fully empowered citizens. These movements insist that the focus of public discourse and policy should be on improving public infrastructure instead of caging women through fears of sexual violation or sexually loose behavior (Roy 2016). Restrictions on (primarily Hindu) women's mobility in the name of their safety and empowerment are ultimately restrictions on their agency, sexuality, and any resistance that they may offer to the Brahmanical patriarchal kinship relations that they are expected to reproduce or uphold. These movements, although urban-centered, help contextualize the rural and semirural campaigns of the NTNB phenomenon as they elucidate competing arguments about the meanings of women's rights to public space without fear of violence and the ways *this*, rather than honor, could (and should) be the locus of state protection.

Given the climate in India today, where a (Hindu) woman's place is being vigorously monitored in various parts of the nation in the name of safety and empowerment, it is not surprising then that in early 2022, Modi stated that the BJP government in Uttar Pradesh had restored the "true honour of women. . . . CM Yogi Adityanath's government freed women from that fear. We gave women their true honour" (ANI 2022). Uttar Pradesh is today gradually replacing Gujarat as the laboratory of Hindutva under Adityanath, a Modi protégé and a saffron monk who represents the ugly face of Hindu nationalism. The "fear" evoked in Modi's speech is women's fear of being harassed and molested by men in public. And the "freedom" from that fear that the state of Uttar Pradesh has seemingly delivered refers to the anti-Romeo squads, groups of men that Yogi Adityanath has formed to control street harassment and prevent young men from loitering around women in public spaces such as colleges and parks. In effect, however, anti-Romeo squads have engaged in the moral, sexual, and religious policing of female bodies and their right to choose their partners, even when consensual couples are involved (Bhandare 2017). The activities of anti-Romeo squads have heavily intersected with the policing of "love jihad." Specifically, the "hope" signified by such squads has helped the BJP in western Uttar Pradesh, where the Vishva Hindu Parishad and Bajrang Dal, both right-wing Hindu nationalist groups, and the BJP have alleged harassment of Hindu girls by boys of a particular community—implying Muslim communities (Verma 2017). These squads are given names such as Operation Durga, referring to the iconic Hindu goddess Durga, which again underscores that it is the "protection" of the Hindu woman (idealized as a goddess) with which the squads are concerned. The Hindutva agenda of such anti-Romeo squads is further revealed as they are nowhere to be found when Dalit women are raped by upper-caste Hindu men; in fact, reports indicate that Uttar Pradesh witnesses the most rapes of Dalit women.[22]

I have provided details of this contemporary climate to aid the reader in seeing how the discourse of women's honor and safety in the NTNB phenomenon reproduces the contemporary and highly charged heteropatriarchal, casteist, and anti-Muslim security logic that powers the Hindu nationalist imagination and its underlying Hindu modern governmentalities—in the name of women's empowerment and modernity—where the nation is gendered as a Hindu woman whose honor must be protected, especially through regulation of her movements outside the home. The discourse of protection of the (Hindu) woman reveals not just the workings of the security feature of the Hindu modern but how it is entangled with the sacralization of land (*punyabhoomi*)—another feature of the Hindu modern. If the national territory is to be regarded as a sacred Hindu space, then controlling and protecting the Hindu woman's body is essential to the purification logic that underlies this sacralization.

This logic, as I explicated earlier, was fundamental to the birth of the nation. Thus, the safety discourse around the Hindu woman is simultaneously a discourse about ensuring her purity (symbolizing the Hindu nation's purity) in the name of empowerment and development—both of which become sacralized in the process.

REWRITING HINDU MASCULINITY THROUGH
A NATIONALIST PROTECTIONIST COMPLEX

I have been arguing throughout this book that the security feature of the Hindu modern, as it plays out in the Hindu public sphere today, is intimately linked to the revival of a Hindu heteropatriarchal, protectionist, and paternalistic subject position whose goal is to protect the nation, heterogendered as a Hindu woman. This subject position emerges in reaction to earlier (seemingly) effeminate expressions of Hindu masculinity: from Partition, which led to the dismemberment of Bharat Mata, to the "soft" Nehruvian era, when India could not protect itself from the likes of China and minorities were appeased too much, to the weak Hindu masculinity signified by the likes of Manmohan Singh, under whom the nation spiraled into corruption and who was constantly managed by a woman (Sonia Gandhi), and who did not counter the 2008 terrorist attacks through a full scale military counterattack but showed restraint and hence did not protect Bharat Mata. Figure 3.4 demonstrates how the BJP framed Singh's United Progressive Alliance government after the 2008 terrorists attacks as "incapable" and "unwilling" to protect the nation.

When Modi came to power in 2014, he promised a shift from a *majboor sarkar* (helpless government) to a *majboot sarkar* (tough government). Since then, Hindu masculinity has become overtly nationalist and security/protection oriented. Modi's own image embodies this, as we frequently see images of him in military uniform.

The national protection complex through which Hindu masculinity is being reimagined today, I would argue, is an expression of *contemporary* postcolonial Hindu nationalism. The BJP's current Hindu nationalist agenda partly rests on *reforming* the Hindu masculine subject position in which developing the nation is linked to protecting the nation imagined as a (Hindu) woman. Arjun Appadurai argues that "Modi is likewise a Hindu reformer, committed to purging it [Hinduism] of its effeminate, antitechnological and tolerant elements to install a patriarchal, developmentalist

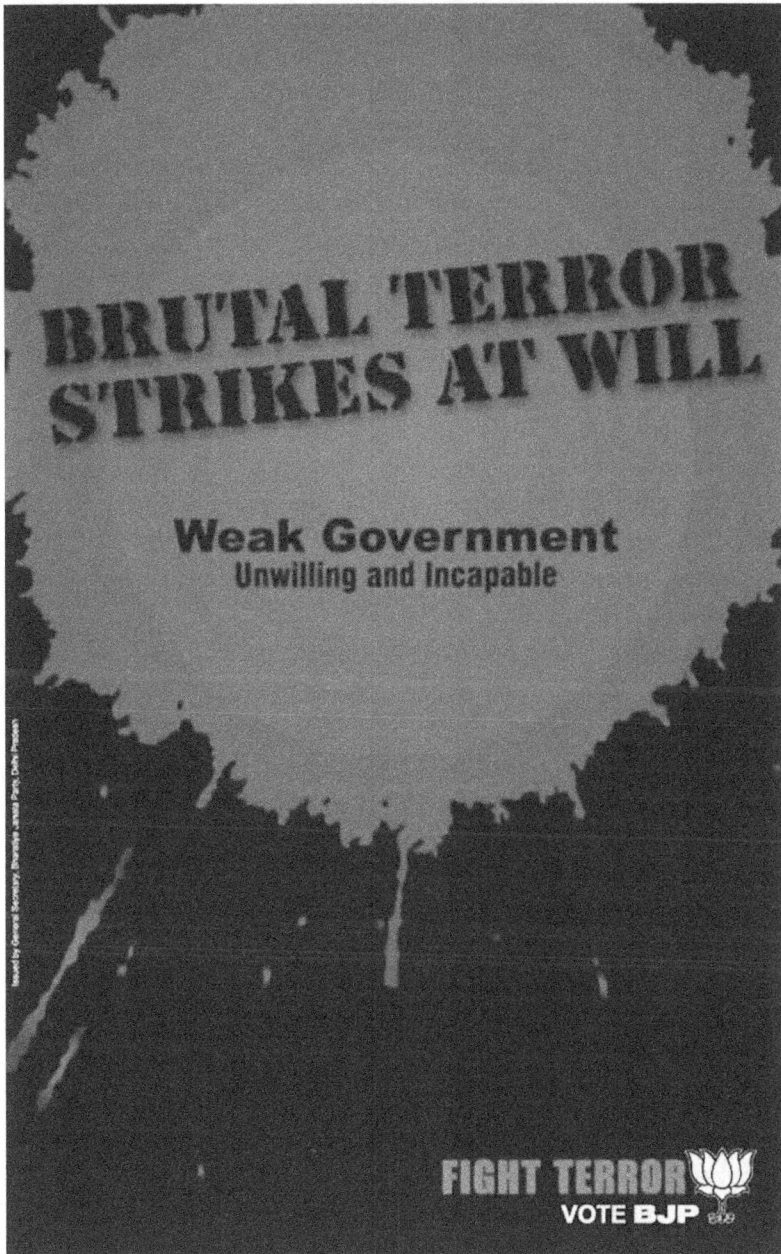

FIGURE 3.4 BJP ad depicting the UPA government of Manmohan Singh as weak and incapable of protecting the nation, produced after the 2008 terror attacks.

and masculine version of Hinduism in its place" (Appadurai 2021). As part of the SBA program, NTNB plays an important role in advancing the narrative of a reformed protectionist Hindu patriarchal masculinity that fuses with national development in the name of (Hindu) modernity.

There are various renditions of this reformist Hindu masculine protectionist position being advanced by recent Hindu nationalist discourses that have been explored by scholars. One concerns the militant Hindu "foot soldiers" (Banerjee 2006, 69) who take it upon themselves to engage in everyday vigilante acts to protect and securitize the Hindu nation.[23] Closely related to this is the second position of militaristic masculinity (Tapscott 2020) that, while not necessarily vigilante, is always concerned about any hint of terrorism toward Bharat Mata, and always ready to adopt a war-like position for the nation.[24] Then there is the third position, that of the "warrior monk" (Banerjee 2005, loc 1598 of 2549), embodied by leaders with sage-like appearances such as Yogi Adityanath, Yati Giri, and at times Modi himself when he strategically represents his persona through ascetic images.[25]

But there is a fourth, and a more benign and virtuous, reformist Hindu masculinist national protectionist position on offer in the BJP's Hindu nationalist discourse. It is more nebulous and has been less explored, but it comes to the fore by centering SBA and other recent development schemes. These four positions are not fixed but fluid and porous; and, while their underlying logic is the same—national protection—their avatars are different. This fourth position is the "common man" (always Hindu) protectionist subject position reflecting a development mindset. This common man is not part of the swanky, Westernized elite that Modi likes to hate. In contrast, he is found primarily in rural and semirural Hindi heartlands as well as among the nation's middle and lower sections of the middle class. He is often of humble origins (like Modi himself). This common-man position today is being discursively recruited to a virtuous and development-oriented (that is, modern) masculinity that can empower the nation but through Hinduized logics.

Modi regularly reaches out to the "common man" via social media and his *Mann Ki Baat* radio program, in which he emphasizes the need for national security, development, and empowerment. This common man, articulated into a national development and protectionist masculinity, exhibits a Hindu modernity where his masculinity is apparently not trapped in regressive superstition and rituals. In the film *Toilet: Ek Prem Katha*, this regressive mindset is found in Keshav's father, the orthodox Hindu priest,

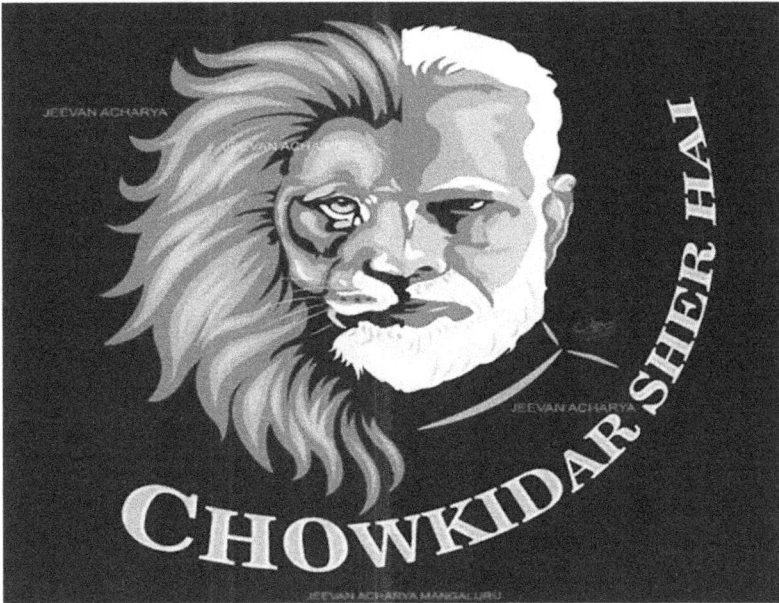

FIGURE 3.5 A Graphic design of Modi created by a Mangaluru-based artist in 2019. The design soon went viral.

whereas Keshav, the hero of the film, represents the common man with a development mindset. This development-oriented common man advances and protects the nation through acts of service that are, however, situated within Hindu kinship and familial logics. This is the masculinist position that we witnessed in chapter 2 in the figure of Akash who stops littering when he awakens (that is, is reformed) to recognize the importance of cleaning Bharat Mata (thus engaging in acts of national service). It is the same positionality that we also witnessed in the sweeper who wakes up from his dream and vows, as a son, to protect, preserve, and clean Bharat Mata.

This protection narrative focused on the common man is also reflected in Modi's own *chowkidar* (guardian) metaphor, referenced in the epigraph of this chapter. Although this metaphor can be applied to the militant Hindu masculinist position, I suggest that it best encapsulates the (Hindu) common-man position. In fact, Modi's own protector image oscillates between aggressive Hindu masculinity and benign common-man masculinity. A viral image of Modi, initially created by a Mangaluru-based artist, shows this split: one side of his face is the common man through which he likes to position himself; the other side is a lion, signifying aggression (figure 3.5). As the images states: Chowkidar sher hai, "the guardian is also a lion."

A *chowkidar* is a common man, typically from the lower class, like a neighborhood or house watchman. He is not the idealized muscled-up soldier fighting on the borders or the Hindu vigilante who does not hesitate to unleash violence on the "other" to protect Bharat Mata. A *chowkidar* guards not the external borders of the nation but the ordinary everyday spaces within it—a neighborhood, a home, a family, and so on. Consequently, when the nation is gendered as a Hindu woman/goddess, the *chowkidar* by default becomes the guardian of (Hindu) women as well, guarding their safety *within* the nation. Modi himself emphasized this common-man national protector position in a tweet: "Your *chowkidar* is standing firm & serving the nation. But I am not alone. Everyone who is fighting corruption, dirt, social evils is a *chowkidar*. Everyone working hard for the progress of India is a *chowkidar*" (*Indian Express* 2019). As "dirt" and "social evils" are undefined here, they can be easily extrapolated, in the current climate, to refer to certain populations and their cultural practices that are positioned by BJP nationalist discourse as threatening the nation.

Modi's *chowkidar* metaphor has inspired millions of common Hindu men in rural and semirural (and even urban) parts of the nation, and fueled a national protectionist impulse that has been channeled in specific directions and not others. The following comments from Anil Baluni, a BJP media head and former MP, reflect this well:

> By saying "Main Bhi Chowkidar" [I am also a *chowkidar*], and inspiring others to say so as well, Modi has single-handedly created a social movement that is not about political messaging but about a positive call to action, to take ownership of the country's *development*. Lakhs of people have said "Main Bhi Chowkidar" along with Modi" (Baluni 2019).[26]

Baluni's reference to "lakhs of people" is an unspoken reference to the implicitly Hindu common man of the nation, for Muslim and Dalit men can never protect the nation imagined as a Hindu Rashtra in this Hindu nationalist logic. This form of a new Hindu masculinity, which invites the common man to be part of a "movement" to "take ownership of the country's development" (where the country is gendered as a Hindu woman, Bharat Mata), has been directly articulated to SBA, and SBA has been staged as a proving ground for *chowkidar* masculinity. In his comments, Baluni additionally noted that "the people are playing the role of *chowkidars of cleanliness with pride. 'Main Bhi Chowkidar'* has evoked this feeling of ownership and pride in Indians" (Baluni 2019, emphasis added). Here, cleanliness is seen as something to be guarded and protected, and since cleanliness is equated with the (Hindu) female body, the *chowkidar* is to guard her body as well. This is unfortunately happening today with the rise of vigilante Hindu masculinity, explored in chapter 4.

In many of Modi's development initiatives, including the SBA campaign, this common Hindu man becomes heroic and virtuous by engaging in *everyday* acts of national empowerment that are explicitly linked to women's empowerment. A few are worth noting in order to provide a broader context within which to situate the NTNB discourse. One is Modi's initiative Selfie With Daughter, which has flooded the internet.[27] With this initiative, he called upon parents to post selfies with their daughters in order to foreground the importance of daughters in developing the nation. While looking at several such selfies on X and Instagram, among other sites, I observed that it is disproportionately fathers who post pictures with their daughters.[28] And they are primarily Hindu fathers. I realize that it is not always possible to recognize a Muslim man *as* Muslim. However, as a critical media scholar, I understand that when representations are geared toward inviting recognition of a cultural/religious identity, that identity is often highlighted through visible cultural (and often stereotypical) markers so as not to blend it into a monolith. None of this was predominantly present in the Selfie With Daughter mediascape. Additionally, if social media handles are anything to go by, then in my analysis I primarily found handles of official posters (disproportionately fathers) largely carrying Hindu last names.

There was, however, one remarkable disturbance that occurred when a Muslim young woman, Nishin Jafri, the daughter of Ehsan Jafri, a Congress MP who was murdered in the 2002 Gujarat pogrom, posted a selfie on Facebook with the statement: "SelfieWithDaughter: This one will haunt him for ever" (*New Indian Express* 2015). The post became viral, appearing on many social media sites. "Him" refers to Modi (although Nishin Jafri does not directly use his name) for he was the chief minister of Gujarat at the time of the pogrom and was seen by many to have allowed it. There were no responses from the prime minister to the post, even though some media outlets covered it. This, again, was an important moment that could have yielded a larger conversation in the nation about the precarious lives of Muslim fathers and their daughters, and thus the Muslim family itself. But that did not occur. Media reports merely covered this factually, and simply noted that there was some dissent toward the Selfie With Daughter campaign.

There was also an attempt at coopting Muslim girls as, for instance, when a Muslim girl from Mewat Haryana was expected to be the brand ambassador of the campaign, although it is not clear whether this finally happened. Overall, however, the campaign resulted in an unmarked *Hindu* father-daughter celebration in the social mediascape. On one level, this is not surprising. When Muslim families are being positioned as a threat to the Hindu cultural order of the nation, or Muslim women are being put up for sale on internet platforms, a Muslim family would probably not leap at the idea of posting a selfie with their daughter and showcase a Muslim daughter in an online space—today that is a risk. The Selfie With Daughter phenomenon reflects the everyday (reformed) Hindu man now exhibiting a *modern* mindset by asserting the value of daughters in their (Hindu) family, and thus the nation.

The other related initiative, Beti Bachao Beti Padhao, is Modi's clarion call to combat female infanticide or female feticide—which is legally criminalized but still prevalent in some parts of the country. This initiative emphasizes to parents (read: fathers, since it is more often men or their families in rural and semirural India that compel wives to engage in femicide or feticide) that daughters must be saved and educated instead of being killed at birth. Yet, reports note that 56 percent of government funds for this initiative has been used for media promotions and only 25 percent disbursed to states for actual implementation (Menon 2019). The hollowness of this protectionist position becomes evident when we remember that the BJP government has at the same time tried to ease or revise dowry and domestic violence laws and refused the criminalizing of marital rape. How will the girl child (*beti*) be saved (*bachao*) in these instances? Today there are twenty dowry deaths every day in India.[29]

But how is this common-man positionality, which is articulated into a protectionist narrative through visions of development, connected to the security logic of the Hindu modern? I stated earlier that security has become intimate today, operating in and networked through familial spaces that connect to larger security ideologies of the nation. The development-oriented common man, as we saw in Baluni's speech, is invited to be proud of participating in national development through the protection of girls/women in his family. Yet, this familial intimacy of protection, operating subtly in discourses of development, also functions to normalize an attitude toward any violence (state and nonstate) that may occur in the name of protecting and securitizing Bharat Mata, for what is ultimately being normalized is a logic of protecting the Hindu woman, whether she is conceived as a wife, daughter, or Bharat Mata. This is why it becomes urgent at this moment to examine and "disrupt sites"—and my focus is on development sites—where the "Hindutva male ideal assumes the role of the protector and the chowkidar" of women, the family, and the nation (S. Subramaniam 2019, 11).

It is also worth remembering that in the BJP's discourses, development and security sit side by side, collapsing the opposition between development and security, which demonstrates that development and security are not operational and ontological opposites in contemporary authoritarian nations.[30] For the nation to become an economic giant (as Modi keeps reminding people) and a powerful Hindu Rashtra, internal and external threats have to be suppressed or managed. Thus, the discourse surrounding the development-oriented common man can also neatly fold into the discourse of the militaristic (or even vigilante) Hindutva solider, striking against (in)securities and instabilities that can interfere with the powerful growth of the (Hindu) nation.

THE COMMON-MAN PROTECTIONIST POSITION
IN SBA DISCOURSE

This Hindu heteropatriarchal, protectionist, and developmental common-man subject position, in which building in-home toilets functions as an act of women's empowerment, is a core ideology that shapes much of SBA discourse. While my focus in the following sections is specifically the NTNB phenomenon, I first reference examples from larger SBA discourses that invite men to gift a toilet to the women of the family, thus positioning men through a logic of chivalry and protectionism, and ultimately positioning the act as a benefit to *their* hetero-masculinist, familial, casteist honor.[31]

Especially noteworthy is how the Hindu family ceremony of Raksha Bandhan has been mobilized by the SBA campaign and sutured to a development logic that coheres around the Hindu woman's protection. This once again reveals how minute operations of the SBA program tend to be attached to Hindu frameworks manifesting the governmentality of the Hindu modern, where developmentalism is connected to Hindu referents and rituals organized around essentialist and hierarchical gender categories. Raksha Bandhan is a Hindu family ritual where a sister ties a *rakhi* (a string or thread) on her brother's hand as a symbolic act, thanking him for his protection of her (*raksha* means "protection"). In return for her gratitude, the brother gives a gift to the sister. This ceremony takes place on the full moon of the Hindu month of Shravana (Shravan Poornima),

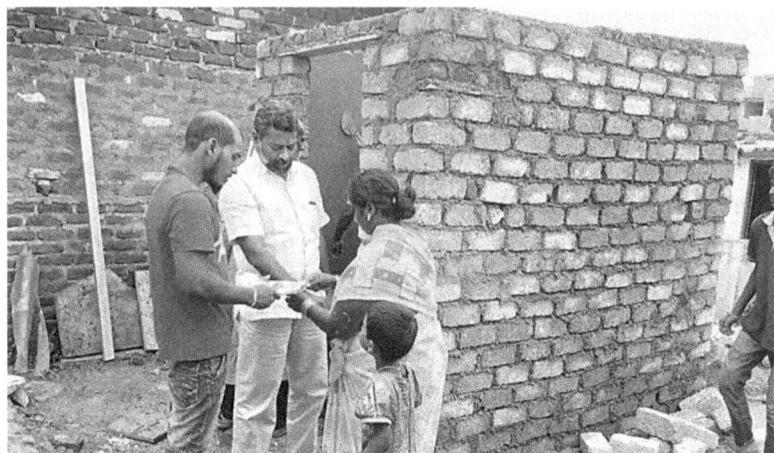

FIGURE 3.6 A sister tying a *rakhi* on her brother's wrist in front of a toilet under construction on the day of Raksha Bandhan. *Deccan Chronicle*, August 5, 2017.

around July and August. Many Hindu boys and men, inspired by the SBA campaign's call for protecting (primarily rural) women from open defecation, are now reportedly gifting sisters with toilets on the day of Raksha Bandhan, where the toilets symbolize their sisters' honor and dignity. Media discourse is rife with reports of this. For example, a photograph accompanying a newspaper article about the phenomenon (figure 3.6) shows a sister tying a *rakhi* and, in the background, prominently displayed, is a toilet under construction, which, we are to understand, is the brother's gift to her.

Local districts in various states have launched competitions for which brothers can register to win prizes and awards for the best toilet constructed by any of them from the local district or town. The Varanasi District Administration in 2017 launched a toilet-construction competition on Raksha Bandhan named Bhai No. 1. *Bhai* means "brother," so the brother who wins the competition is the "number 1" brother, the *shresta* (supreme) brother. The chief development officer of the district stated to a reporter, "For ages the brothers are responsible for providing security and protecting their sisters' dignity and health, and what better gift than giving a toilet which will respect her privacy and dignity" (Karelia 2017d). Modi frequently tweets congratulatory messages to such brothers. These stories represent rural or semirural Hindu boys and men being articulated into a reformed modern development mindset of the Hindu common man who protects his sister by empowering her (via toilets) and who also keeps alive but (seemingly) "modernizes" Hindu patriarchal rituals such as Raksha Bandhan. We can conclude that from such acts, he also learns the importance of protecting the purity of Bharat Mata/the nation, which in turn is focused on affirming and protecting his own (Hindu) heteropatriarchal value.

In the NTNB phenomenon more specifically, instead of a brother gifting a toilet to his sister we have scenarios of Hindu husbands or grooms—who were seemingly unaware of women's challenges with open defecation—now reforming themselves by realizing the need of building an in-home toilet for their wives or potential brides. It is rare to find among reports of the phenomenon stories about a Muslim husband. Figure 3.7 is from a newsclip about the story of Neha, referred to at the opening of this chapter. In this newsclip, we see a few men from a local NGO telling the reporter that after Neha walked out of her wedding, the problem before them was a matter of protecting her dignity and honor (see *India Today* 2016b). A bride already prepared for a wedding from which she then walks out *must* find a groom, for it is a matter of her (and her community's) "honor"—not to be left without a man to marry—as the men from the NGO recognize. Thus, they had to immediately find a groom whose home had a toilet. They finally found Sarvesh, whose home not only had a toilet but who was impressed with Neha's bold moves and thus wished to marry her. The wedding was organized by members of the local NGO. Sarvesh is presented as a groom with a progressive mindset just as the local NGO members (all men in the newsclip) are presented as honoring Neha's decision. Sarvesh is depicted in the news report as virtuous and chivalrous. And, unlike the first groom who betrayed Neha by not building a toilet, he agrees to wed her despite knowing that she walked out of the earlier wedding. His virtuosity, we are to understand, reflects his modern mindset. Yet the discourse of the local NGO men seeking to protect Neha's honor, and Sarvesh putting his hand up to marry her, remains enmeshed in a heteropatriarchal Hindu familial *rescue* framework. What if Neha had not found another groom after she walked out from the first wedding? Would her honor have been tarred forever? In Hindu traditional logics—especially as practiced in rural areas—a bride left without a husband on her wedding day can signify "bad luck." From the newsclip we learn that the local NGO members found Sarvesh, the new groom, that *very* day, and in the video the bride Neha is still resplendent in her original wedding attire. The local NGO men save her honor not simply by ensuring her safety by finding a groom with a toilet but also her family's honor by getting her married on the same day.

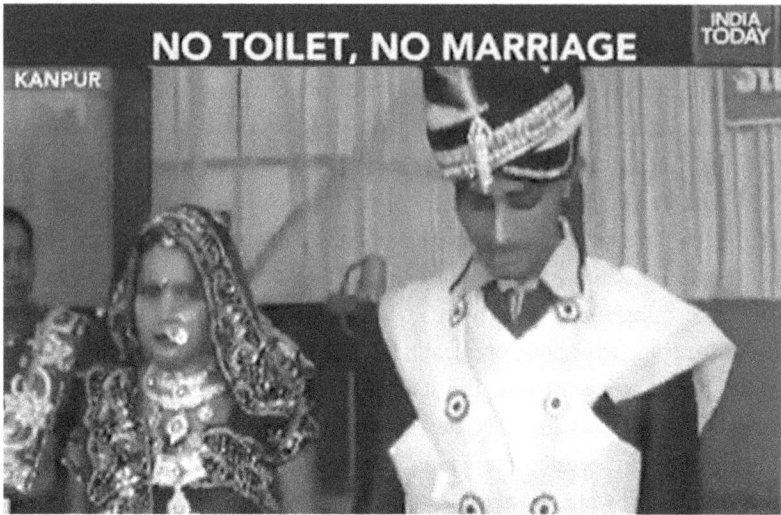

FIGURE 3.7 Neha with the second groom, Sarvesh. India Today TV-newsclip posted on Facebook, April 18, 2016.

On the one hand, the NTNB discourse critiques the (unstated Hindu) family for not safeguarding women's honor when it compels women to open defecation; on the other hand, it also offers Hindu hetero-familialism as the framework within which women's protection (that is, empowerment) is to be imagined. That is, instead of rejecting the Hindu family, it asks for a *reformed* ("modern") Hindu family that is aligned with the development and security goals (of guarding the Hindu woman) of the Hindu nation. Here again we see the workings of Hindu modern logics. Developmental aspirations are attached to the Hindu family, and conjugal structures are securitized through a "progressive" Hindu hetero-male protectionism that uses a toilet to protect the safety of the bride.

Figure 3.8 is from a newsclip about the village of Brahmaputhi in Uttar Pradesh, where members of the *panchayat* (village council) determined that they would not marry "their daughters" into homes without a toilet, for that would render them unsafe.[32] Again, we see the common *reformed* Hindu male protection narrative at work. This reformist position is marked because typically *panchayats* have not been the bastions of progress where women's issues are concerned. Thus, when news reports highlight such *panchayats'* emerging progressive mindset, what we are supposed to be glimpsing are images of reformed (that is, modernizing) rural Hindu common men exhibiting a (seemingly) gender-sensitive progressive mindset.

बेटियों की कसम... शौचालय नहीं तो शादी नहीं

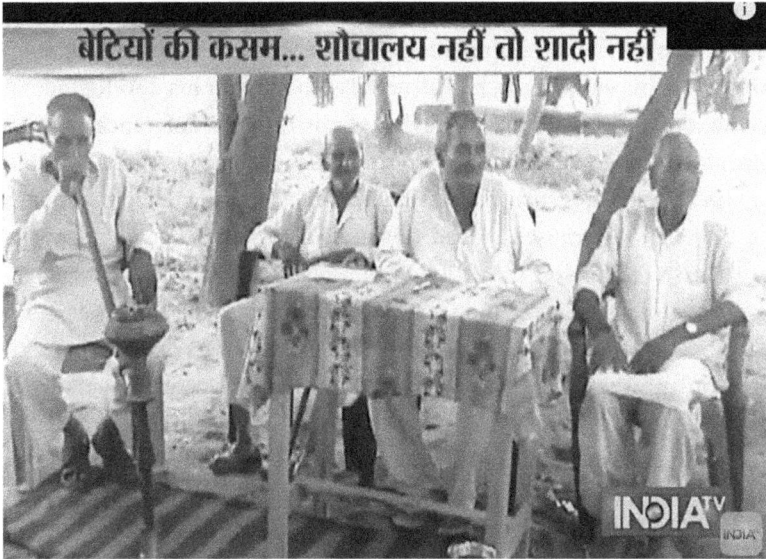

FIGURE 3.8 Interviewed *panchayat* men revealing their commitment to keep their "daughters" safe. IndiaTV, September 26, 2017.

As the use of phrases such as "we will not allow our daughters" reveal, their sensitivity still rests on a hetero-familial Hindu male protectionist logic. In idealizing the heteropatriarchal Hindu family as the site that will protect and empower women, the NTNB discourse renders invisible so many relations that escape this logic of protection, such as, but not only, domestic sexual and physical violence, the impact of compulsory heterosexuality, and the unequal labor relations women are forced into at home.

This development-oriented reformed masculinity is best embodied in the character of Keshav, played by Akshay Kumar, in the film *Toilet: Ek Prem Katha*. In a charged scene in the film, Keshav addresses the *panchayat* leaders (all men), imploring them to build toilets in villages to guard women's *izzat*. The leader of the *panchayat* invokes the ancient Hindu text the Manusmriti, which is supposed to contain all appropriate codes of conduct for Hindu Brahmins, and which is exceedingly patriarchal and casteist in its attitude toward women and caste outsiders. He argues that this text endorses open defecation, for building a toilet inside a home sullies its purity. Keshav, exhibiting his own expertise regarding the Manusmriti, retorts by reminding the *panchayat* leaders that this reverent text also tells us that open defecation should take place far away from water bodies, and that hands should be cleansed after defecation. Yet villagers regularly flout this and twist the scripture for their own purpose. Although Keshav is represented as a development-oriented reformed Hindu man bent on protecting his wife's *izzat*, he still seeks authority for his developmental aspirations, however, from a regressive Hindu text. The difference between him and the *panchayat* leaders is that he argues that the instructions found in Hindu scriptures such as the Manusmriti *can* be aligned with modern developmental purposes. Indeed, this could almost have been Modi or any BJP minister reminding the nation, as they often do, especially when invoking science, that ancient Hindu texts *are* compatible with progress and modernity. Keshav reveals the (regressive Hinduist) limits of "women's empowerment" when he invokes the Manusmriti and attaches it to a narrative of progress. Again we witness the operations of Hindu modern governmentality in the SBA context as logics of developmentalism are sutured, in this case, to the authority of an ancient (but now resurgent) Hindu text.

It is important to recall that the social reformer B. R. Ambedkar, as an act of protest against the caste system and the gender inequality it secures, had publicly burnt the Manusmriti in 1927. This event resulted in the ceremony of Manusmriti Dahan Divas (Manusmriti burning day), which is celebrated by Dalit Bahujans annually. Ironically, even as some BJP leaders try to coopt Ambedkar to soften the party's image, they never engage in Manusmriti Dahan Divas, one of Ambedkar's signature acts of protest. The large amount of public and state attention that the film *Toilet: Ek Prem Katha* received, including from Modi personally, was for its seeming commitment to "women's empowerment." What this also symptomizes is the dangerous return of the Manusmriti's authority in the current Hindu nationalist landscape. Members of the Hindu nationalist bloc Sangh Parivar frequently draw on the Manusmriti in their public speeches. In 2019, a Dalit MP, Savitri Phule, quit the BJP to join the Congress Party, claiming that the Hindu nationalist organization Rashtriya Swayamsevak Sangh (RSS) and its many followers, including Modi and his party officials, were attempting to replace the constitution with the Manusmriti (Sharma 2019). There have also been recent attempts by some members of the RSS to whitewash the Manusmriti, claiming that is not anti-caste or anti-women, so as to align it with a (seemingly) more inclusive and modern Hindutva.

Toilet: Ek Prem Katha ends with Keshav's father—an orthodox Hindu priest who thus far has prohibited Keshav from building a toilet at home for his new wife—realizing his own narrow-mindedness. The father, thus far an upholder of regressive customs, states that it is now time to lift the veil from a backward mindset (*soch*) and focus attention on a toilet

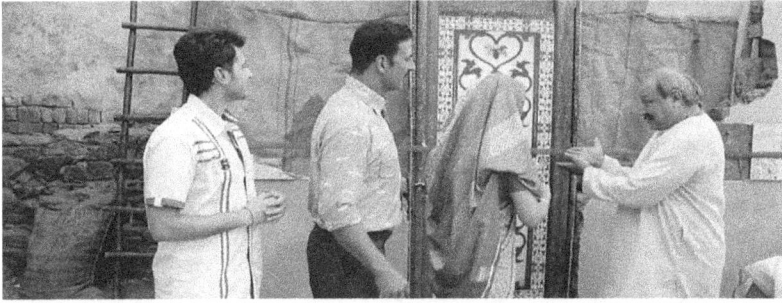

FIGURE 3.9 Still from the film *Toilet: Ek Prem Katha.*

(*sauch*)—that is, to accept technology and modernity. The film ends with Jaya, the bride who had walked out of her marriage to Keshav, now returning to his family and inaugurating the new toilet in her husband's home by cutting the ribbon while her father-in-law (now accepting the modern mindset), along with her husband and his brother, stand at her side applauding (figure 3.9).

Jaya, however, is still covered with her *ghunghat,* even though her father-in-law, the now-reformed Brahmin priest, tells her that it is not necessary for her to do so—demonstrating the limits of this now reformed Hindu family, where the (seemingly empowered) wife continues in the traditional role of a Hindu *bahu* (bride) covered with a *ghunghat* that emblematizes her subordinate role to male family members. The family is now happily united through a toilet (technology/development) that will guard the wife's and, thus, the family's (and thus the nation's) honor. The image of a Hindu wife in her home surrounded by the three Brahmin men reinforces the narrative of developmental-protectionist masculinity of the (reformed) ordinary man that is situated in casteist Hindu hetero-familialism.

SECURITIZING ENDOGAMY

Given that one of the ways in which the security feature of the Hindu modern works is through the intimate—for example, policing interreligious and intercaste relations that often manifest through (vigilante, familial, and even state) violence, as in Adityanath's aforementioned anti-Romeo squads—it is disconcerting to find that the visual field of the NTNB

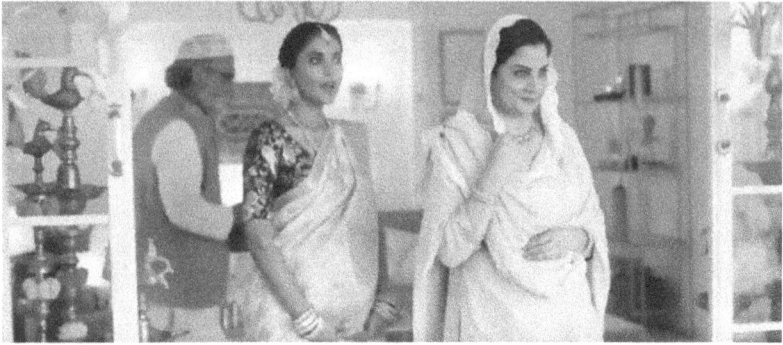

FIGURE 3.10 Still from an advertisement for Tanishq's Ekatvam campaign.

discourse primarily normalizes and shores up Hindu marriage and tends to exclude other marital frameworks, including interfaith and intercaste marriage, from its visual regime. I could not find reports about interfaith or intercaste marriage in the NTNB phenomenon. But this overall absence was not surprising to me. This illustrates how developmentalism is advanced today through Hindu (in this case familial and marital) logics. And that advancement further evinces the twinning of development and security, so that endogamy itself, in today's heightened anti-Muslim and anti-Dalit climate, functions as a security ideology.

Ambedkar argued that endogamy is the core, or the mechanism, of the caste system: "Caste in India means an artificial chopping off of the population into fixed and definite units, each one prevented from fusing into another through the custom of endogamy" (2013, 84). The constant representations of endogamous marriage in the visual field of the NTNB campaign reveals it not just to be about the governance of cleanliness and the production of (toilet) modernity through logics of women's safety, but about the invisible governance of caste and interreligiosity itself.

The visual foregrounding of Hindu marriages in the NTNB campaign at the exclusion of other forms of marriage is troubling at a time when alternative visions of marriage are being violently rejected and attacked by Hindu nationalists today. Not only are anti-conversion laws being passed in states as noted earlier, but even the realm of popular culture has been subject to such hateful sentiments by Hindu nationalists. In 2020 the jewelry company Tanishq launched an ad as part of a campaign called Ekatvam (coming together, or unity), in which a Muslim family is shown organizing a baby shower for their pregnant Hindu daughter-in-law (figure 3.10). The

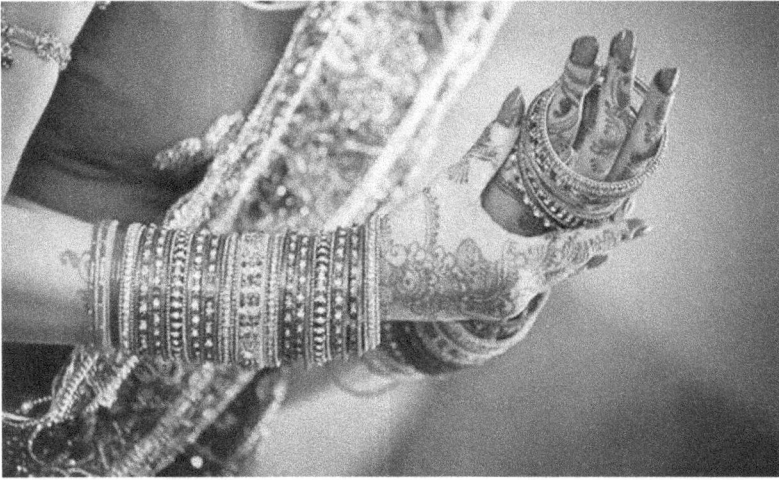

FIGURE 3.11

ad, which celebrates interfaith marriage, soon found itself embroiled in a Twitter storm, with vile comments from Hindutva people that played on "love jihad." Hashtags such as #BoycottTanishq trended, and Tanishq capitulated to the pressure and removed the ad. If the SBA campaign was serious about women's empowerment, this was an opportune moment to represent NTNB, and SBA more broadly, through government-funded, or government-encouraged, publicity campaigns that include exogamous and interfaith marriages as well as same-sex partnerships. In fact, around the same time as the Tanishq controversy, an ad that featured a lesbian couple celebrating the festival of Karva Chauth incited homophobic and Hindu nationalist outrage and had to be immediately removed (*Times of India* 2021).

Many news videos about the NTNB phenomenon that I have watched primarily showcase Hindu weddings. There are almost no images of *nikah* (Muslim marriage) or Christian weddings. Images such as these (figures 3.11–3.13) constitute the media coverage that typically represents the marriages from which brides are walking out or entering if the groom's house possesses a toilet. All these images evoke a Hindu bride or a Hindu-looking bride, sometimes signified by the *mehndi* (henna designs) on her hands, or a Hindu wedding. I say "Hindu-looking bride" because the aesthetics adorning the body of the bride evoke a Hindu bride. Sometimes the face is cut off in the image, so the focus is on the adornment of the bride. While *mehndi* is also applied by some Muslim women as a fashion statement, generally,

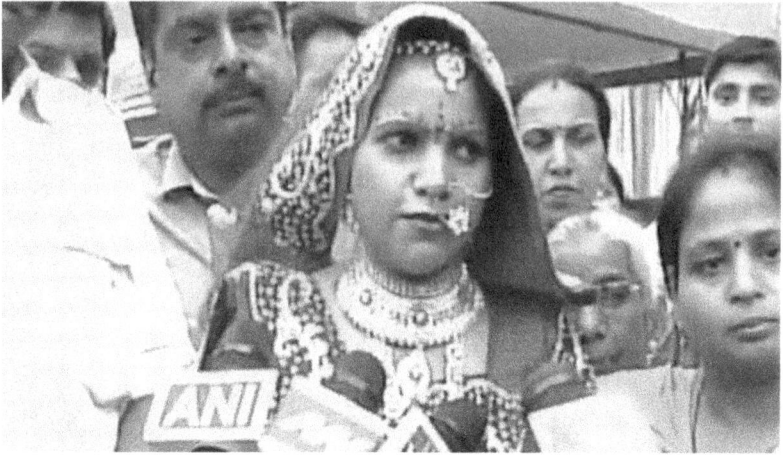

FIGURE 3.12

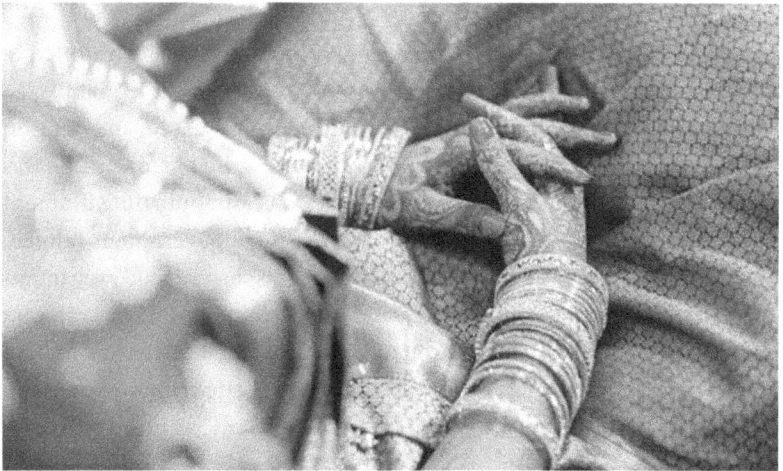

FIGURE 3.13

however, *mehndi* (despite having a complex cultural history) adorns a *Hindu* bride's palms, especially in northern India. In many media images that represent brides in the NTNB phenomenon, the visual focus is frequently on the *mehndi*-adorned hand covered with heavy bangles. We often do not see the face of the bride—a feature that takes away from the individuality of the woman and simply stamps her as a bride (thus again inscribing her in a kinship framework) by visually pointing to bridal signifiers.

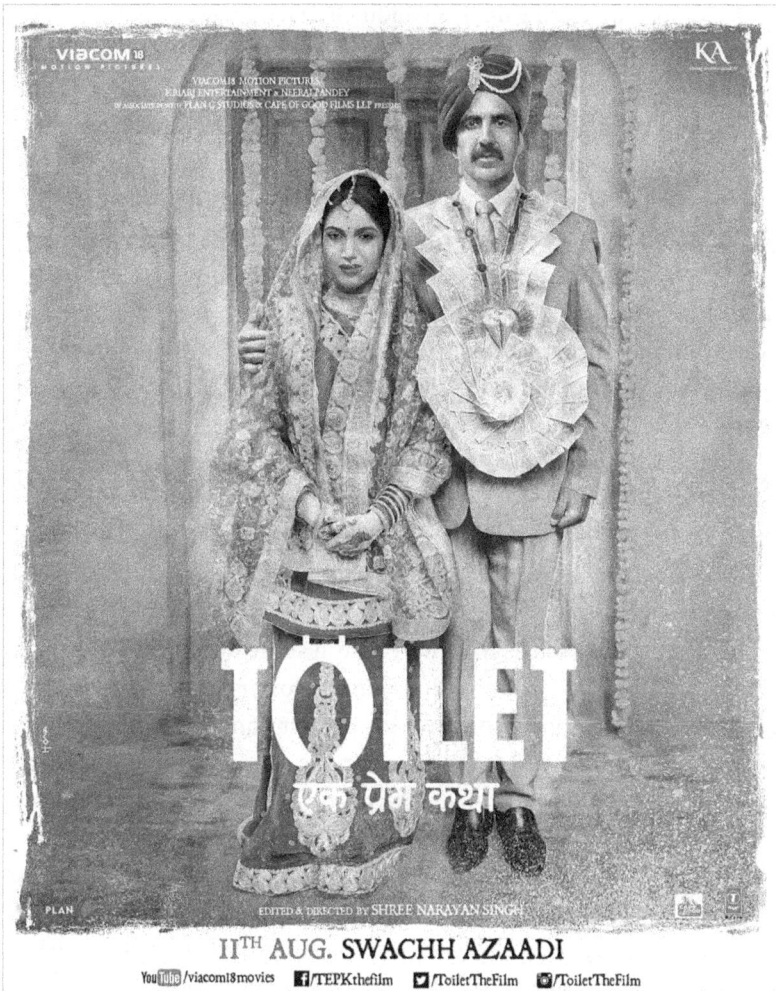

FIGURE 3.14 Poster for the film *Toilet: Ek Prem Katha*.

And then there is the poster for the film *Toilet: Ek Prem Katha*, which was highly circulated on social media and has become a major part of the visual field of NTNB and SBA more broadly (figure 3.14). The poster shows a Hindu married couple and is framed by the slogan "Swachh Azadi." In India, *azadi* means "freedom," and it is associated with national freedom as the term was deployed during the nationalist struggle against the British. This links building a toilet for a bride—thus freeing her from open defecation—with national freedom, once again equating a Hindu (in this case married) woman with the nation.[33]

This constant shoring up of a Hindu marital framework becomes even more explicit when we learn that in certain districts in Uttar Pradesh, district officials asked husbands to gift a toilet on the day of Karva Chauth to their wife. Karva Chauth is a highly heteropatriarchal Hindu ceremony performed primarily in the Hindi heartlands of north India, during which a wife fasts the whole day and prays for her husband's long life. Only Hindu married couples perform Karva Chauth. The local administration asked husbands to make the day of the ceremony special for their wives by giving them a toilet. The husband was to send a selfie to the local administration that displayed a toilet under construction at their home. They would then be rewarded with financial assistance from the government toward the cost of building a toilet at home. In Varanasi District in Uttar Pradesh, the chief development officer represented the purpose of this financial assistance scheme in the following way: "Wives will demand '*Izzatghar*' [toilets] in place of sari or jewelry on Karva Chauth as token of love and affection from their husbands" (quoted in Karelia 2017c).

In other states such as Madhya Pradesh some local governments require would-be-grooms from economically lower classes to post selfies of toilets (or toilets being constructed) in their homes as "proof" of their marriage eligibility—and to send them to the state government as part of an application for funding toward marriage. On receiving such selfies, the government, after the completion of other paperwork, grants 51,000 rupees to the would-be-bride (and not the groom)—again in an attempt to empower the woman for help with marriage expenses. Without this selfie, there is no assistance available. Newspapers report that "'selfie with loo' has become a marriage ritual" in Madhya Pradesh" (News18 2019). One positive aspect of this scheme is its naming: the Mukhya Mantri Kanya Vivah/Mukhya Mantri Nikah Yojana scheme, which explicitly recognizes Muslim marriage (*nikah*), even if visual representations of Muslim marriages are hardly present.

THE GOOD MUSLIM?

As suggested throughout, there are minimal representations of Muslims in the SBA visual regime. However, I found one image under the selfie-with-toilet initiative in Madhya Pradesh that is worth commenting upon. The photograph, which accompanies a news article, is of a young Muslim groom-to-be posing inside a toilet. This is a small, cramped, squat toilet, and he is standing with his two legs on either side of the squat hole. We see him from the side in the photograph, standing tall and straight with shoulders back. His white skullcap and beard identify him as Muslim. The image is underlined by a caption that states: "A groom poses for a 'toilet photo' so that his bride can apply for the financial aid" (Ayub 2019).

What is one to make of this image of a Muslim man standing upright—a posture suggesting bodily discipline—in a toilet posing for a selfie to legitimize his marriageability and cleanliness in the eyes of the state? When most images are of Hindu men in this selfie-toilet regime, this image gives us pause. It discloses something about the terms under which the Muslim male body—which the Hindu state has constructed as a threat—acquires legitimacy. This Muslim man pictured in a toilet has submitted himself to the surveillance of the Hindu modern regime of cleanliness. In doing so, he has declared himself to be a "clean citizen." This is a "good Muslim." Mamdani (2005) reminds us that in Islamophobic regimes one is never just a Muslim. One is either a "good Muslim" or a "bad Muslim." In current Hindu nationalism, while most are framed as "bad Muslims," there also "good Muslims." "Good Muslims" do not exist a priori; they are discursively constructed by the state and populist discourses to contrast them with undesirable Muslims in accordance with current politics. Good Muslim men are those who can be aligned with the imperatives of contemporary Hindu nationalism—such as protecting Bharat Mata. Pondering over this image, I found myself asking: But what if this Muslim groom-to-be, declaring his modernity and cleanliness through a toilet-selfie, is marrying a Hindu woman? Would the state of Madhya Pradesh award a bride 51,000 rupees for marriage expenses when it screens a Muslim groom's application? One can reasonably speculate that since no interreligious disturbance was unleashed by this man's application to the state, this "good Muslim" is marrying a Muslim woman. Endogamy has not been disrupted.

Selfies, as suggested in chapter 2, are very much a part of the SBA campaign's ethos. The selfie culture of NTNB, in particular, provides an example of "informational Hindutva" (Basu 2020, 157) combined with logics of neoliberal development—all integral features of Hindu modern governmentality. What the NTNB phenomenon illustrates, however, is how, as its selfie imperatives gather data about the Hindu protectionist, development-oriented common man, it functions as a surveillance assemblage (Haggarty and Ericson 2003) that regulates the intimate realms of the family and (potential) marriage. We see here the fusion of the logics of security (as in surveillance and data gathering), development, and informational mediation that reveal specific workings of the Hindu modern.

The imperative of sending selfies of oneself in a toilet or a toilet under construction to the local administration also unsettles the binary "between the patriotic and the intimate" (Kuntsman and Stein 2015, 16), or, we could even say, the state and the intimate. In enabling the state to visually enter the toilet of one's home, such selfies represent a fusion of self-surveillance *and* state surveillance—where the self's gaze at itself, in taking the selfie, refracts and reproduces the state's gaze at the (potential) clean citizen. At the same time, it also puts the personal household toilet under the regulation of the state, thus normalizing its—that is, normalizing the state's—expanded purview of governance. On the former point, the groom-to-be internalizes the gaze of the state and surveils himself accordingly. As he does so, he is recruited into a development- and protectionist-oriented masculinist position, for in taking a selfie with a toilet, he is announcing to the state, and submitting to its development sublime, that he is capable of protecting the honor of his wife-to-be. This exemplifies again how the security logic of the Hindu modern operates through intimacies—it surveils and invites self-surveillance of "clean citizens" in the toilet (one of the most intimate spaces for the body). In doing so it forces a Hindu heteropatriarchal, masculinist, protectionist subject position on the common man, for if you cannot pose with a toilet that will "protect" the honor of your wife-to-be, she will not receive financial assistance.

On the point about citizens' selfies broadening the purview of what the state legitimately governs, this reinforces the idea that the state can legitimately intervene in all realms related to cleanliness and intimacy, as has already happened in the expansion of laws patrolling interreligious marriages, for instance. A campaign like NTNB, in essence, opens new directions for state surveillance and regulations to potentially unfold at the site of the home. The intimacies of home become securitized just as security becomes more homely. And as Hindutva forces have historically characterized Muslim Indians as pollutants of the purity of the nation, and have been engaged in stereotyping individual Muslims as unclean, this may render their homes and other intimate spaces more susceptible to state power.

Kuntsman invites us to ask under what conditions a selfie can do political work (2017, 21), or, as I am asking, a particular form of Hindu nationalist work? And "what are the regimes of in/visibility in which such work operates?" (2017, 21). "Who has the ability—and the safety—to star in a selfie?" (2017, 20). When transferred to the NTNB scenario, these questions provoke us to confront, for instance, that a Muslim man as a potential groom can only star in such a selfie if his claim to "clean citizenship" is not disturbing the endogamy structure that is being enforced by the Hindu nation today and replicated in campaigns like NTNB. Similarly, Dalit men often cannot construct toilets due to upper-caste harassment, or because they do not own land, or because as Dalits they can never be coded as clean and thus cannot perform the citizenly work of responding to a (state directed) selfie regime's (Althusserian) "Hey, you!" and declare themselves (and their family) to be clean citizens. Certain political conditions need to be in place to respond affirmatively to the "Hey, you!" in order to submit to the selfie's call and be recognized by the state as a (clean) citizen-subject. Such required acts of producing and sending selfies with toilets continue the shift toward biometric governance that is alarmingly on the rise in contemporary India under the BJP regime that, in routinized ways, is excising from citizenly belonging swaths of populations who, for various political and historical reasons, are unable to enter, or are being disappeared by, the panoptic regime of data governance, which will be addressed in the following chapter.

When I first began analyzing the NTNB discourse, I approached the task with some enthusiasm—thinking that women in semirural and rural parts of the country demanding a toilet for their safety certainly has some political value that cannot be dismissed. But the more I studied this discourse of "women's empowerment"—and particularly the narrativization of a particular version of female safety that functions as a rationale for toilet building—the more I found that it mobilizes a moral panic around women's safety that converges with, and shores up, a larger ongoing national anxiety about protecting a Hindu woman' honor as a way to protect and securitize the Hindu national family. If there was room available in the NTNB discourse to offer a subversive and intersectional vision of female agency, that possibility was foreclosed the moment women's empowerment became located in a logic of honor and hetero-familialism. Beneath the equation of women's empowerment with *izzat* (always attributed to Hindu women) lie violent relations of caste and communalism that have a long genealogy. These relations, as we have seen, are tied to the enablement and even promotion of certain forms of Hindu nationalist heteromasculinity that can be, and have been, utilized to enact violence in the name of cleansing and protecting Bharat Mata, and thus Hindu women.

But most important, the NTNB discourse leaves unanswered the following question: When toilets are built to guard a Hindu woman's *izzat*, who will clean them?[34] Especially, but not only, in rural villages in the Hindi heartlands of the nation, the family's *bahu* (bride) is expected to be clean and pure; hence the task of cleaning a toilet in Hindu homes is performed usually by Dalit women, as latrine cleaning is one of the prime occupations to which they are subject. In SBA discourse as evidenced in the NTNB phenomenon, the masculine protectionist logic of development is explicitly *not* extended to protecting those who are really the most vulnerable to harm. The life worlds of the Hindu woman who is to be "empowered" via toilet building, and the protectionism of the development-oriented Hindu man, converge in the "death worlds" (Mbembe 2003, 40) of the Dalit female latrine cleaner. Unrepresented in typical NTNB coverage, the Dalit (female) body functions as the sacrificial and disposable infrastructure that makes possible the various hetero-gendered Hindu familial subject positions of contemporary Hindu modernity advanced by development imperatives such as, but not only, the SBA campaign.

This point is further supported at the ground level when we remember how little has been spent in the SBA budget on solid and liquid waste management, which was addressed in chapter 1. Equally important, while the Indian government outlawed the practice of manual scavenging through two acts in 1993 and 2013, its definition of manual scavenging continues to be narrow and conservative, offering plenty of loopholes to subvert it. The focus is only on dry latrines and carrying fecal waste in bare hands "rather than on any act which pertains to direct human contact with faecal waste" (Shekhar 2023, 140) and not just in dry latrines.

The SBA campaign provides an explicit materialized instance of a development initiative of contemporary Hindu nationalism that is simultaneously situated in biopower and necropower. Mbembe (2003) taught us, through his reading of Foucault, that biopower is about the management of life to enhance life; thus, it also functions by producing states of exception—"death worlds" for those who can be potentially killed by the state in order to manage the life of those (in this case Hindus) considered worthy of living. As toilet building increases in rural villages and semirural towns in order to ensure the safety of (that is, manage the life of) the (Hindu) woman, it further confers upon Dalits the "status of *living dead*" (Mbembe 2003, 39–40, original emphasis). This entanglement of biopolitics and necropolitics in the SBA campaign reflects yet again the mutual operation of the developmentalism and security features of the Hindu modern. Developmentalism through toilet building purportedly aims to enhance (securitize) the life of the (Hindu) woman against unknown dangers in public space. This securitization, however, is reliant on the "slow death" (Berlant 2007, 754) of Dalit labor. Indeed, it would be simplistic to say that this is just a problem of *contemporary* Hindu nationalism: Dalit bodies have always being killed in cleanliness cultures of upper castes. But what this does reveal is the reluctance of SBA narratives (and corresponding practices on the ground) to confront how keeping the (Hindu) woman safe through a hetero-masculinist, protectionist development logic of increased toilet construction is only going to further condemn Dalit bodies to states of abjection. This has been noted by Dalits themselves. In 2015, one year after the SBA campaign was launched, Dalit workers led by the Safai Karmachari Andolan, a human-rights organization, launched a countrywide march to tell citizens and the government, "Stop killing us" (Sabrang 2015). The Dalit activist Bezwada Wilson asked: "If you add another 12 crore toilets, how many more Dalits will die?" (Us Salam 2016). The march did not seem to have much, or any, impact on the SBA program.

This chapter leaves us with an urgent question: When "women's empowerment" is used by ethnonationalist fantasies to advance a rhetoric of cleanliness and female protection that is promoted through a logic of developmental modernity, what types of expulsions and dispossessions become possible, what kinds of anxieties, violences, and terrors are then reinforced as well as unleashed?

FOUR

SWACHH VIOLENCE

THE WILL TO PUNISH

A pradhan (village leader) in Uttar Pradesh believed that it would be essential to give severe punishments to people who do not use a latrine. [He stated that] "It should be such a punishment that people remember it, it should hurt. . . . If you hit them hard, then it will sting for a while."
—NIKHIL SRIVASTAV AND NAZAR KHALID

"[W]hat we see here is a working model of fascism in the neoliberal era."
—ANAND TELTUMBDE

This chapter advances our exploration of the governmentality of the Hindu modern as it plays out through Swachh Bharat Abhiyan (SBA) by revealing how the enforcement of cleanliness has been largely predicated on a public culture of violence and coercion organized around a "will to punish" offenders in the name of protecting the nation.[1] It also examines how the neoliberal majoritarian Hindu nationalist public sphere that enacts punishment is cleansed of culpability for its dirty deeds.

The culture of violence that underlines the execution of cleanliness, particularly in relation to toilet construction and the eradication of open defecation, as well as other campaigns such as anti-littering, is part of a larger architecture of violence—symbolic (representational), physical, infrastructural, statist, and ideological—that scaffolds the Hindu modern today. This architecture of violence, as alluded to in chapter 1, consists of both statist and nonstatist realms, where the latter functions as a counterpart or supplement to statist violence. This architecture symptomizes a broader culture of punitive populism, or what Didier Fassin (2018) calls a "will to punish," that marks authoritarian public spheres today. Contemporary Hindu nationalist India offers a powerful case study that demonstrates how, as Fassin (2018) observes, punishment has become a contemporary passion in majoritarian cultures, one which I show is often consummated through acts that are framed as cleansing.[2] In the case of India, this passion is typically situated in the affective interlocking structures of gender, caste, class, and religion, the integrity of which in all cases can be (and has been) framed as imperiled by various forms of contagion and pollution.[3] I think here of the recent promise by the BJP Home Minister Amit Shah (Modi's second-in-command) to pick up illegal immigrants (whom he has also called "termites") who have entered India from Muslim-dominant Bangladesh and hurl them one by one into the Bay of Bengal (Reuters 2019a). Not enough to mark or restrict them, they have to be punished (through some form of violence, and note here specifically a watery form, associated with cleansing) for violating the body of Bharat Mata.

Shah's comment provides us with a glimpse into a Hindu nationalist India that is dominated by a will to punish anyone seen to be deviating from the dictates and desires of the neoliberal Hindu modern state. The punishment typically expresses itself through modalities of violence that often but not always operate outside the law (vigilantism)—ranging from "soft" violence, if one can even use that phrase (such as harassment and intimidation) to "heavy," in-your-face, brute violence that can even lead to death.[4]

Who enacts this violence? There has been an increasing growth of non-state actors (primarily male and upper caste) engaged in vigilante acts who, mobilized by majoritarian sentiments, have taken on the task of executing punishment on behalf of their leaders and their nation imagined as Bharat Mata. Jaffrelot notes that "the moral and political economies of these arrangements" are sophisticated for the "state cannot harass the minorities openly, but by letting vigilantes do so, it keeps majoritarian feelings satisfied" (2017). Hansen further argues that the violence expressed by such nonstate actors gives them a sense of power, a sense of inclusion (or at least the promise of inclusion) in the majoritarian sphere; they feel that they have been given permission by their leaders "to act, to hit, and to abuse" (2021, 39). So, when Amit Shah promises to throw illegal immigrants into the Bay of Bengal, he is already mobilizing a (casteist Hindu) will to punish that can be easily exercised by people (usually, but not always, Hindu men, often without an adequate job, who may feel disenfranchised because of the presence of "others"). The governmentality of the Hindu modern that

I have been tracing throughout this book is reliant on this kind of violence, which is mobilized by a will to punish, and often specifically one that is framed as a mandate to protect, cleanse, and purify. The violence of cow vigilantes or "love jihad" vigilantes are cases in point although, as I will show here, often this violence *does not* acquire such extreme mob-oriented expressions but remains disguised as citizenly practices performed by individuals who purport to protect the modernizing projects of the current Hindu state by engaging in unlawful violent practices against perceived offenders of the state.

It is not a new observation that neoliberal or authoritarian development projects are potentially also projects of violence producing unfreedoms instead of enabling development to produce linked political, economic, and social freedoms (Escobar 2004; Sen 1999). What the SBA case reveals, alongside other state-led development projects, is the entanglement of development, religion, violence (and thus security, for expressions of violence are justified in the name of security), and neoliberalism in contemporary Hindu nationalist India that is a modus operandi of Hindu modern governmentality. There abound instances of "routine violence" (Pandey 2006), such as the building of the Kashi Vishwanath Temple complex that threatens the Gyanvapi Mosque, where conditions are being set up for future violence that could further injure the Muslim community, which is already being kept from praying publicly here (Suta Dogra 2023). Where physical violence has not yet occurred, situations can be pregnant with that possibility (if we remember Ayodhya), and charges of impurity or the impulse to cleanse can trigger the transition.

Violence has always informed the Indian nation; it was the ground upon which the nation was birthed, as discussed in the preceding chapter. So, marking a culture of violence in India is nothing new and there is plentiful literature on this, in which the focus has largely been on communal violence. But what makes today different is that the targets of violence are not simply, although they are largely, religious or caste minorities. The targets are also anyone who deviates from or questions the desires of the Hindu neoliberal authoritarian heteropatriarchal state, which are not framed as desires but rather as proactive or protective development initiatives: dissenters, activists, journalists, educators, international nonprofits, and more. The will to punish that drives Hindu modern governmentality frequently *creates* the "crime," the "criminal," the "threat," or the "problem," as we saw with the National Register of Citizens (NRC) exercise where "illegal" immigrants were created overnight. The criminal does not always exist a priori. Nor is the criminal produced just by the state but also by nonstate actors who have taken on, with encouragement, policing functions. In the case of SBA, this policing occurs in the name of protecting development and cleanliness—which is ultimately about protecting a cleansed Bharat Mata by producing and excising abject bodies who violate upper middle-class/caste norms of cleanliness through which the land that Bharat Mata symbolizes is to be sanitized—made into a *punyabhoomi* (at least in its ideology). Thus, one never knows who will end up being a threat or an inconvenience to the state (or to "the people") and its desired moral and social order. Consequently, one never knows what punishment might be meted out, for one does not know what law if any has been broken or what crime if any has occurred. As chapter 1 discussed, this has occurred on many occasions such as the arrest of "antinationals" or, as we will see below, in the informal criminalization of open defecation and the punishing of offenders in brutal ways that directly impact their conditions of living. In the culture of violence fanned and enabled by (Hindu) majoritarian neoliberal culture (Patel et al. 2022), the lines between "law" and "morality" have blurred, just as the lines between crime and what is not a crime have blurred. It would not be a stretch to say that in contemporary India, it is morality—rooted in some sense of Hindu, upper middle-class/ caste, civilizational discourse that is entangled in a neoliberal ideological complex—that has run far ahead of law in punishing those seen as threats to the nation or as inconvenient subjects for the fulfilment of its projects.

Further, the will to punish and the embedded violence that is expressed increasingly by nonstate actors purporting to serve the state's desires also reveals a particular shift in the working of sovereignty that was briefly addressed in my discussion of the Hindu modern in chapter 1. We are increasingly witnessing, especially in the Global South, the practice of what Willis calls "shadow sovereignties" or "informal sovereignties," where the right to kill, punish or discipline is being displaced from the formal structures of the state (2015, 10).[5] Hindu modern governmentality, as this book has been suggesting, is enabled and fortified by such informal expressions of sovereignty that are protected with impunity by the formal structures of the state. The current workings of Hindu modern governmentality certainly challenge or invite revisions of some contemporary theories of sovereignty, such as Agamben's thesis about the state of exception (2004).[6] True, Agamben's theory was conceptualized primarily in terms of Western democracies, but it has taken on a rather universal character in contemporary political and cultural theory. If, for Agamben, the sovereign power of the state is revealed in the state of exception—that is, in the state's power to suspend law, constitutional rights, and freedoms in conditions that the state believes require the execution of violence outside of the law—what we have in India today is something different. The suspension of rights and law is increasingly *not* an expression of a state of *exception*; rather, it is the state of the normative, where the "exception" ironically *enters* the law by being protected by its authority.[7]

The SBA campaign has emerged as a significant arena where the architecture of violence is being enacted across the nation on grounds that tend to not only deflect critique but even garner global praise. I use the term *violence* broadly here—to mean acts and practices ranging from physical attacks on the vulnerable, the dissenting, the marginalized to their harassment and intimidation as well to describe erasures of populations, discursive or material, including via the digital sphere (as we saw in the NRC exercise and in the shutdown of communications in Kashmir in 2019). I also include here majoritarian ideological violence that functions to erase or regulate any counter-ideology of Hindu nationalism and the neoliberal state, such as the excising of Mughal history from the school curriculum that is going on now, although I deal with this aspect less in this chapter. Additionally, I include "infrastructural violence"—a notion advanced by anthropologists Rodgers and O'Neill, who remind us that workings of infrastructures can be "substantially deleterious" and that "processes of marginalization, abjection and disconnection often become operational and sustainable" via infrastructures (2012, 403).[8] Further, I do not mean only "illegal" violence at the margins of the law/state, but as addressed earlier, also violence that acts outside the law in order to paradoxically strengthen the force of the law.[9] In some cases, such violence even calls for new laws or the strengthening of existing laws (such as cow protection legislation, which was enforced as cow vigilantism and became pervasive). Indeed, violence that operates in a tenuous area between legality and illegality, and between state and nonstate realms, is especially relevant to SBA and its operation as Hindu modern governmentality.

Finally, I mean violence that has *not yet* occurred though its possibility is very much there. Veena Das suggests that violence does not always have to be "transparent" (2007, loc. 1737) for it to be violence.[10] Violence deferred is also violence. The very possibility that violence *can* occur is enough to damage or injure the potential subject (typically vulnerable) of violence. While much of this punitive violence is intentionally willed in India today, some of it is an outcome of thoughtless policy planning, which also reveals a particular kind of will of the neoliberal development-oriented Hindu state that is focused on securing the desires of the middle and upper class and castes (as we saw with the demonetization program and COVID-19 control endeavors that drastically affected the poor, migrant, Muslim, and lower-caste populations).

Many engaged in, or enamored by, SBA at an official and even nonofficial level will refuse the description of acts and practices that I identify in this chapter as violence, or may even be enraged by my naming them as such. But my goal precisely *is* to intervene in such refusals, as these examples, I argue, open a window onto the larger architecture of violence that scaffolds Hindu modern governmentality in India today. My argument is that by focusing on various acts of violence (which create their own potentialities for repetition) through which cleanliness is enforced in SBA culture, we are able to learn something about the extent to which the nation—its everyday citizens/nonstate actors (especially from majoritarian groups) and government officials—are gripped by a will to punish that is justified through notions of moral righteousness or, as in SBA, through notions of citizenly actions and ideologies of civilizationalism that are sutured to a (majoritarian) neoliberal national protectionist complex.[11] Needless to say, this will to punish expresses the entangled power of class, caste, religion, and gender through which punitive populism is being shored up in India today.

Morality figures in all this significantly, for the will to punish aims to protect something sacred or coded as sacred. While the sacred is the nation of course, I want to be more specific about what exactly in the nation is to be protected (for not everything in the nation is seen as sacred and worth protecting). In the current national context, as previous chapters have illustrated, the sacred can be anything from the aesthetics of purity—and practices of open defecation violate this—to the purity (and sexuality) of the Hindu woman who is to be protected from "love jihad." Whatever it is, the sacred today ends up being anything that can signify national purity and development itself as development has been sacralized while reflecting the desires of the Bhartiya Janata Party (BJP) and the upper and middle caste/class.

Clearly, the will to punish that marks the Hindu-dominant neoliberal polity is an outcome of the security feature of Hindu modern governmentality, particularly as that governmentality regulates modernizing and national purification initiatives that in turn enhance its power. Punitive populist sentiments become normalized in a nation when insecurities are generated for the majoritarian culture that result in demands for security not just from the state but, as I have been arguing, from nonstate actors as well. This of course further heightens the surveillance culture on which states rely to enact security. This is a global trend. One recalls here Emmanuel Macron's recent calls for a "society of vigilance" to fight and report on the Islamist "Hydra" in France and every French citizen is to be vigilant about Islamic terrorism for, as he stated, state services alone cannot tackle this (Reuters 2019b). Macron's comments clearly show how the production of shadow sovereignties and the creation of "watchful citizens" (Walsh 2014, 237) are encouraged directly or indirectly by the state today—which is an increasing feature of populism, including in India.

Loïc Wacquant makes the point that today social problems are treated less as social problems; rather, they are subject to penalization, which results in their "invisibilization" (2009, 23). In other words, social problems are reframed through security and protectionist frameworks (and constructed as threats or disorders to be managed). So, instead of seeing the disenfranchisement that Muslims and others feel in India today, which may result in expressions of dissent, as a *social problem*, the Hindu nation reframes it as a security problem, thus rendering the social problem invisible. For instance, take the recent farmers' movements. Instead of the government listening to the farmers' demands, it subjected the farmers—many of whom live below the poverty line—to "unlawful force and prevent[ion] [of] free movement as well as access to essential facilities" (ICJ 2021).[12] The government explicitly inserted the national protection angle when it claimed that the farmers' movement (which has a huge Sikh presence) has been "infiltrated by Khalistanis," pointing to the "presence of Khalistan flags and separatist slogans" in the Sikh community's solidarity protests in the United States (Khosla and Milliff 2021). I offer these examples to set the stage for my ensuing analysis of similar patterns in SBA that reveal a larger will to punish that powers the violence of Hindu modern governmentality and that calls forth and normalizes *punitive* scripts. These scripts, as in the case of SBA, are often targeted at the bodies of the poor (which largely tend to be Dalits, Muslims, and Adivasis but can also be very poor Hindus).

It is valuable to remember here, as evidenced by a 2018 report on multidimensional poverty by the United Nations Development Programme (UNDP) and the Oxford Poverty and Human Development Initiative (OPHI), that every second person in the Scheduled Tribes and every third person in the Scheduled Castes (that is, one-third of Dalits) remains poor (Tewari and Mishra 2019). Every third Muslim is multidimensionally poor, just as two in five children under the age of ten are (OPHI 2018). The report deals with poverty as a multidimensional phenomenon, highlighting the fact that poverty is not just based on income but on health, nutrition, education, assets, and living standards (Tewari and Mishra 2019). This means that, as another report avers, these three groups—Scheduled Tribes, Scheduled Castes, and Muslims—constitute around 66 percent of the poor in India (*India Tomorrow* 2019). Poverty is disproportionate among women as well. Let us also remember that to be poor in India is to be extremely poor, to be in abject poverty where survival is a daily struggle. As we encounter stories of poor people being violated and punished for open defecation in the next sections, we need to remember to which groups these poor people most likely belong. Thus, whether always directly intended or not, the will to punish becomes directed at the lowest caste and class and Dalits, as well as Muslims, who also dominate populations in poverty.

I use the term Hindu *majoritarian neoliberal* (Patel et al. 2022) culture more explicitly in this chapter than I have in others because what we will see here is how it is the poor who are penalized and sometimes even disposed of—rendered invisible—by the cleanliness-enforcing culture of SBA that is executed not only by the government but by myriad "private" citizens, and this is also linked to the flow of global capital that plays a role in producing a shining and gleaming India for the upper and middle classes. The above point becomes especially relevant because it is a normative upper- and middle-class/caste notion of clean that powers the will to punish cleanliness "offenders"—typically those living in poverty or migrant workers, Adivasis (tribals) or the homeless or Dalits, many of whom have not been able to construct in-home toilets for financial or other reasons that will be explored later, and thus seek far away fields and land for open defecation.

Gender relations—including their embeddedness in caste, class, sexuality, and religion—constitute and are being (re)constituted by this punitive culture, which dominates the public sphere today and underlines Hindu modern governmentality. The will to punish—whether expressed by the state or by nonstate actors—calls forth a punitive heteromasculinist script of masculinity. However, it is a masculinism that is not equally available to all men, "only to those who accrue particular forms of power" (Grewal 2020, 183) or those who can advance and/or protect the majoritarian neoliberal imperatives of the state. Sometimes this can constitute even those who are being left *behind* by the neoliberal policies of the current government but who aspire to the dreams that those polices promise. This thus also mobilizes some poor Hindus even as they are constantly being disenfranchised by the neoliberal state. For the most part, however, Dalit men, Muslim men, gay men (especially if they are Muslim or from "backward" castes) or other lower-caste men fall outside this punitive hetero-masculine script today, although there are times when their insecurities are co-opted and they are seduced by the state to serve Hindu casteist hetero-nationalist neoliberal desires in return for expansive political rights and protection.

While scholars examining Hindu nationalism and masculinity have variously focused on themes such as the rise of muscular masculinity (Banerjee and Williams 2018), armed masculinity (e.g., Banerjee 2005), Modi-masculinity (e.g., Srivastava 2015), anxious masculinity (e.g., Anand 2007), ascetic masculinity (e.g., Chakraborty 2022) and so on, I argue that what needs to be added to these important insights is an *explicit* recognition of the rise of a will to punish (embedded in the authoritarian classist and casteist Hindu neoliberal patriarchal structure) that is today producing an explicit *punitive* majoritarian hetero-masculinity in the name of national protection, which is frequently framed through logics and practices of cleansing. The label "bulldozer Baba" that symbolizes "strong governance" or "bulldozer justice" (Banerjee 2022) recently given to Yogi Adityanath, who wears it proudly, metaphorizes this. Adityanath is seen as someone who will bulldoze (clean out, level) anything or anyone that threatens order (that is, his sense of order).

A contemporary popular and charged-up image that captures this script of punitive majoritarian masculinity is that of Angry Hanuman (figure 4.1). Hanuman is a benign, lovable figure in the Hindu epic the Ramayana. Children often embraced him as a protector figure. He is devoted to Lord Ram and plays an important role in rescuing Ram's wife Sita, who had been abducted by the cruel Ravana (a demon king, who incidentally is claimed as an ancestor and figure of worship by many Dalits and Adivasis). The lovable figure of Hanuman has broadly symbolized protection to the common person. In 2016, however, two years after the BJP came to power, Hanuman, under the brushstrokes of a Kerela artist, underwent a makeover and emerged as an angry dark figure symbolizing a dark script of Hindu masculinity—angry and ready to punish. The writer Dewan, who has written many books and biographies about Hanuman, tells us, drawing on Ravana's spy Shuk, that "when Hanuman gets angry, he can wipe out entire oceans" (quoted in Bamzai 2018). This image not only became

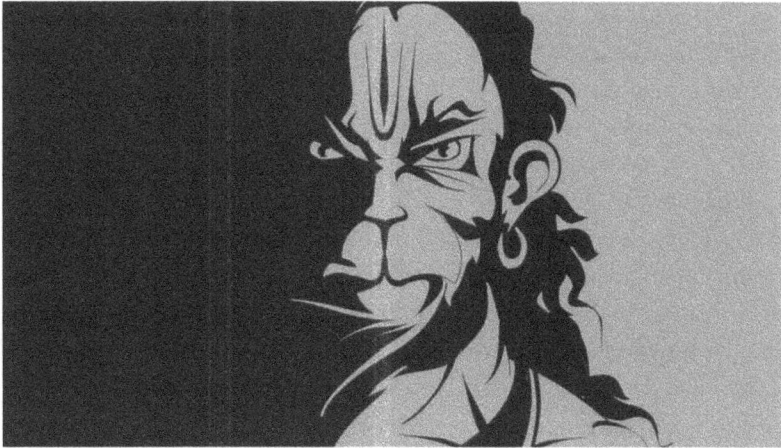

FIGURE 4.1 Angry Hanuman, created by graphic designer Karan Acharaya in 2015.

viral quickly but found itself on T-shirts and stickers on cars, scooters, and more. Modi hailed the image. During my own visit to Delhi in 2016, I witnessed this angry Hanuman image on many cars just as I witnessed the same in Bengaluru a couple of years later. Hanuman is angry, we can speculate, because his role has always been to protect Ram Rajya. We can reasonably surmise that the image expresses his wrath at the (perceived) demise of Ram Rajya and the values that need to be recovered—which is consistent with the concept of Ram Rajya that Modi and the BJP aim to institute (and doing so quite successfully) in the nation. Pande notes that what we have here is a "transformation of a genial, well-loved icon into a militant killer" (2018)—an image that potentially awakens killer instincts in the majoritarian population.[13]

This script of a punitive majoritarian masculinity powered by a will to punish has also become attractive to many Hindu women, including those who have begun to see themselves as warriors of the state (Bacchetta 1999a, 2004; Banerjee 2006; Mazumdar 1995; Sarkar and Butalia 1995; Sen 2007). In SBA we find women, including trans women, who have taken on, or are given, policing functions by the state or local municipalities to surveil those (typically poor) who violate cleanliness protocols. In fact, trans women performing scripts of punitive upper-caste heteromasculinity constitute important even if small moments in the SBA text that teaches us something larger about how the Hindu nationalist neoliberal state is being negotiated and managed through a gendered politics of inclusion that extends protections to some and not others, while often making this protection contingent on performative participation in majoritarian culture.

Given this wider context, the tools of violence employed in SBA and the arenas where disciplining and punishment are being promoted and enacted can serve to obscure the Hindu modern's intensifying governance over intimate bodily realms and the social and politic relationships that are mediated through the policing of bodily functions and cleanliness more generally. In particular, digital devices deployed for the purposes of SBA, from individual cell phones to government-controlled drones, increasingly provide capabilities for the enactment of forms of Hindu modern governmentality capable of enacting violence as cleansing.

THE RISE OF CITIZEN VIGILANTISM

Vigilante violence became a common occurrence to prevent open defecation and enforce toilet construction in the SBA program in the first phase. Scholars have pointed out the rise of vigilantism in contemporary India (e.g., Banaji 2018; Cook 2019; Jaffrelot 2017, 2019; Jaffrelot and Gayer 2010; Mukherjee 2020), especially under the BJP government. This rise of vigilantism in India, while it has its own specificities, is part of what Jean Comaroff (2021) discusses as a global resurrection of vigilantism. Recent discussions of vigilantism in Modi's India have largely focused on communal vigilantism, understandably. What has been less explored is how vigilantism has gone beyond its typical realms (communal violence) and has begun to inform "modernizing" projects such as the SBA program. Gupta et al. (2019b) have noted the expansive use of coercion in SBA by local officials and citizens in accomplishing the goal of toilet building. While noting the coercive tactics used in the SBA campaign, this otherwise important report does not link it to the larger architecture of punitive violence that pervades the nation today, nor how these tactics are folded into a Hindu neoliberal majoritarian nationalist complex.

Abrahams, a pioneer in vigilante studies, discusses vigilantism as a phenomenon extremely difficult to pin down but that typically involves an "organized attempt by a group of 'ordinary' citizens to enforce norms" (2008, 423), often by taking recourse to violence. Similarly, Gardenier reminds us that vigilantism often aims to "preserve a social or moral order"

(2022, 10). While scholars describe vigilantism in various ways, there is agreement that it typically involves nonstate actors, and it is typically extralegal in its operations (Bateson 2021). If vigilantism is about acting outside the law by nonstate actors (sometimes to further the law), what SBA reveals is a kind of vigilantism that is becoming banal in India today, where we often see both nonstate actors and state actors such as the police (or local SBA officials of a state) acting outside the law or engaging in vigilante behavior that operates outside modes of human decency (that any moral or legal order is meant to protect) to punish offenders of open defecation.[14] In fact, what is most disconcerting about the kind of vigilantism—both soft and hard—that we see in the SBA context is that it is being represented in many dominant media outlets and by local SBA officials as a *citizenly practice*.[15] As Banaji argues, this kind of practice is often endorsed as "civic action" (2018, 337). This is different from what De Jong (2023) examines as "vigilante citizenship" in Amsterdam from 1980 to 1990, where vigilante groups emerged as victim support groups and neighborhood watch teams to prevent neighborhood crimes, as the police department was failing the city. These kinds of groups—even though De Jong terms them "vigilantes"—seem to be more *vigilance* groups that operate *within* norms of civil society and cooperate with the police to raise civic awareness about neighborhood crime prevention. They are not gripped by a vengeful will to punish. In contrast, I am concerned with the kind of citizen vigilantism that is inherently tied to *majoritarian* violence and *majoritarian* (nationalist) logics, and whose goal is to protect the *majoritarian* public sphere through (violent) punitive practices.[16]

It is important to underline that the enactment of illegal authority and coercive power including violence outside the law is not a new phenomenon in modern states. Extralegal violence has always been "sovereignty's constitutive outside" (Comaroff 2021). In India in particular, the enactment of violence outside the law is neither "unexpected or exceptional" (Brass 1997, 274; see also Hansen and Stepputat 2005). It happens frequently. And it is not always collective in expression, as for instance when a neighborhood goon thrashes someone for some perceived violation or for challenging his authority. Or, when some upper-class person humiliates a poor, typically lower-caste person through physical or verbal abuse (such as a domestic servant in the house, or a local electrician who did not show to an appointment, or a male lower class and caste worker who dared to look at someone's daughter). The tremendous cultural and economic inequalities that exist in India provide the conditions for the normalization of this kind of unlawful behavior. Similarly, communal violence that has a long history in India has often been protected with impunity (if it is the violence of the majoritarian class). Those of us who grew up in India grew up with all this around us.

But I want to suggest that the current kind of vigilantism—of which we see a partial glimpse in SBA—may be different. First, it is not *only* communal vigilantism that is the problem today; as the SBA context shows, vigilantism has now expansively spilled over into other realms, such as infrastructure development, media (seen for instance in the killing of the journalist Gauri Lankesh), and education (seen for instance in attacks on students and professors at Jawaharlal Nehru University). Second, while many growing up in India in the past are familiar with assertions of authority outside the law—in local neighborhoods for instance—these were not pervasively about protecting Bharat Mata and middle- and upper-class/caste Hindu populations that power the neoliberal state. I do not suggest that this has never happened in the past. Of course, it has. Rather, I am pointing to the pervasiveness and the stabilization of this today. Third, the strengthening of vigilantism (in all its guises) today is visibly *lopsided*. In the 1980s or even in the 1990s, if an upper-class group or person harassed or beat up a lower-class or a marginalized individual for some alleged uncitizenly act or violation in a neighborhood, sooner or later one would see groups of individuals from that marginalized class gathering steam and ready to lash out at the upper-class person or group—for instance gathering outside their house and demanding an apology or threatening to harass their family and so on. But today, it is *majoritarian* vigilantism that is "allowed" (via being coded through a national protectionist complex) and any resistance, however feeble, is quelled and deemed traitorous and subject to the nation's will to punish. The SBA context, I argue, does not just provide examples of the rise of this type of violence, but also helps to explain its frequent operation as a citizenly practice linked to particular modalities of governance, ones that SBA reflects and also institutionalizes along with other realms of governance (such as the governance of "love jihad" in the Hindi heartland, in states such as Uttar Pradesh, or the governance of COVID in 2020).

All this raises the following questions: When boundaries of citizenly practice begin to openly accommodate with impunity soft and hard violence that operates outside the law in the name of national protection, how should we rethink citizenship in these illiberal contexts? If liberal notions of citizenship (which, since Independence, India has officially subscribed to) guarantee protection of rights against, and freedom from, violence, what does it mean when the enactment of an alleged citizenly practice is based on the performance of illegal violence? And whose violence then counts and is excused as an act of citizenly practice, and whose violence (or acts coded as violence) is then marked as an uncitizenly act that must be repressed or punished? At the heart of these matters simmers a larger issue: the blurring of (majoritarian) vigilantism and citizenship in authoritarian times.

While scholars have attended to communal-inflected vigilantism in India, there is limited exploration of the gendered dynamics of vigilantism, including its intersections with class and caste and how these dynamics express themselves in noncommunal arenas, including the development arena.[17] I understand of course that in a society such as India everything ultimately is communal in some respects, but for now, I wish to retain a focus on vigilantism that is not as explicitly organized around communal lines of group membership but is rather deployed in the name of citizenly practice. The following section focuses on how scripts of punitive masculinity, that are typically upper caste in orientation, are being deployed in acts of vigilantism in the arena of development such as SBA and that end up targeting poor bodies (typically Dalits, poor Muslims, or people from lower castes).

STRIPPING FOR A CLEAN NATION: VIGILANTISM, EMASCULATION, AND THE SUBJECTION OF THE POOR

In 2017, Ranchi Municipal Corporation (RMC), responsible for the civic administration of the city of Ranchi in Jharkhand, launched a campaign called Halla Bol, Lungi Khol (HBLK) in order to meet the upcoming deadline by which the city was to be declared "open defecation free" (ODF) by the government.[18] *Halla bol* is a Hindi phrase that roughly means "raise your voice" and is typically used to protest some injustice, while *lungi khol* roughly translates as "take off your lungi." A lungi is a piece of clothing resembling a skirt or wrap that is worn around the lower part of a man's body. While in middle-class and upper middle-class families men may wear lungis at home for comfort, the garment typically has a lower- or working-class association (unless one is from the southern part of India, where one may see fashionable lungis worn on formal occasions). The lungi thus is typically a marker of class. Additionally, it is important to note that lungis with a checkered design are associated with Muslim men (especially working- or lower-class Muslim men), a style that has a long history into which I am not able to dive here for constraints of space. Generally, for lower-class or poor men, the lungi is often a daily piece of clothing, worn in public.

In SBA, ODF recognition is granted following an annual survey conducted by the Indian government. This survey, known as Swachh Survekshan, is now touted as the world's largest cleanliness and sanitation survey. It assesses the performance of cleanliness in cities, ranks them, and determines if the city has achieved ODF status (Drishti 2022). The survey began in 2016. The findings are publicized on government websites as well as other media forums, and awards are given in public functions hosted by the government. These rankings play a role in establishing claims by the government about the nation's overall ODF status, which is then also linked to overseas funding. Understandably, competition to achieve ODF status and gain high rankings has been intense among cities. Local officials are under pressure from their states (and sometimes threatened with job loss) to achieve ODF status for their cities, towns, and municipalities. Although some nongovernmental reports have questioned the mechanisms used in the survey to award ODF status to a city (Trivedi 2019), pursuit of this status is widespread and attaining it is generally celebrated domestically and within the global development community. [19]

The Halla Bol, Lungi Khol campaign was enacted by "enforcement teams" that were formed by RMC to catch and punish people caught defecating in the open. So, when the campaign was named Halla Bol, Lungi Khol, it had already determined which bodies were to be subject to surveillance and then punished for open defecation. Such people—typically the poor, migrants, slum dwellers (all men, and one can also reasonably assume that many were poor Muslims given that they often wear lungis)—were picked up, stripped of their lungis, and fined 100 rupees. The men's lungis were only returned after the offenders had paid their fine and pledged never to defecate in the open again. For a poor person, who may earn 500 rupees a day, a fine of 100 rupees is steep. Although the campaign is called Halla Bol, Lungi Khol, it does not mean that if a poor person engaging in open defecation but not wearing a lungi will be spared. So the lungi really functions as a sign for lower-class or poor people who go outside to defecate, signaling the classist and even casteist ideologies already informing the campaign, for there is no parallel associations made with men in trousers (typically signaling the upper and middle classes), who often do not hesitate to urinate in the open or even defecate if needed.

The state urban development minister of Jharkhand, C. P. Singh, defended the campaign, stating that the aim is not to harass people. "The idea is to create some sort of deterrence" (*Wire* 2017). On the other hand, Deputy Mayor Sanjeev Vijayvargeeya acknowledged that it was not necessary for the enforcement teams to remove men's lungis, but he noted that "people are so robotically programmed in their minds since ages that they will go to defecate in open even after you build dozens of toilets attached with their homes" (S. Jha 2017). Thus, it was important to adopt various harsh methods through which such people caught openly defecating could be turned into "civilised citizens" (S. Jha 2017). And to turn them into civilized citizens was to first visualize them as noncitizens by stripping them, rendering them primitive, exposing their semi-naked body to the disciplinig upper- and middle-class hetero-patriarchal gaze of the state. What we see here is the operation of a will to punish whereby in order to enforce a "bourgeois environmentalism" that is embedded in a project of "disciplining the poor" (Baviskar 2003, 92) , the poor are (quite literally) stripped of any dignity, ironically at the same time that the Modi government has linked toilet construction to dignity. A report conducted in 2020 by the Center for Policy Research in India, which focused its attention on the state of Odisha, noted that while such practices of coercion are gaining ground, the marginalized (from lower castes and minority religions) who are often the targets of such coercive acts are left out of local decision-making processes, such as around how ODF status might be regulated (Dwivedi and Singh 2020).

One image of an underprivileged man being stripped by RMC officials went viral, being published in many newspapers, including the *Times of India*, as well as circulated on X (figure 4.2). Here, the man's lungi has been removed by the RMC official and he is left standing in his underpants. He is rendered semi-naked by an agent of the state who is ready to punish him. One of the officials, who has a baton in his hand on which the lungi hangs, is looking down at the man in his semi-stripped state. And in that look is revealed the power differential between two masculinities—the violent, statist, vigilante, upper-caste masculinity embodied by the official, and the poor man's (possibly lower-caste and/or Muslim) masculinity, which is feminized as he is emasculated through that stripping. One could even read an erotic homosocial relation into this gaze. While indeed homosocial logics cannot be culturally universalized, there is, however, some value to Eve Sedgwick's famous observation that homosocial relations (under which homoeroticism falls) can be not "that of brotherhood, but of extreme, compulsory, and intensely volatile mastery and subordination" (1985, 66).

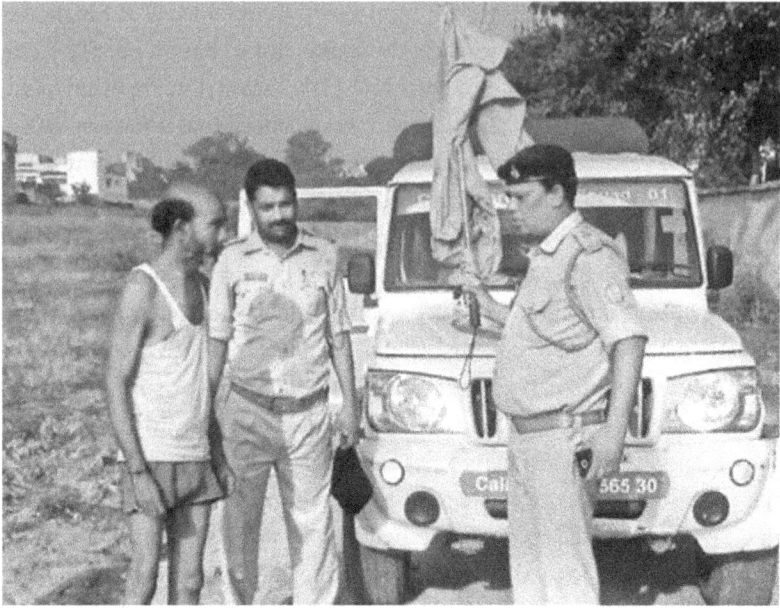

FIGURE 4.2 A man stripped of his lungi by officials of the Ranchi Municipal Corporation as part of the Halla Bol, Lungi Khol campaign. *Times of India*, X, September 24, 2017.

In the penetrative gaze of the upper-caste officials one can read a hint of sexual penetration or castration—both of which may be denigrated as unmanly under heteropatriarchal norms—when we remember the long history of Hindu-Muslim (or "other") men's relations in Indian national culture. Bacchetta (1999b) has addressed how Hindu nationalist men castrated (or threatened castration of) Muslim men in communal riots, thus putting them in place through acts of violence symbolizing demasculinization and thus abjection. Other works such as Misra (2014) have discussed how during Partition (and the Hindu-Muslim "riots" that followed), the male genitals became proof of whether one belonged or not to the Hindu nation and community; thus many men—especially if they were suspected of being Muslims—were forced by Hindu nationalists to strip down to reveal their genitals. The point is that the stripping down of the male body of a lower-caste/class/religious identity in the Indian context is charged with historical associations. While clearly in this image we do not definitely know whether this is a Muslim man (possibly, if we see the beard as a stereotypical signifier that is often commonly used to signify

Muslim men in media images), it is certainly an image of an "other" masculinity.[20] Given that the fear of an "other" (especially Muslim) masculinity taking over Hindu women and diluting Hindu-ness in the nation has been constantly stoked in Modi's India, one could perhaps read into the penetrative gaze of the official (and other similar disciplining gazes) in the HBLK campaign a subconscious (or even conscious) attempt to contain and reverse the fear of "other" masculinities (especially Muslim) by disciplining their bodies and bodily intimacies.

In a *Times of India* article, the image from the HBLK campaign was captioned "Ranchi civic body disrobes those defecating in the open" (Kislaya 2017). The rhetoric of the caption a priori excludes the disrobed man from the "civic" body politic. The word "disrobe" is laden with gendered connotations of honor in Hindu culture—for example, Draupadis's disrobing in the Mahabharata—and it is typically associated with disrobing a woman to strip her of her honor (*izzat*), as discussed in chapter 3. By framing this as a disrobing, the author of the article emphasizes the feminization (and even a perverse sexualization) of the poor (and possibly the Muslim man's masculinity). This classist, casteist (most officials or nonofficials engaged in toilet vigilantism are from upper castes), and Hindu heteropatriarchal gaze of the official replicating the gaze of the state surveys—owns, possesses—the semi-naked body of the man.[21] This image significantly captures the anti-poor ethos (which is entangled with caste and religion) of Hindu modern governmentality as it is focused on enabling the neoliberal logics of the state, which in SBA is about the privatization, securitization, and control of disorder that filth symbolizes.

While the official's uniform may disguise this act from being seen as vigilantism, it is nothing short of that. The official does not have the right under the constitution to engage in devaluing and dehumanizing the body of someone by forcing him to strip as an act of punishment. Here we have an example of what I alluded to earlier—vigilantism performed by state actors operating *outside* the law to enforce the desires of the state, and more significantly to implement a middle-class civilizational order of cleanliness. This example (and many others like it) of "citizenly" vigilante acts reveals the logic of violence—and more specifically vigilante violence—of Hindu modern governmentality working here to terrorize those who do not fit the majoritarian neoliberal order of current Hindu nationalism. In Madhya Pradesh, for example, an elderly man suffering from dysentery who could not control his stomach was slapped, forced to clean his crap with his hands and throw it away using his *dhoti* by men claiming to be from Ujjain

Municipal Corporation (Mekaad 2016).[22] Obviously, intestinal and digestive ailments are more likely to inflict the poor, due to aspects of structural violence they face in terms of food, housing, water, and healthcare.

With SBA, it should be pointed out, the central government issued an advisory to the states that any kind of coercive action taken by private or state officials with respect to sanitation behavior "is unacceptable under any circumstance" (NDTV 2019). At the same time, there is pressure on local officials from their states, who often shift this pressure onto local citizens who volunteer to take on surveillance duties, to achieve ODF status for their state. Despite the central government's advisory statement, such campaigns of violence have continued and there is no known account of perpetrators being punished or such behavior being criminalized. This becomes especially complicated when the perpetrators themselves are frequently glorified in the media, where they have been described as "crusaders" acting to prevent open defecation in their areas.[23]

The HBLK campaign is not the only instance where poor men caught in the act of open defecation are being stripped. Sehore is another town in Madhya Pradesh where this happened. Not only was the poor man who was caught openly defecating reprimanded and stripped by the chief municipal officer, he was also made to hold his ears and do squats. All around stood other local men witnessing this humiliation. The man was so devastated that his family reported that he stopped leaving his home and ceased interactions with anyone, pointing to the kind of social death that can result from such vigilante actions.[24] Figure 4.3 is from a video that captures a similar incident that was screened on Jansatta Network—a Hindu channel—that has over 2 million online subscribers (Jansatta 2017). While I cannot be sure that this particular image refers to the Sehore incident, it exactly captures the kind of punishment that occurred in Sehore and that is probably happening in other places as well. In this video, the poor, male (and possibly lower-caste) body is infantilized through the act of punishment (the man is seen holding his ears while being directed to do squats, as though punishing a wayward child). In this infantilization he is rendered an incomplete citizen, an infantile citizen, whose body cannot symbolize the modern Hindu nation being forged through initiatives such as SBA. In the video from which this image is taken, the official (or he could be a local volunteer—it is not clear from the image) directly invokes this infantilization when he yells at the man for his "childlike" behavior.

This kind of infantilization and the emasculation that accompanies it has unfolded in other health-related contexts. It was seen during the

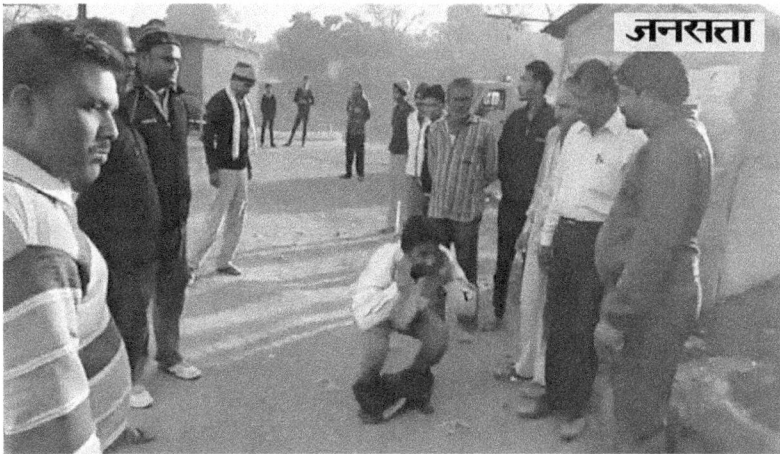

FIGURE 4.3 A man doing squats while holding his ears for flouting open defecation protocols. Jansatta Network, YouTube channel, February 24, 2017.

COVID-19 pandemic (Sharma 2020), when poor people who took to the roads to find a job were punished for not staying at "home" by being made to hold their ears do squats numerous times (figure 4.4). In another instance, internal migrants were forcibly sprayed with a chemical in a bus station in Uttar Pradesh in order to disinfect them, risking their health. The pattern is the same—"citizenly" vigilantism and the infantilization of offenders whose agency over their own bodies is suspended as they are subjected to humiliating public punishments.

What we find in Sehore or even in the HBLK campaign is a kind of public torture or lynching in that the punishments being meted out invite witnessing and even popular enjoyment, as can best be seen in figure 4.3. Scholars have written about state repression of "other" masculinities in which corporeal, including sexual, humiliation works as an instrument of power, seen for instance in acts of sexual hazing or torture during times of war, whippings during slavery, and lynchings. In the act of humiliating open defecators in a process that infantilizes and feminizes them, the poor men's bodies are reduced to a primitive object, or even property, of the upper-class/caste heteronormative state that determines how that body should exist in the regime of the modern that the development-oriented state is obsessed about today. If, for instance, it was an upper-class man caught engaging in public "nuisance," he would never have been subject to such a practice, for his body is already situated in a heterosexual upper-caste/class

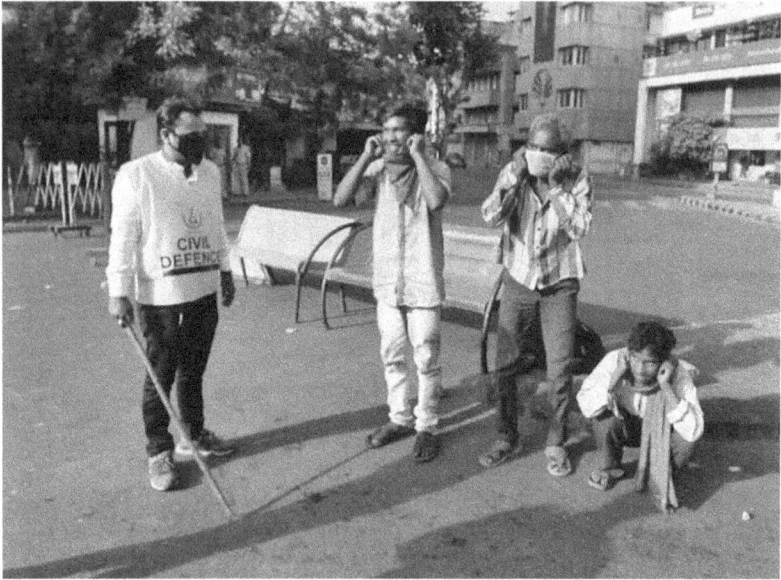

FIGURE 4.4 Men caught defying COVID-19 lockdown protocols being humiliated by police and made to do squats while holding their ears in north India in 2020. *Daily Sabah*, March 24, 2020.

network of privilege that he would have availed of, if needed, to reassert the authority and power of his body.

Something like this happened when a BJP minister was caught on camera urinating in a public place while traveling to remote Champaran District. The photo was posted by an opposing party, and it went viral and he was mocked. But he was not in a semi-stripped position. The photograph showed him from behind, clad in a *dhoti*. The spokesperson for the minister stated, "There is absolutely nothing wrong in what the minister did" and that "one cannot suppress nature's call for long. What do you do if you are traveling long distances and there are no public urinals on the way?" (quoted in Suraj 2017). Nothing happened to the minister. However, if this had been a poor man from a lower-class/caste background, public urinal or not, he could potentially be fined or subject to more spectacular bodily mistreatment. This demonstrates the casteist/classist structural inequalities that inform the will to punish. It also indicates how these practices of enforcing cleanliness can function as disguised acts through which the disenfranchisement of lower castes, the poor, disenfranchised Muslims, and "others" are continuing in the nation.

Both figure 4.2 and figure 4.3 reveal how the will to punish that powers the violence that informs Hindu modern governmentality today often expresses itself in spectacular ways. The punishment is often visually recorded—by the punisher or an onlooker—and is circulated on social media. Just as the lynching of Black men in the Southern United States was undertaken as a deliberate public spectacle so as to remind other Black men of the fate they might meet if they performed a (perceived) transgression of the racial order, here too the highly mediated and circulated images of cleanliness offenders being punished—humiliated or beaten—performs the effective function of spreading terror among the vulnerable and the poor, while inviting enjoyment from the upper-class/caste who view these "uncivilized" bodies and applaud the punishment meted out to them, which keeps them in "their place." Celebrities such as the author and actress Twinkle Khanna—whose picture of a man defecating on Juhu beach went viral—are increasingly normalizing these practices, making spectacles of such poor bodies for the whole nation to see. This not only reinforces bourgeois upper-middle-class scripts that regulate the punishment of cleanliness offenders, but it can also work to bring attention to already privileged citizens such as Khanna, although fortunately, while Khanna was applauded by some, she was criticized by many on social media for exposing a poor man in such a manner.

Rahul Mukherjee discusses this kind of phenomenon as "vigilante virality," which is on the rise in contemporary India (2020, 80). We have seen this in the flogging of Dalits in Una in 2016 or the attacking of Muslims by Hindus, where the attack is often filmed and goes viral on social media.[25] With SBA, however, vigilantism and the viral spread of images of it have even been encouraged by many state governments under the guise of citizenly duty. People in different towns and villages are asked by local municipalities or states to take photos or make videos of those they see openly defecating and share them on social media with the express intent of humiliating the individual. In Rajasthan and some other states, teachers have been forced to surveil the fields for open defecation, take pictures of it, and send their photos via WhatsApp to their senior officials (*Deccan Chronicle* 2016), who presumably forward them to local officials. In Chandol *panchayat* in Budhiana District, Maharashtra, a decision was made to put in place a more mercenary scheme in 2017: whoever took a selfie with a person defecating in the open was to receive a cash award of 500 rupees (Nair 2016). And in Gwalior, a scheme encouraged people to take selfies of open defecation, send them via WhatsApp to a government-associated

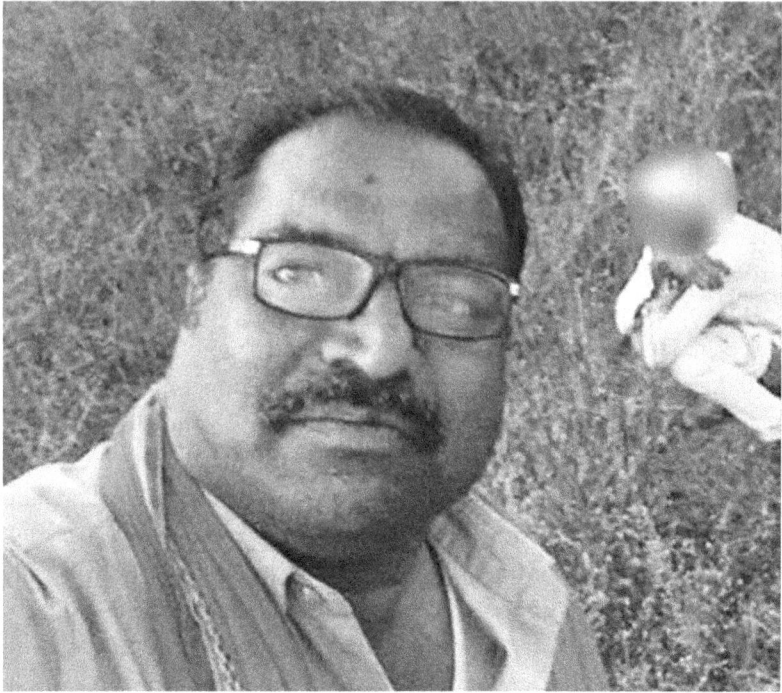

FIGURE 4.5 A selfie posted by a local corporation official on his Facebook page showing a truck driver in the background defecating in the open. *New Minute*, January 23, 2018.

number, receive 100 rupees, while the defecator would be fined 250 rupees (Tomar 2017). One selfie from the scheme taken by a local corporation official and shared on his Facebook page shows him in front of a lorry driver in Hyderabad, who is defecating in the fields (figure 4.5). In some cases, photos are shared only on WhatsApp networks of administrators; in other instances, they are posted to (and reposted on) social media platforms. Through constant mechanistic (and bureaucratic) circulation—where such images become data—they produce a detachment from the violence itself that further conceals the caste, class, and gendered intersections that inform networked relations of viewing that ensue. As Kuntsman and Stein note of digitalized violence, "the patina of the digital everyday can minimize and banalize this violence, obscuring its visibility and mitigating its impact" (2015, 24). Moreover, the constant WhatsApping of photos of cleanliness offenders by local officials and everyday citizens makes these images data items that "prove" to local states and those in central government that the *swachhagrahis* (or local volunteers and teachers) *are* doing their job. The violence toward the cleanliness offender ends up becoming an informational item for tracking cleanliness and its enforcement, which contributes to the dehumanization and the technicalization of the initial punishment.

What we see here is the explicit entanglement of three important features of Hindu modern governmentality. First, there is the securitizing of cleanliness via violence toward poor bodies. Second, there is the distribution (and thus routinizing) of that violence through sophisticated informational networks whereby that violence becomes part of a larger architecture of punitive violence of a neoliberal Hindu order through which digital hate is networked through online channels and spaces. Third, the violence becomes part of the neoliberal digital *Hindu* casteist order because the vigilance committees meting out punishment and taking photos for circulation tend to be from the upper caste, and those unable to build a toilet and caught in open defecation tend to be poor and lower caste, Adivasis, tribals, or poor Muslims.

The HBLK campaign in Ranchi has been paralleled by similar campaigns in others states, such as the formation of the Dabba Dol Gang (DDG) in Madhya Pradesh, which also evidences punitive vigilante masculinity. The DDG received positive media attention, including becoming the subject of a short celebratory film (Cherukupalli 2016). Made by WaterAid India, which is a global nonprofit network that aims to improve access to clean water, toilets, and hygiene for everyone—the film follows a group of young boys, ten and more, who formed a gang to prevent open defecation in their village. They wake up at the crack of dawn and go outside to chase and whistle at those openly defecating or walking toward the fields used for defecation. They spill the water from people's *lota* (wash bottles) so that the offenders cannot wash themselves and thus will stop open defecation from then on.[26] This becomes especially cruel as many poor people lack water in their homes from which they might have saved a small bottle for their toilet functions. The targets of the DDG's actions are left in a semi-exposed state as they are unable to wash themselves when their *lota* is kicked over by the boys. Phrases like "crusaders" (Cherukupalli 2016) or "whistling in change" (Anima 2023) are approvingly used by the media to refer to this group's "unique method" by which they serve the nation (Cherukupalli 2016). In one image that captures a scene from the short film about the DDG, it is noteworthy that the camera shot is from a low angle, thus making the young boys look powerful as they look down at the man defecating—a position that renders him vulnerable to the visual stature given to the boys (figure 4.6). The boys ask, "why are you

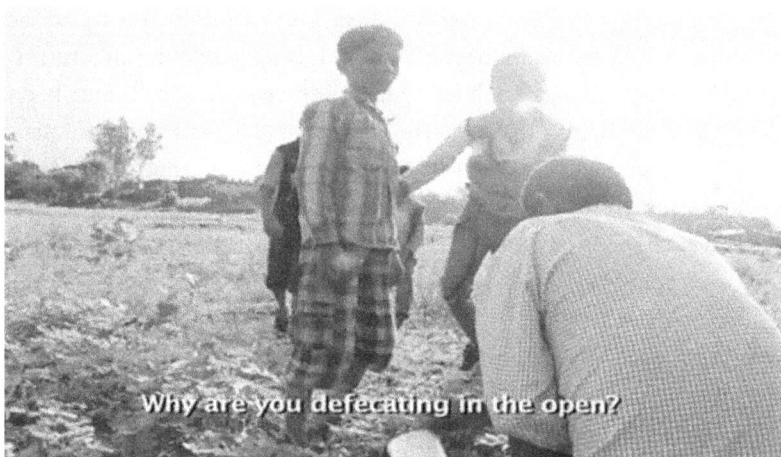

Why are you defecating in the open?

FIGURE 4.6 Still from the short film "Dabba Dol Gang."

defecating in the open?" One of the boys lectures the man on the fact that the government is providing subsidies for toilets. This group is one example among many, where children—especially young boys—are engaged in acts of surveillance, harassment, and humiliation that replicate vigilante practices. With DDG we have a situation of young boys being socialized into a script of punitive (vigilante) masculinity that is targeted toward poor men's bodies. These kids are learning at an early stage which kinds of bodies are valuable and can signify the (Hindu) national modern, and which bodies are primitive and uncivilized, and thus need to be targeted. The kids are also learning at this early stage the value of a punitive masculinity in protecting the nation, while the youthfulness of those disciplining the defecators shows the latter to be below even children.

What is disconcerting is that the script of punitive casteist/classist masculinity that the children embody is, however, concealed by their innocence. The use of children to institutionalize shaming and abuse of poor people engaged in open defecation has been a significant feature of SBA campaigns. In the village of Lolad, children went around whistling and shaming those engaged in open defecation (Doshi 2017). In Gardwara village in Madhya Pradesh, a team of children referred to by the media as "commandos" engaged in whistling at open defecators till they abandoned their act (Pareek 2015). In Maharashtra, "good morning squads," composed of students (and self-help groups), were created to surveil, report on, and impose fines on those openly defecating.

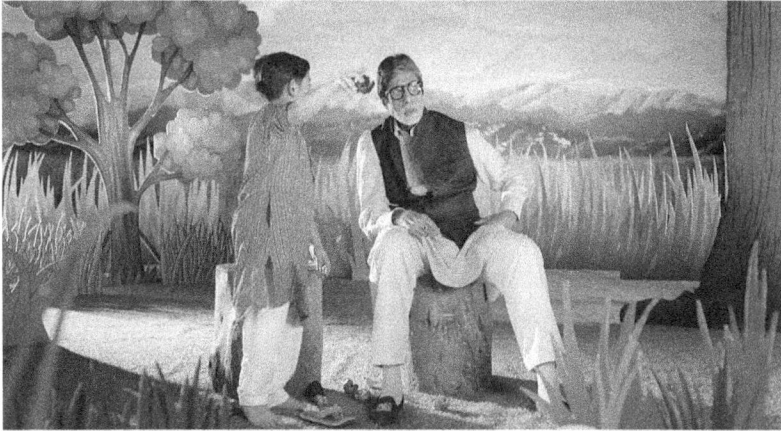

FIGURE 4.7 Still from a video for Swachh Bharat Abhiyan's Jadugar campaign. Created by Ogilvy and Mather ad agency, 2016, for the government's SBA initiative.

Additionally, ad campaigns have run that have paired children, particularly boys, with prominent celebrities who serve as spokespeople for SBA. A famous one is the Jadugar (Magician) campaign created by the advertising agency Ogilvy and Mather that features Bollywood male icon Amitabh Bachchan with a young boy from a well-to-do background, signified by his clothing (SBM 2016a). Bachchan and the boy are sitting in an area with trees, bushes, and fields set against a mountainous background. The little boy asks Bachchan to perform some magic. Bachchan says, while pointing to a tree, "Fine, I will throw stones there and you will see birds emerging." This happens, but the boy is not too impressed. He then says, pointing to some bushes, "Now let *me* show you, *my* magic. I will throw stones there and people will appear" (figure 4.7).[27] After the boy throws stones into the bushes, men emerge from behind the bushes with their *lotas*. They were defecating. The boy has a good laugh that the stones he threw resulted in this. Those poor men are then lectured by Bachchan. Once again, the use of a child renders innocent the act of throwing stones at poor men. The little boy is scripted into a punitive, classist/casteist, vigilante masculinity—throwing stones at the poor (as he already knew that the offenders were defecating behind the bushes)—and this vigilante act is glamorized through the presence of a celebrity figure like Bachchan. The use of such ad campaigns by SBA created by major advertising companies also point to the coming together of two important areas of neoliberal capital in India—entertainment (with the use of Bollywood celebrities) and development—that fuel domestic growth (and play a significant role in reforging national identity) through the infusion of transnational capital.

The discussion above reinforces Imogen Tyler's argument about how the production of national abjection functions as a mode of governmentality, and that state power relies on the "production of abject subjects to constitute itself and draw its borders" of civility and belonging (2013, 4). As neoliberal state policies continue to disempower populations—particularly already vulnerable populations—these populations are constructed as abject by the state. By being made abject they are made responsible for their conditions. This conceals the structural challenges that produce the conditions within which such (usually) vulnerable populations have to survive. The making of abjection, then, is a strategy of national concealment, in that it helps to conceal the various forms of violence (material and representational) and the underlying "will to punish" through which populations—those already marginalized—are constantly excluded from the protection of the state. Tyler suggests that stigmatization of particular populations is one way in which abjection is produced that legitimates and justifies social inequalities. Through protocols and judgments offered about cleanliness in the SBA context, and the ensuing disciplining of bodies who are seen to violate them, we see how "stigmatization operates as a form of governance" (2013, 8). In her discussion of "hygienic governmentality," Lauren Berlant further argues that such abject populations function as examples of obstacles or threats to a "good life" and a "felicitous image of a national future" (1997, 175).[28] Little wonder then that in the Swachh Survekshan surveys, some populations are "disappeared" as I discuss shortly—their toilet-less existence threatens the promise of "good life" in a town or city that is to be declared ODF by these surveys, which produce national rankings of cleanliness. So it is no surprise that during the G20 summit recently held in Delhi, many slum areas were curtained off from the road, and many homeless shelters were demolished so that dignitaries driving by could not see them(Aafaq 2023). These populations were simply erased from the visible cityscape; they were made nonpublics.

Throughout the SBA campaign there has been a systematic violation and degrading of poor people and an emasculation and even criminalization of poor men, who we need to remember are typically lower caste, Dalits, migrants, the homeless, or Muslims. This recurring pattern teaches us what scripts of masculinity—a middle- and upper-class/caste, majoritarian, and punitive—are being willed by the neoliberal, heteropatriarchal

Hindu nationalist state and its modern development imperatives. So far, the analysis of the intersections between SBA, vigilantism, and violence has focused primarily on men (and boys), both as vigilantes and as victims, and on the ways spectacles of punishment demarcate proper masculinity. However, citizens of all genders are engaging in these campaigns.

FEMALE VIGILANTISM

Women are also taking on the punitive vigilante script in enforcing cleanliness. There are videos available on the internet that present activities of local female volunteers—members of *nigrani samitis* (vigilance committees) or *swachhagrahis*—regulating open defecation. Many of them work along with men to stop open defecation. Figure 4.8 is a still from a video posted by Shri Krishna Studios on YouTube (SKS 2017). The exact location of the incident is not identifiable. The video itself shows women *swachhagrahis* (and again, members of such committees and teams tend to be upper caste, as addressed earlier) forcibly dragging a poor woman, possibly from a lower caste. The image suggests that they are either working under the supervision of male *swachhagrahis* (in the background in the image) or working with them. They have chased the woman from the nearby field where she was going for open defecation. They pull her to a nearby official-looking vehicle. In the video, we see the poor woman screaming and resisting as she is captured, but to no avail. The torture continues and she is forced into the car. What we have here is a kind of kidnapping: picking people up, and in this case a helpless poor (most likely lower-caste) woman, forcing them into cars and taking them somewhere where they will probably be further disciplined. As I was watching the video, I was most disturbed by the intense screams of the poor woman trying to resist the cleanliness enforcers who are pushing her into the official-looking vehicle.

What to make of this female vigilantism and its expression of a will to punish (which here looks like torture!)? Where does it fit into the larger architecture of violence that powers the nation today? Although this act, when seen in isolation, is not an explicit expression of *Hindutva* violence, I want to suggest that it reflects a growing trend in the nation where (especially upper-caste Hindu) women are being recruited into discourses of security-driven nationalism that "enacts Hindu mythological archetypes of strong womanhood as protectors of the nation, albeit a nation underlined by a patriarchal order" (Banerjee 2019).

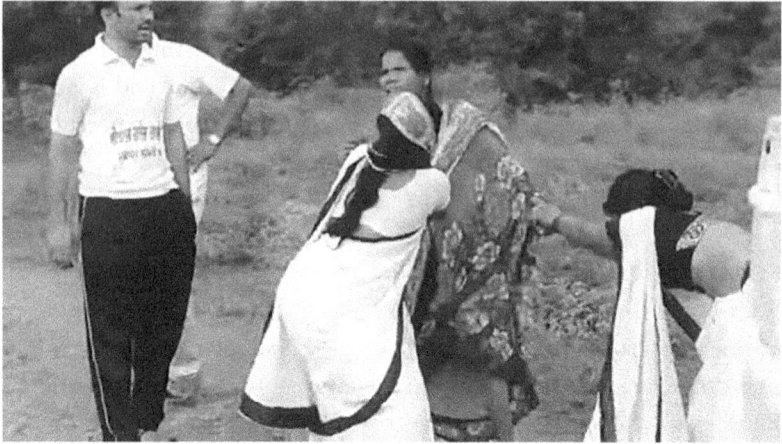

FIGURE 4.8 Still from a video of a woman caught by *swachhagrahis* for open defecation in the fields and being forcibly led toward a car. Shri Krishna Studio, YouTube, August 29, 2017.

Scholars have already written about the long history of women being recruited into Hindutva outfits and engaged in martial training and vigilante activities. More recently, this strong national protector role for women in Hindutva politics can be seen in the career of the former BJP Defense Minister Nirmala Sitaram, an upper middle-class Brahmin who became the first full-time woman defense minister of the nation.[29] Moreover, since 2022, women have been allowed to train at India's National Defense Academy (BBC 2021). What we have today in addition is something more nuanced (that is, not just an overt expression of Hindutva training) that nonetheless continues this logic. Especially since Sitaram became defense minister, more women have been recruited into formal military and other security positions. These positions allow women to express a commitment to protect the nation; simultaneously, this new appearance of women in these arenas helps the state present itself as modern and committed to women's empowerment. Bollywood has in recent years pushed this kind of militant women's empowerment narrative by showcasing stories featuring strong, modern (typically Hindu) women in security positions, where they often act outside the law to secure the nation.[30] This is occurring at the same time that fewer women from the lower strata of society have decent paying jobs, and discrimination and violence toward Muslim, Dalit, Adivasi, and northeastern women are at an all-time high.

If the previous chapter illustrated how "women's empowerment" was being touted in SBA through "(Hindu) woman's *protection*" then this section illustrates the flip side of this women's empowerment logic: (Hindu) women as *protectors* who don upper-caste masculine and vigilante scripts to securitize cleanliness as a service to the nation. Women have visibly participated in vigilante activities in postcolonial India since the early 1990s. Many Hindu women were actively involved in the violence related to the demolition of Babri Masjid in Ayodhya in 1992. In addition, women were also present among the Hindu mobs that attacked Muslims in the 2002 Gujarat pogrom, and many urban Hindu women participated in the violence underlining anti-Mandal Commission protests in 1990. While this pattern has been addressed by others (Bacchetta 2010; Basu 1993, 2011; Ghosh 2002; Sarkar and Butalia 1995; Turner 2012), women's vigilantism in SBA is different in scope, context, and goals. Unlike these earlier instances, where women explicitly occupied unlawful vigilante positions, in the SBA context, women (particularly upper-caste women) who take on the role of *swachhagrahis* function *within* state registers and engage in statist acts—like their male counterparts. To that extent, their positions are not unlawful. Yet their actions are potentially unlawful and violate people's civil rights, including their right to safety and dignity. This is what is demonstrated by the example offered earlier of the vulnerable poor (possibly lower-caste) woman being pulled about and terrorized by women *swachhagrahis* who force her into an official car. Do these *swachhagrahis*—state ambassadors or volunteers—have the right to do so? What "law" if any has been broken by this poor woman? How can she be forced into a car (in a way that looks like a kidnapping) by state-appointed volunteers of SBA? Yet their actions are nothing short of a kind of vigilantism that is now safeguarded by the state as these vigilante women present the women-friendly face of the state in enacting SBA surveillance protocols. Their vigilantism is concealed by their statist positions. This Hindu female vigilantism in SBA, while different from earlier times, nonetheless points to a larger strengthening of a heterogendered casteist patriarchal architecture of violence in the nation through which women (of a particular group) are often being officially recruited as national(ist) subjects—and thus seemingly being empowered—in the name of securitizing various realms of the nation.

Yet the use of women for these vigilante policing functions does not disturb the heteropatriarchal casteist structures underlying them; rather, being able to present a "woman friendly" face communicates SBA's apparent modern logic. In the case of women policing open defecation by other women, there is no serious reflection on why a poor woman (possibly from a lower caste) defecates in the open, what gendered/casteist structures promote this, what infrastructural violence results in that, and what social injuries are continued when women from upper castes or those scripted into protocols serving the upper-caste patriarchal state express a will to punish by forcibly dragging a helpless poor woman into an official vehicle (signifying the state). In the light of all this, when the government keeps praising women's involvement in SBA, one must ask which women's lives are not captured by this and *how* are women being recognized as citizens by the state today?

I do not mean to diminish the work that many women have done to engage in cleanliness activities. But that is not the focus of this book. Rather, I am once again interested in the terms of women's inclusion (and which women are included) in SBA and how that conceals the (class/caste) violence that women are encouraged to perform toward "other" women in the name of securing cleanliness for the nation. The women's empowerment narrative that powers the BJP ethos and that is too often folded into a logic of security and surveillance can never enable the *production of solidarity* among women across caste, class, and religious lines that is so badly needed today. This is because its very arrangement pits women from different strata of society against each other. As discussed in chapter 1, this is one of the ways in which right-wing populist movements in the world are hijacking gender movements and reframing feminism through an individualized narrative of women's empowerment that celebrates "strong women" serving the nation—even as the nation's purported commitment to women's empowerment is highly circumscribed regarding which women and which forms of power are supported.

What is interesting is that the practice of surveilling people and educating (or disciplining) them into "clean subject" positions is performed not just by (upper-caste) men or women. Media celebrations of the SBA program have highlighted with enthusiasm the role played by gender-variant populations in surveilling and persuading people to build toilets, especially in small towns and villages—signaling SBA's seeming inclusionary and modern nature.[31] Recent scholarship has noted how Hindutva discourses are assimilating queer and trans people (Bacchetta 2019; Dutta and Roy 2014; Upadhay 2020). While the disciplining, surveillant discourses of SBA that I have been charting in this chapter are not always *explicitly* Hindutva discourses, as state discourses they do reinforce the logics of Hindu modern governmentality as I hope to have amply demonstrated in earlier sections.

Media coverage of the SBA program has frequently celebrated the work of gender-variant populations—particularly those they label as transgender individuals, and specifically trans women—in persuading villagers to use toilets via singing and dancing, a practice or skill that is stereotypically seen by the media (and much of the straight population in India) as somehow unique attributes of trans people, thus reproducing age-old stereotypes about this population as though "singing and dancing skills" (Dutta 2017) are inherent to their identity.[32] In frequently using the term "transgender," media reports on SBA also end up reinforcing the hegemonic use of transgender that is common in many development and state discourses (Dutta and Roy 2014), which frequently subsume (or render invisible) local expressions of gender variance, including in gender-variant lower-caste populations such as Dalits. This again shows how the media, in relation to SBA, performs for elite, urban, and even international eyes.

Although a fuller and more complex account of the provisional absorption of gender-variant populations into SBA is beyond the scope of this project, nonetheless I wish to gesture toward the fact that SBA, as an allegedly modern discourse, is another site through which gender-variant populations are being recognized by the Indian state, a recognition that however rests on their serving the Hindu state. Notably, there is no focus on potentially nonnormative or therefore disruptive sexualities/sexual orientations, or disruptive intimate/family formations in these discourses, which signals the limit of the state's rhetoric of inclusion for nonnormative populations. Moreover, it is also crucial to recognize that trans (and other gender-variant as well as sexual minority) populations continue to face harassment and violence on an everyday level, including in public bathrooms. While there has been a push at the central government level to allow trans populations to use any public bathroom of their choice, many trans activists argue that this does not go far enough, for there is no mechanism or government intervention to address the harassment or sexual or physical violence that trans and other gender-variant subjects encounter in bathroom spaces and other spaces (Manral 2018). Additionally, the recognition of trans populations (especially trans women) in SBA discourses is reliant on the nonrecognition of other gender-variant populations, who are not only excluded by the (colonizing) term "transgender" in SBA, but also in the visible media spaces that represent transgender activism in SBA. Underlying all of this, of course, is the continued socioeconomic marginalization that gender-variant and sexual minority populations face in India and the ways that this marginalization tends to intersect with their disproportionate vulnerability to forms of not only personal but also infrastructural violence.

INFRASTRUCTURAL VIOLENCE

A few words need to be said about the *infrastructural violence* that SBA vigilante practices conceal. Infrastructural violence manifests in and through structures and services developed to support society and its operations but in reality unevenly serve or even harm and disempower particular people or groups of people. While the harms perpetuated by and through large-scale infrastructure projects such as dams in India have rightly received much attention, the more subtle material infrastructures such as those related to SBA also enact various forms of violence. One place this can be seen is in the classist and casteist nexus underlying the logics of toilet construction.

How SBA funds are distributed is often a matter of local/state policies and arrangements (Agarwal 2018). In the case of the HBLK campaign, one female individual who was caught defecating in the open stated that her family had applied for government subsidy, but the application was rejected (*Wire* 2017). Independent reports have noted several reasons for such rejection that has occurred in many other places. One reason is that SBA has taken the 2012 baseline survey to identify households without access to toilets and then disbursed funds. However, the nature of the households often changed after that time—for example, a son may have married and moved out of his parents' house (and thus he fell out of the baseline survey, for his family is no longer counted as a household).[33] In other words, only village households that were listed in the 2012 survey were eligible, while households established after 2012 were not. This also includes those who may have moved to a new village after 2012 (Agarwal 2018).

Investigative reports done in cities such as Brabanki, Meerut, Lucknow, and Shamli found that village leaders (*pradhans*) sometimes favored those who belonged to their caste, and thus funds were easily disbursed for that population. One resident in Chinhat, Lucknow, stated that "toilets have been built only in that part of the village where the Vermas live" (Agarwal 2018). Reports have also revealed that sometimes the *pradhans* or *panchayat* officers in villages pocket the government subsidy instead of placing it in people's accounts, and then get toilets constructed using the cheapest materials, which do not last.[34] Further, most toilets that have been built are single pits. Many owners are uneducated about twin pits, which are being pushed by the central government. In the twin pit model, fecal matter in the first pit decomposes while the second one is used; the decomposed material turns into compost and is then easier to clear out (*Wire* 2019). One study states that twin pits mean people want to build large pits so that they do not fill up easily. But that costs more than the amount of money given as the government subsidy (Jain et al. 2020).

Many poor Indians do not have sufficient land on their property to build toilets, especially double pits that require more space (Kedia 2022). For migrants who do not have permanent homes and live with landlords for a short duration, or Dalits (who have the least access to land), homelessness becomes a huge problem. One report notes that rural villagers perceived an anti-rural and anti-poor bias on the part of the government, claiming that it only builds proper waste and water infrastructure in urban areas (Jain et al. 2020). Most centrally, water needed to maintain and clean toilets is in short supply. In India, water is a classist luxury that among the middle and upper class is taken for granted. One poor rural man claimed that "One *lota* [wash bottle] of water used to be enough (with open defecation in fields), now we need one bucket of water (to clean toilets)" (quoted in Jacob et al. 2021, 101). The man asked how they were supposed to get so much water when poor people struggled to secure water for household chores and bathing. Water levels are often low in many areas, especially where the rural poor live, which makes it further difficult to access water. Thus, the imposition of toilets without connection to sewers or a piped water supply reveals the classist violence that water infrastructure in India is informed by, something that has been explored by Nikhil Anand (2017). Additionally, reports show that even if people use community toilets, the charge may be 5 rupees for each visit. For a poor family of four, that is 20 rupees, and when we multiply that by several toilet visits, it can add up to 100 rupees a day and 3,000 rupees a month—amounts completely out of reach for many (V. Jha 2017). Additionally, the subsidy for toilet construction given by the government is often provided *after* construction has begun or completed by an individual family, and often selfies of completed toilets are required as proof (Venugopal 2014). Most poor people do not have sufficient money for the upfront cost of building a toilet, disqualifying them from accessing the government subsidy.[35] For example, Dalit women in the "Harijan" Basti in Toolera, Rajasthan, earn 750 to 1000 rupees a month and live on a few rotis a day. As they cannot afford to begin constructing a toilet, they go to the fields for open defecation early in the morning (Yadav 2018).[36] There have also been incidents where a poor family initially paid some amount to the corporation for a toilet to be built, but then no work was done. A report on the city of Indore, for example, noted that, "as soon as the families paid, the IMC [Indore Municipal Corporation] followed up by digging pits, one for each house. But then there was nothing—no officials showed up" (Shantha 2017). Later, just before the Swachh Survekshan team was to visit Indore, a "team of twenty IMC officials and eight police personnel descended" on one family's doorstep and orders were given "to raze the house to the ground" because it did not have a toilet (Shantha 2017).

There have been many such instances of demolition, and often poor Dalits who are unable to construct a toilet for financial or other reasons have experienced this vigilante-like demolition of their home. Such families are then moved to makeshift shelters away from the city that further enhance their abjection and precarity. One report notes that in 2015 over one hundred Dalit families working as waste collectors in the city of Indore were evicted and shifted several miles away to the outskirts of the city. They were "disappeared," rendered out of sight, and this also affected their source of income. This was done so that the city's ranking did not fall when the Swachh Survekshan committee arrived for evaluation (Shantha 2017). In the case of Indore, the officials were under pressure not to lose Indore's top place in the rankings. So, every home without a toilet would have cost them points (Shantha 2017).

This case of disappearing populations—who are typically vulnerable—is part of a larger ongoing pattern in the nation in which some populations are simply being rendered out of sight, becoming nonpublics (even if temporarily) and ceasing to exist in lists and databases. And as they cease to exist in lists and databases, they also cease to exist in the political community (Ather 2023).[37] In Toolera village in Alwar District, Rajasthan, the very poor (often Dalit) households that have not been able to construct a latrine have simply been "edited out" of the residents list by officials so that the village can claim ODF status (Yadav 2018). Not only does this call attention to the violence, in this case infrastructural violence, in which Hindu modern governmentality is embedded, it also emphasizes how one of the ways in which Hindu modern governmentality operates today is by disappearing populations in pursuit of cleaning the country. This brings SBA into direct contact with similar cases of this pattern, as occurred with NRC, with Adhar identification systems, and with Kashmir (where the internet was shut down by the government for three months, literally removing Kashmiris from communication systems). It is also happening with the increasing demolition of Muslim homes and property (often based on claims of "illegal construction") and the expulsion of Muslims from their towns due to claims of "love jihad." This "disappearing" of populations is intimately linked to the logic of the Hindu modern, especially its commitment to a *punyabhoomi* that must excise "others" who represent disorder in this neoliberally etched sacred land. Today's regimes of development in India as manifested in SBA reveal what Bhan calls "development as depopulation" (2022, 279) that once again challenges the official narrative that SBA is a "people's movement." Perhaps it is better to think of the SBA program as a *majoritarian* people's movement, as well as a minority depopulation movement.

What we encounter in the examples offered above is what Nikhil Anand, Akhil Gupta, and Hannah Appel term "infrastructural abandonment" (2018, loc. 103). Infrastructures, they recognize, are "critical locations" through which "accumulation *and* dispossession" are performed (2018, loc. 119; emphasis added). At the same time that infrastructures promise distribution and safety, they also deliver "ruination, and abandonment" of certain lives through breakdowns and absence (2018, loc. 123). In India, infrastructures have always been situated in a class/caste nexus that, in the SBA case, is directly related to why so many (especially the poor, migrants, slum dwellers, Dalits, and others) continue to resort to open defecation (see also Truelove and O'Reilly 2021)—for instance, due to the lack of an adequate water supply. This kind of infrastructural abandonment produces a disconnect that constitutes an "active process through which *subjects are 'thrown down' or cast out' of the social and political systems*" (Anand 2017, 235; emphasis added) and rendered noncitizens or nonpublics. In SBA as with other realms in the nation, those "thrown down" or "cast out" are typically Dalits, poor Muslims, migrants, and tribals. The zealous will to punish cleanliness offenders that is celebrated in media and government coverage of SBA as citizenly action conceals this infrastructural violence and makes cleanliness offenses a matter of individual, primitive, or uncivilized pathologies instead of outcomes of infrastructural abandonment and disorder.

DEADLY (DIGITAL) INTIMACIES

On June 16, 2017, in the Pratapgarh District of Rajasthan, a lower-middle-class Muslim man, who was also a Communist Party of India (Marxist) activist, found himself in a scuffle with some local male *swachhagrahis* appointed by the municipal corporation. These appointees were doing their morning rounds and taking photos of people defecating in the open in order to track and curtail cleanliness violations. On this morning, they started taking photos of women from the Bagwasa Kachi *basti* (a slum area made of infirm materials), who had no option but to relieve themselves in the open. The woman came from one of the poorest pockets in Pratapgarh. The *basti* had residents from different castes and communities. Ninety percent of the houses in the *basti* did not have a toilet, one reason being that the promised government subsidy to build toilets had not been transferred to people's accounts (Jain 2017). One woman from the *basti* said, "I've written to the municipality several times to provide me money for constructing a toilet, but they never listen and instead threaten to demolish my home" (quoted in Jain 2017). There was only one community toilet for three thousand households, and it lacked basic standard features including adequate water and flushing capacity (Jain 2017). Perhaps this lack of infrastructure, some have speculated, was due to the fact that the *basti* had been targeted for demolition by the local government in order to build a posh residential development on the land.

One report on the events of that day notes that a team of local municipality cleanliness workers got too "close to where the women were, encroaching on their privacy, [and] they also started kicking their water containers and to top it all started taking photographs of [the] women in a state of undress" (Counterview 2017). All this happened in the presence of the chairperson of the municipality, Ashok Jain. Apparently capturing photos of women in compromised states as they defecated in the open had been a pattern of the municipality officials. As the women started resisting and yelling, men came out of the *basti*, including Zafar Khan, who asked the team to stop taking pictures. Khan's daughter Sabra, who was present at the scene, claimed that the municipal chair told his men, "Yeh roj roj ki pareshani hai, isko dekh lo aaj (He [Zafar] creates problem every day, teach him a lesson today)" (quoted in Jain 2017). The problem that the municipal chair was possibly referring to had to do with Zafar filing written complaints against the municipality with the *nagar parishad* (city council), demanding the disbursal of SBA funds for the *basti*, and criticizing the regular sexual harassment of women (who belonged to different castes and communities) by the municipality team taking photos of them in states of undress. Clearly Zafar was seen as a troublemaker.

Sabar Khan described seeing members of the municipality team then inflict severe violence on her father, which was accompanied by threats to her and her family. She stated: "[They] began hitting his stomach and pushed him on the road. They didn't let us intervene to save *abba* [father] and said, 'Tere baap ko jala denge, teri maa ka thobda todh denge, tujhe utha le jaenge (We'll burn your father, break your mother's skull and abduct you)'" (quoted in Jain 2017). Zafar was beaten, punched, and kicked. And then he died. He was taken to hospital. Official reports deny this account, stating that Zafar's death was of "natural causes," but numerous witnesses from the *basti* who were present counter this. Official statements also deny that members of the municipality were engaging in obscene acts of photographing women. Zafar's death led to local protests and protests in other parts of the nation, pointing not only to the failure of SBA where the poor and minorities are concerned, but also to the intersections of SBA and state violence against the people it purports to represent and protect. The fact that Zafar was a Muslim man was not lost on many of the protesters, for just a few months back, Pehlu Khan (another Muslim man) was lynched in Rajasthan by cow vigilantes, who suspected him of transporting cows.

The Zafar Khan incident highlights important issues relevant to the scripts of vigilante punishment, the gendered dimensions of surveillance and control, and the intersections of SBA enforcement and infrastructural violence. It also calls particular attention to the ways in which traditional modes of violence meld with contemporary digital technology. Cell phone cameras in particular play a pervasive role in the enactment of state and nonstate violence in India today, and are part of *how* citizens today encounter state and nonstate violence (via the digital realm) that purports to serve the state. This pattern comes to the fore in SBA when we look for it—and we should look for it, because it is important to understand the ways, in SBA and elsewhere, that the neoliberal majoritarian Hindu nationalist public sphere and the will to punish offenders through violence and coercion often coproduce one another.

These digitally enabled forms of violence also refute the thesis of the retreat of the state under neoliberalism. The use of digital devices as a dimension of vigilante surveillance and punishment in the SBA context rather demonstrates how the state ironically has become more intimate in its enactment of violence through new technology. The cell phone camera has become a biopolitical and even a necropolitical machine as there are increasing situations in India where such devices are used to capture (and then share on various social media platforms) images of the lynching of marginalized people by vigilantes. While work on social media has been burgeoning, there is still limited work on the relation between witnessing and documentation with cell phones, and new expressions of state power (and its biopolitical/necropolitical gaze). Of course, cell phone witnessing and recording can also be, and has been, used to record the violence of powerful groups on the marginalized to challenge the authority of the state and majoritarian culture, a phenomenon that scholars term "sousveillance" (Mann and Ferenbock 2013), where the gaze is reversed. This has been seen, for instance, in the Black Lives Matter movement, which took off because onlookers' recordings of the brutalization of Black men by the police were circulated on social media, or as in Arab Spring protests. But in the context of India today, sousveillance is becoming increasingly difficult. In addition to obvious issues of poor people's access to digital technology (especially in villages), or their lack of sophisticated digital literacy, digital recordings made by sympathizers of the victims of religious, caste, or other majoritarian acts of violence are not legally admitted in court. They are also quickly deleted on the internet as internet space under the BJP increasingly functions as a *majoritarian* internet space—another form, we might add, of infrastructural violence. As digital platforms are heavily monitored today, whose digital witnessing of whom ends up functioning as *data* for statist and nonstatist forms of governance is an important question that reveals the limits of the celebratory "Digital India" narrative. As Gitelman and Jackson (2013) have explained, data is always spoken for. It never speaks. Cheney-Lippold further argues that "who speaks for data, then, wields the extraordinary power to frame how we come to understand ourselves and our place in the world" (2017, xiii).

Zafar was not merely fighting the men taking photographs—that is, the men who were "shooting" photos and video (and the shooting of photos with a phone can be seen as a metaphoric act of shooting with guns that underlines how these digital intimacies are simultaneously often necro-intimacies). Zafar was also fighting the right of the state to engage in digital vigilantism, which in this case involved digital (sexualized/classist/casteist) intimacies *without consent*, and was performed with an explicit will to punish. He was challenging the state's right to digitally circulate those intimacies that would function as data through informational networks—the semi-exposed bodies of women from lower castes and Muslim women being viralized and datafied, as in that *basti* poor people from various castes and communities lived. Zafar died fighting the digital security gaze of the state, which was trying to govern intimacies in the name of protecting cleanliness, a governance that was localized through the cell phone cameras of the civic officials, most of whom as indicated earlier tend to be upper caste. Zafar was a victim of a deadly digital intimacy.

It is concerning to note that, whether intended or not, a necropolitical classist/casteist strain has made itself present in the SBA program's formal (the state) and informal (nonstate vigilante actors) cleanliness governance. In chapter 1 I mentioned the killing of two Dalit children in Shivpuri District by two Yadav men (from the lower castes rank but part of the Savarna castes). But there are other cases as well: the killing by fifteen people, including both men and women, of a man who wanted more time to build a toilet in Chhattisgarh (Drolia 2016); the killing of an e-rickshaw driver in Delhi when he tried to stop two men from publicly urinating in an area where he and others ate (Angad 2017); the withholding of rations in some states from poor families dependent on state food aid because they have not built toilets (Jitendra et al. 2018); and the death threats issued against open defecation via hoardings, as in Meghnagar Nagar *panchayat* in Jhabua District, Madhya Pradesh (H. Sharma 2017). What this once again literally evinces is the deadly anti-poor impulse of SBA. But perhaps more importantly, it raises the questions: Why such an intense affective investment in cleanliness that one can be killed for it? Is it really cleanliness that is the issue here? Or is it a (purified, cleansed) image of the nation that people are being encouraged to invest in and that the cleanliness narrative seeks to uphold? In addressing these questions, it is worth plumbing the ways that SBA's reliance on digital infrastructures, such as cell phones, social media accounts, WhatsApp networks, and so on, function to both fan the vigilante will to punish and masks the hierarchical, violent nature of state power that expands into the governance of homes, bodies, and other intimate arenas.

Tragic in itself, the Zafar case mentioned above raises some important issues. There is an overt sexual/casteist/classist voyeurism that is being sanctioned here by the state, by the (majoritarian) publics who applaud cleanliness governance, and by the mainstream media when people are encouraged, and in many cases forced or required (as part of their job) to click and forward digital photos of cleanliness offenders on social media platforms. The unspoken and intersectional sexual/classist/casteist dimension of this digital witnessing and photographing of open defecators is inadvertently folded into the work of cleanliness patrols that disproportionately comprise upper-caste men. The Zafar incident was not the only one. The pervasiveness of this digital witnessing is indicated by another case from 2017, when the broadcaster CNN-News18 directly encouraged citizens to take pictures of open defecation and send them to the network (figure 4.9). The aim presumably was to exhibit such photos on their programs.

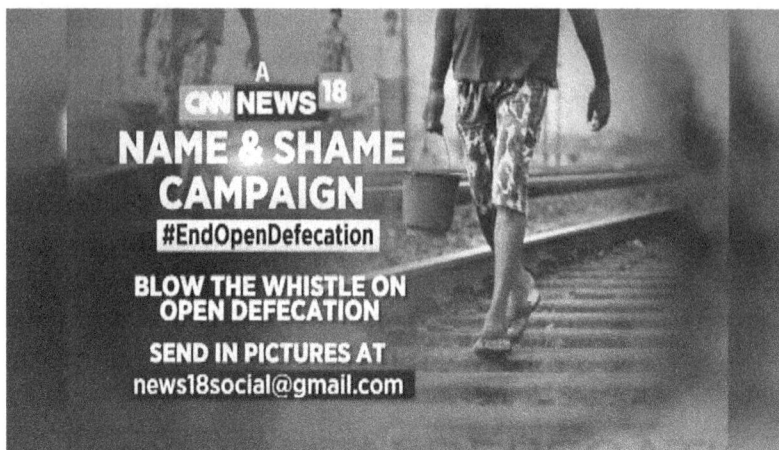

FIGURE 4.9 CNN-News18 Name and Shame campaign.

In the Zafar situation, we had (upper-caste) appointed male officials attempting to photograph women (typically lower-caste or Muslim) from the *basti* on their cell phones. But the reverse has also occurred that also shows how women are being forcefully exposed to unwanted sexual encounters—a phenomenon that ironically contradicts the "securing women's honor" theme of SBA. In Rajasthan, where teachers were asked to patrol their neighborhood in the morning and send photos of open defecators (or face disciplinary action), many female teachers have been unhappy as they often encounter men (typically poor and thus predominantly from marginalized communities) in states of undress openly defecating during their "forced" vigils. This sexualizes their "work" of catching open defecators, which is ignored by their local districts or municipalities just as it sexualizes men from marginalized communities openly defecating as they come under the vigilant eyes of (typically upper-caste) women teachers.

Perhaps the most extreme instance of this kind of digital witnessing of everyday intimacies is in the use of drones to apprehend cleanliness offenders from above. In Karimnagar town of Telangana, in Khyora Khatri village in Kanpur, and in six villages of Bilsapur block of the Yamunagar District in Haryana, drones have been used to curb the practice of open defecation (*Times of India* 2016). In Karimnagar, forty-one-year-old Sudhakar Palli, after relieving himself near a dam, was returning home when two officers from the Karimnagar police station confronted him. They showed him a

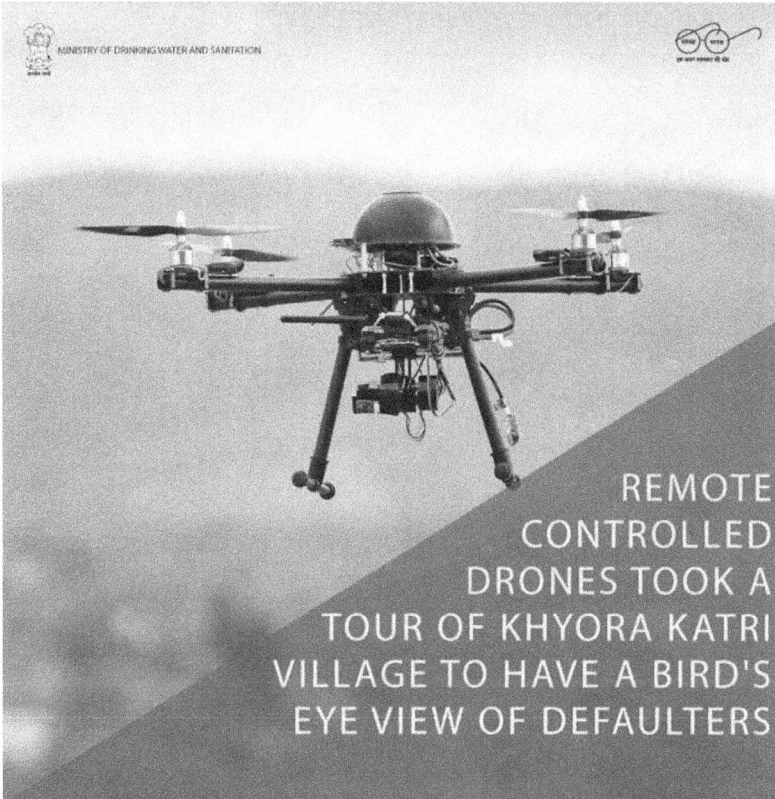

FIGURE 4.10 A government poster for the Swachh Bharat Abhiyan campaign in the Swachh Bharat Abhiyan Mission Facebook page.

picture of him defecating that was captured by drone (Karelia 2017b). Such use of drones has been applauded by the central government—seen again as another feature of SBA's (seeming) modernity. On the Facebook page of the government's Swachh Bharat-Gramin initiative is an image posted by the Ministry of Drinking Water and Sanitation (figure 4.10).

I am struck by the use of drones in SBA, which I believe captures something broader in the nation and in the workings of Hindu modern governmentality. If, as Derek Gregory (2017) and others (e.g., Parks and Kaplan 2017) have noted, drones are not simply products of a technical imaginary but very much a part of a cultural imaginary, we must ask what current cultural imaginary in India makes local officials so easily think of drones as means of capturing cleanliness offenders in order to cleanse Bharat Mata. It is important that we recognize here that the use of drones in SBA is not

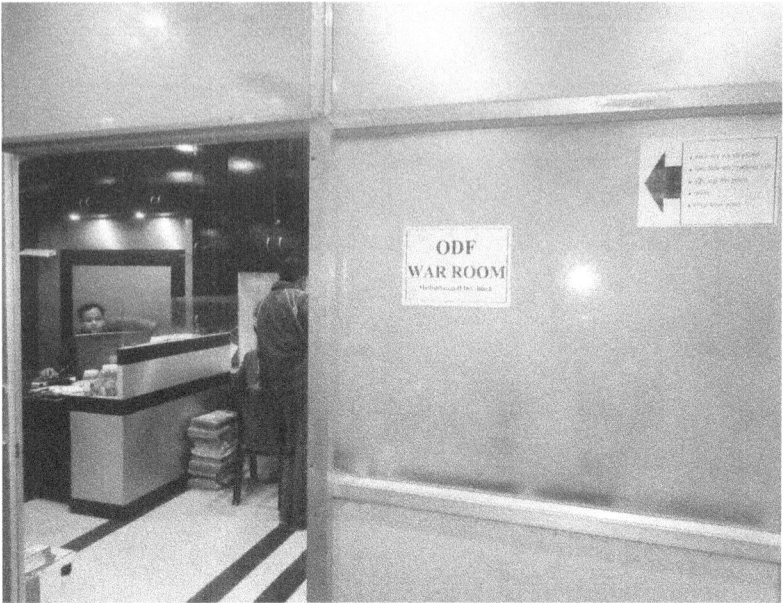

FIGURE 4.11 ODF War Room, Cooch Behar. *Swachh Bharat (Grameen)* (blog), December 21, 2016.

an instance of the commercial use of drones. Here, the drones function through logic of a war machine (war or a crusade against filth, as Modi has framed SBA, as discussed earlier) or a security machine, for they are surveilling and aiding in the catching and arresting of open defecators (and we cannot forget that most of these open defecators are from marginalized cultural and economic groups). It is perhaps not surprising then that some cities and districts—such as Bareilly, Cooch Behar, and others—have ODF "war rooms" (figure 4.11). The district magistrate of Cooch Behar, explaining the war room, stated that it "ensures that we implement our plans [against open defecation] on [a] war footing" (SBM 2016c).

The drones monitoring cleanliness from above further demonstrate the heightened ways in which India has turned into a neoliberal "security economy [that is] premised on the regulation of bodily movement" (Parks and Kaplan 2017, 16), except that now this regulation occurs from above, through remote control. Contrary to the common-sense notion that drones are "unmanned" and that the view from above is somehow "precise"—as in "precision killing" (neutral, objective, and so forth), Kaplan reminds us that "drone sight is always embodied" (2013). Indeed, the images that drones capture are being produced and processed by an embodied gaze that is gendered and sexualized (and situated in relations of caste, class, and religion in the case of India). Here, my cynical self begins to wonder: When drone operators at a "remote" distance process images, perhaps of a Dalit body or a young Muslim woman defecating in the open on a big screen, perhaps watched in a "war room," do they laugh at those bodies, perhaps hurling expletives? Do they shudder in disgust? Do they visually fragment the body and minutely analyze it for its "uncivilized" difference? Do they sexualize these "other" bodies, especially female bodies? Does all this activate and intensify their casteist and religious disgust toward such bodies? I am reasonably assuming that those in a room "manning" the drones and taking the images are for the most part (at least in the context of India) male, from upper castes or the middle class, and typically Hindu. Of course, one cannot always tell what group a body belongs to (although sometimes one can if someone has clothing or other markers that signify that they are from a particular group or religion). But this point is irrelevant at one level to my larger concerns here: that the use of drones in the SBA context points to the workings of a "visuality that is produced in collaboration with a set of militarized and racial visualities" (Nath 2017, 247) that are born out of a logic of war and conquest (of "others"). What we also see here is an extension of the use of spy craft that, under the Modi government, India has been very invested in, especially as its relations with Kashmir, Pakistan, and China have become more problematic. Now these crafts have been adopted for patrolling everyday intimacies, but not everyone's intimacies—only the intimacies of the marginalized who are increasingly being left behind by Hindutva neoliberalism.

I asked earlier what kinds of cultural or national imaginaries would lead one to easily think of using drones to govern cleanliness. I want to suggest that it is a cultural imaginary that *already* sees the nation as engaged in a battle with its "others," a battle in which Bharat Mata (in all her iterations) must be rescued and preserved by excising and disciplining others who symptomize the filth on her body that makes the production of a gleaming neoliberal India a challenge. It is this war mentality—already prevalent— that easily enables one to transpose a military imaginary to the regulation of cleanliness. In this militarization of cleanliness (and drone warfare is characterized as "*clean* warfare" in many parts of the world, such as the United States) and its "technopolitics of visuality" (Grewal 2017b, 343), the logic of the citizen and the soldier, cleanliness and security, intimacies and algorithms, body and data become intimately entangled.

This section's focus on deadly intimacies has attempted to foreground particular features of the Hindu modern that demonstrate how its logics are pervasive and repetitive in different realms of the SBA program and its mediation. Specifically, it has emphasized the entanglement of the digital or informational realm with security and violence and how that once again regulates and governs everyday intimacies that are often sexualized in particular ways. Although the digital violence in SBA's cleanliness enforcement is not always directly an expression of Hindutva violence, as posited earlier it ends up contributing to it for the poor bodies that the enforcement of cleanliness through the digital punishes are for the most part from lower castes and are often poor Muslims. Thus, it augments "informational Hindutva." Digital mediation in SBA, particularly in practices of cleanliness enforcement by state or nonstate actors—and even in the case of drones, whose actors appear disembodied—exemplifies (as others have also demonstrated [Banaji et al. 2019; Mirchandani 2018; Mukherjee 2020; Nizaruddin 2022]) how the sphere of the digital functions to expand the majoritarian public sphere and has become charged with necropolitical intensities where the lynching of "others" become viralized, functioning both as spectacle and as surveillance data. Additionally, this section has called attention to how deadly digital intimacies related to "cleanliness offenders" are intricately connected to infrastructural violence—as we saw with *basti* people who do not have water or the state subsidy for toilets despite applications—that disappears on the digital screens that capture the offenses of open defecators.

Let me summarize explicitly what my discussion in this chapter has revealed about the workings of Hindu modern governmentality. The central issue I have addressed is how cleanliness enforcement in the SBA context is powered by a security logic that plays itself out through violence (a feature that underlies all aspects of the Hindu modern) by state and nonstate actors. This violence is expressed through a classist/casteist masculinist will to punish that is directed toward "offenders" of the cleanliness regime, who are typically from the lower castes and classes of society. I have illustrated how this once again demonstrates how the security logic of the Hindu modern pervades spaces of intimacy, regulating and surveilling intimacies—which in SBA becomes the regulation of open defecation and toilet use, and punishment of poor cleanliness offenders by exposing the intimacies of their bodies to the gaze of the majoritarian state. In contrast to the last chapter, this chapter thus shows another side of the intimacies of security and securitization of intimacies that underlie Hindu modern governmentality and the brutalization of poor (lower-caste) or poor (Muslim) bodies in the nation in the name of security.

Additionally, I have illustrated how the violence performed by various local officials, *swachhagrahis* (sometimes called "clean-up marshals"), and *nigrani samitis* (vigilance committees) capture the point made in chapter 1: that state violence and nonstate/social violence mediate each other today in order to fortify the Hindu neoliberal state.[38] I have also shown that security is not simply enacted by the state but by nonstate actors, unmarked everyday soldiers, who complement the security desires of the state by presenting their actions as citizenly or patriotic duties. This reinforces again how today in the Hindu nationalist state, violence from below (localized violence) has become an increasingly pervasive phenomenon (which is also a sign of penal populism) that fortifies (state) violence from above.

The discussion has further made visible the fusion of security and morality in Hindu modern governmentality, which I argued is a significant way in which security logics are beginning to function in the postcolonial Global South and in India in particular. Chapter 3 already offered some glimpses of this. Because cleanliness has been moralized and given a (Hindu) civilizational ascription, those enacting violence toward offenders in the name of citizenly duty or patriotism see themselves not just as securitizing cleanliness but securitizing the underlying *moralities* (purity, patriotism, *punyabhoomi*, protecting Bharat Mata, upper- and middle-class civilizationalism) that have been associated with cleanliness in SBA.

Further, this chapter's analysis has foregrounded the neoliberal logics and anti-poor thrust of the SBA campaign that mirrors what is going on in the nation at a higher level, often in the name of development. Vigilante violence toward poor bodies (who are typically from marginalized cultural groups of society) reinforces a neoliberal logic where the poor are made responsible for their acts of open defecation and their inability to build toilets, instead of attending to the infrastructural violence (including its casteist nexus) that produces such situations. The poor are seen as not being "entrepreneurial" in constructing toilets; yet the politics and inadequacies of fund disbursement, issues around water shortage, caste politics, lack of land, the disappearing of some populations, and more are rendered invisible.

The discussion has additionally emphasized how the will to punish those who engage in open defecation (or other violations of cleanliness) is intimately expressed through a digital order, where selfies and social media postings of cleanliness offenders (who are, again, largely from marginalized communities) are viralized as acts of humiliation and punishment, and sometimes even lead to death. The bodies of the poor are further degraded and devalued—turned into a visually commodified spectacle, a visually grotesque body—in this viralization. The poor man's (or woman's) anus and what pours out of it circulates through social media as a sign of the primitive, the repulsive, the non-modern that must be excised, while at the same time it ironically also eroticizes such bodies—for the grotesque (the "other" body) as we know is linked to the erotic, where the erotic is not simply sexual but embodied pleasure or desire expressing primal instincts. Such viralizing, where the poor person's bottom or anus moves rapidly across screens, produces a mediated disgust, a disgust that unsettles "us" for at one level it reminds us of the *similarity* between us and the pictured openly defecating body. What that body does outside is the very same thing that we do inside—the couching, the pressure in the belly, what emits out of our anus: they are all the same. This kind of viral vigilantism, which digitizes and constructs the primitive and invites disgust toward it, while attempting to enhance the gap between us and that body by denying community with it, has to be seen as part of a larger architecture of online violence and hate where perceived transgressions by Muslim, Dalit, and other poor and vulnerable bodies begin to function as "data" that signifies a postcolonial *disorder*, a postcolonial grotesque if you will that must be quelled, online and offline, where both mediate each other.

Finally, I have suggested that the digital order through which violence is executed in SBA sometimes begins to function like a war machine where cleanliness becomes more than itself: it becomes a battlefield that is drenched in military vocabularies that makes us forget that a national cleanliness exercise must be about public good: it cannot function as a warring machine. My hope is that this chapter, with its focus on how violence powers the SBA program, sheds some light on how a will to punish grips the Hindu majoritarian state today in ways where violence toward the "other" is normalized and protected with impunity, and where violence that is outside the law is often framed as citizenly duty. This is a signature of penal populism in our times and the SBA case provides a rich example of this in India.

FIVE

FROM CLEANSING TO CLEANING

AN ALTERNATIVE (CLEAN) INDIA

Only a Swachh [clean] India can become a Swasth Bharat [healthy India].
—AMITABH BACHCHAN

The ecological crisis is glaringly missing in public discourse. . . . We have to change perceptions, draw the links between forests and water, environment and health.
—PRERNA BINDRA

In this chapter, I turn to the challenge of conceptualizing a national cleanliness program that is not governed by (Hindu) nationalist neoliberal logics whose associations with Hindu modern governmentality this book has explored. While my focus remains on the case of India, this inquiry can be extended, more broadly, to other authoritarian or majoritarian regimes. How might a national program focused on democratizing cleanliness conceptualize cleanliness so that it can ensure minorities equal benefits as well as protections from more insidious forms of cleansing? What would it mean to clean a nation (such as India) while giving full consideration to the fraught local histories and complex global contexts structuring health, hygiene, pollution, and other indicators of cleanliness? These are complex questions because, as this book has demonstrated, ideas of cleanliness are woven into social hierarchies and thus into everyday structures of power. These are also complex because cleanliness, widely understood as an indicator of modernity and development, is enmeshed in an entire way of life that a state delivers (or not) to its citizens. To rethink cleanliness is to rethink the operations of a network of relations and systems that sustain (or not) a nation's way of life. On the surface, such operations may seem to have nothing to do with cleanliness; yet as this book claims, they are intimately entangled with the production of cleanliness (or the lack of it). Drawing on my in-depth study of the Swachh Bharat Abhiyan (SBA) campaign, this theoretical chapter invites the reader to rethink cleanliness from the margins of the nation and beyond it, something which also involves, I argue, rethinking the nation itself.

The discussions in this chapter are informed by two underlying recognitions. First, that national cleanliness is intimately linked to issues of democracy, citizenship, and national belonging, and thus must be tied to a spirit of welfare and social justice (with a small *j*). Otherwise, cleanliness can easily slide into a cleansing—and history provides enough evidence of this—characterized by disturbing necropolitical and ethnonationalist tendencies. And second, that cleanliness constitutes a *resource* or *capital* (rather than simply being a behavioral or aesthetic matter) that must be *redistributed*. This redistribution must happen downward and outward—that is, toward the margins of the nation and beyond it, in ways where the marginalized become empowered to shape, and primarily benefit from, its allocations. In India, there are people (including those in the administration) who would likely argue that SBA, like other schemes such as Ujjwala Yojana and Jan Dhan Yojana *are* welfare (anti-poverty) schemes and thus committed to redistribution. But as I have addressed in this book, and further elaborate in this chapter, such schemes are too often framed and operate *within* (and not against) neoliberal logics of self-help, entrepreneurialism, and privatization. Without redistribution guided by a democratic spirit of welfare and social justice, and from the margins, cleanliness cannot be substantially advanced in any nation.

As this book has indicated, a major problem with the SBA campaign is that it takes cleanliness as a known phenomenon, as a given, and as a stable and settled thing instead as a site of cultural, economic, and political struggle. The SBA campaign frames cleanliness through a behavioral change and a pedagogical/civilizational model (we just have to teach "these" people, show them how to be clean) that repeats colonial logics. The focus instead should be on structural and infrastructural issues (such as access to water, land, shelter, and so on) that could direct attention to the systemic and historical inequalities of a Brahmanical heteropatriarchal structure that position groups differently along the cleanliness ladder. Further, in consistently tying the issue of cleanliness to the Hindu nation, imagined as Bharat Mata, SBA forecloses the possibility of a secular, democratic, and human rights–oriented imagination of cleanliness and instead makes cleanliness a sacred thing, a part of the current Hindu nationalist logic of purifying the nation and creating a *punyabhoomi* (purified territory). Consequently, cleanliness is only thought of and mediated within (and not without) a Hindu framework. In addition, instead of identifying cleanliness merely with *individual* bodies, habits, practices, and aesthetics that make it easier to punish or "civilize" bodies, SBA should include the entire ecosystem of environmental pollution that is so intimately connected to cleanliness. This would have demanded accountability from the state by (possibly) compelling a more systemic approach to cleanliness that would offer an opportunity to examine the role of state policies (that also precede the Modi administration) in contributing to an "unclean" and "unhealthy" India.[1] As SBA has made cleanliness a narrow behavioral issue, it has made and makes possible the ignoring of these urgent environmental matters—ones that are entangled with corporate greed—absolving the state from responsibility. This again invites the question: What really is the purpose (and effect) of SBA? Who does it ultimately benefit?

What has been especially disappointing about the implementation of the SBA program is the exclusion of disempowered voices and people who are on the receiving end of cleanliness. In taking urban upper-class/caste Hindu ideas about cleanliness as normative, SBA foreclosed the possibility of a larger national conversation that could have invited a *critique of the dominant (Hinduist) national wisdom* about cleanliness (and its associated attributes of pollution and purity, health and hygiene, class, caste, and gender). Cleaning a nation, any nation—as opposed to merely cleansing it—requires *multiple* conversations and approaches, especially ones that draw upon experiences of disempowered groups, for they are the ones who tend to be on the receiving end of governmentality through cleanliness. There were ample opportunities for the administration and various sponsors of SBA to use media platforms such as national television and even social media through which to foreground Dalit and lower-class/caste perspectives and voices on cleanliness and filth, and how they are violently positioned in relation to them. While simply listening to the voices of class and caste (and even sexual and gender) outsiders is certainly not enough to redistribute cleanliness in democratic ways, it *is* a beginning that one can only hope will educate people to imagine and (possibly) demand changes in the systemic structures and the casteist/classist/hetero-gendered ideologies that bind them in ways that inhibit the flow of cleanliness downward. But all this requires the existence of a sufficient democratic political will that does not exist in India today. We can only hope for the return of such a will in the near future, one that can be mobilized toward a more egalitarian distribution of cleanliness through casteist and classist structural interventions.

RECONCEPTUALIZING CLEANLINESS
AS AN ASSEMBLAGE

Implementing a different sort of national cleanliness exercise that is committed to democratizing cleanliness, however, requires *shifting* our conceptual lenses about cleanliness. This is less an empirical matter and more an epistemological (and even political) one that can guide new and alternative knowledge about cleanliness in order to shape its democratic implementation and practice in a nation. Indeed, *how* we conceptualize cleanliness is intimately related to how we see and thus implement it. It is also related to how we see those who are already positioned as "unclean" in society.

Drawing on cultural theory, I want to suggest that cleanliness be conceptualized as an *assemblage*. The concept of assemblage moves us away from seeing cleanliness through a singular lens, as though it is an entity or phenomenon that we can neatly mark and that has clear boundaries. The concept of *assemblage*, initially advanced by philosophers Deleuze and Guattari (1987), has had great purchase in cultural theory over the last three decades. It has generated complex ways of imagining the social. Although today the concept has gone beyond its initial usage by Deleuze and Guattari—with scholars taking it up in various ways—some of the basic features through which it is understood, across its different uses, remain the same. I first describe some of these features, especially ones that are relevant to my discussion of cleanliness. Then I highlight the advantages of reconceptualizing cleanliness as an assemblage, which is a move that could have practical impacts on both scholarly and public discourses around national cleanliness initiatives.

Assemblage—the English term—is an awkward translation of the French word *agencement* that was advanced by Deleuze and Guattari. *Agencement* refers to the design, layout, organization, or arrangement of heterogeneous relations that come together, interplay with each other, to produce an assemblage (Puar 2012, 57). The focus is not on the content but on the connection of relations that make up the arrangement (2012, 57). A wide network of relations and processes hold an assemblage together or create it such that "we cannot presume that what we see is the final product nor that this product is somehow independent of the network of social and historical relations to which it is connected" (Nail 1997, 24). There is no essence to an assemblage because each new mixture or arrangement of heterogeneous elements can produce a different assemblage. An assemblage thus is not about unity but multiplicities. It is always contingent. The relations of an assemblage are not eternal or unchanging; they are always provisional. As Nail (1997) states, one does not ask what the essence of an assemblage is (because there is no actual essence, even if there is some provisional thing that is being stabilized by an assemblage), but rather *what work it is doing* through a particular arrangement of heterogeneous relations that make it up in a particular time and moment. As Deleuze and Guattari (1987) argue, the important thing about an assemblage is *how* it functions. Nail addresses the importance of an assemblage through these questions: "What are the consequences and implications of this assemblage *now*? What can the assemblage accomplish and where are its limits . . . ?" (1997, 26). These questions reveal that an assemblage is political, and what makes it political is *the way in which it is arranged* through diverse relations and holds together (provisionally, not eternally) something, and in doing so, does some work. This means that preestablished assemblages can be reestablished, rearranged, reassembled, and reorganized toward more emancipatory functions.

The idea of assemblage offers a critique of any notion of a pregiven unified subjectivity or identity (for example, a "clean" subject). As Jasbir Puar (2012) suggests, in depriviliging identity and the body as a discrete thing, an assemblage posits that a particular subject/identity *emerges* from a particular arrangement of the relations that make up an assemblage. In other words, cleanliness does not have a fixed identity, nor positionality (Puar 2013). Thus "cleanliness," a "clean body," or "clean citizen" do not have an essence. This moves us away from a behavioral (identity-focused) and universal model of cleanliness and toward a more processual and dynamic approach that is attentive to structural circumstances and power dynamics. Reconceptualizing cleanliness, and in this case SBA, as an assemblage enables us to diagnose and analyze the various heterogeneous relations—which seemingly have nothing to do with "clean"—that become arranged and mixed up to create an ontology or unity around cleanliness in a given time and context. This prepares us to ask the questions this book addresses: What is this assemblage (SBA) of "cleanliness" trying to accomplish? What relations are coming together and "connecting" with each other to produce this assemblage? What are consequences of *this* cleanliness assemblage? And so on.

Further, conceptualizing cleanliness as an assemblage prevents us from falling into a dichotomy of clean/unclean, for the idea of *arrangement* suggests that social phenomena, objects, and entities are not constituted through binaries.[2] They are always mixed up with a whole host of other relations—that is, they are relational. Thus, the notion of assemblage enables us to confront the fact that a national cleanliness exercise *does not* have to be this way; it can be *rearranged and reassembled*. But this also invites us to consider what might hinder and impede such a reassembling (Russell et al. 2011, 580). Additionally, the concept of assemblage compels us to recognize that a national cleanliness assemblage is intermeshed with other assemblages—they are not self-contained with neat boundaries (for example, one can think of a security assemblage or religion as an assemblage). Indeed, it can help us identify and ask about which other assemblages SBA did and did not intersect with.

Keeping this in mind, SBA is a cleanliness assemblage where relations of Brahmanism (caste), neoliberalism (as in the *privatization* of "toilets" and cleanliness), class, national security/violence, modernity, nationalism, gender (for instance, upholding the purity of the Hindu woman), Hinduism (cleanliness equated with Bharat Mata), and corporate media (among others) came together and interplayed with each other in particular ways and through which we were invited to understand and identify cleanliness (or the lack of) and take action in relation to it. As a majoritarian cleanliness assemblage, SBA does the work of ordering and homogenizing the nation by shoring up desires of the Hindu upper-class majority and excising "others" and "other" relations that could have produced a more democratic assemblage.

In feminist and cultural theory, intersectionality and assemblage are often seen as oppositional concepts—one focused on identity and the other on arrangement and the connection of relations. However, I am in agreement with scholars such as Jasbir Puar (2012) who have challenged this seeming oppositionality by arguing that both these heuristics could work in tandem in our analytical and conceptual deployments as they produce more maps for analyzing something. Intersectionality, with its emphasis on identities, teaches us that relations that make up identities always intersect. But *how* they intersect is "always changing" for they intersect only within an arrangement—assemblage—of particular relations (Puar, quoted in Sircar 2021). Assemblage gets to the issue of "what is prior to and beyond" that makes particular intersections possible (Puar 2012,

63). In this book, I have employed (although not always explicitly) both these analytics in tandem to explore SBA as a cleanliness assemblage with particular links to wider assemblages of Hindu modern governmentality. Explicating this approach here provides a summative takeaway that can be utilized to extend this book's research on SBA to other scholarly and practical pursuits invested in reconceptualizing cleanliness.

Where does the Hindu modern fit into all this? The arrangement and interplay of relations in the particular cleanliness assemblage that we call SBA reflects the dominance of Hindu modern governmentality in the nation—a dominance that expands into other development projects as well. Particular external relations (only seemingly "external" to cleanliness) of the Hindu Modern interplayed with cleanliness because the governmentality of the Hindu modern (which itself is a larger assemblage) and the relations that it stabilizes (sacralization, purification, ordering land, security, violence, information, media, neoliberal alliances, and so on) informed the conception of SBA from the very beginning as a state project. In other words, the Hindu modern itself is a larger assemblage that intersects with so many other assemblages, SBA being one. This is evident in public and governmental rhetoric about SBA, as this book has demonstrated. The SBA program is part of a larger Hindu modern assemblage; and its implementation and production of "clean subjects" illustrates the governmentality of the Hindu modern, and also crucially enables it. While it may be argued that relations of Brahmanism, gender, Hindu sacrality, and so on that constitute the SBA cleanliness assemblage *predate* the Hindu modern order of contemporary India, what makes these relations *still new* are the fresh ways in which they have been revitalized and recharged in their *mixing* (their arrangement) with other relations (aggressive nationalism, security, neoliberalism, modernity, and so on) in SBA—but also other programs and projects of Hindu India that are being advanced by the Bhartiya Janata Party (BJP). Equally relevant are the ways the SBA cleanliness assemblage relates to a neoliberal global order within which the BJP positions India and which has often uncritically celebrated SBA.

DELINKING "CLEAN" FROM A NEOLIBERAL AGENDA

If cleanliness can be reassembled in order to implement a more democratic cleanliness assemblage, then part of that reassembling means first considering what relations need to be disassembled from the current assemblage of cleanliness that is SBA. In other words, we have to examine the "prior to and beyond" (Puar 2012, 63). As this book has posited, while there are several relations that need to be delinked from this SBA cleanliness assemblage to enable the reassembling of a different cleanliness assemblage, one that is especially crucial is neoliberalism. Without purposefully delinking cleanliness from neoliberalism, cleanliness cannot be democratized in any nation. It is thus appropriate to briefly recount some of these neoliberal relations in contemporary India to have a better grasp of how they flow into a cleanliness assemblage such as SBA. Finding ways to delink them from the dominant cleanliness assemblage is urgent for accomplishing a *democratic* national cleanliness exercise.

Neoliberal relations today inform every aspect of national governance in India—including the governance of cleanliness, as this book has evidenced. As the upper class keeps getting richer, the poor (largely made up of caste and religious outsiders, tribals, and sexual and gendered "others") struggle with employment, food, land, and water insecurity.[3] These relations of insecurity also interplay with other elements (often in unseen ways) in the cleanliness assemblage called SBA, as they are intimately related to people's inability to produce and practice cleanliness when their bodies are threatened in other ways (for example, lack of land, poor or no housing, low wages, lack of proper food and health). These relations of insecurity have increased and been compounded over the last decade as privatization has become an entrenched mantra in Modi's India, especially since National Democratic Alliance 2.0, the multiparty alliance led by the BJP.

India's neoliberalism, under the Modi administration, is different from its Western avatar, and indeed from its even earlier avatar under the administration of the Congress-led United Progressive Alliance (UPA). The BJP has social welfare schemes, but their welfare agenda is of a peculiar kind. It is recrafted within and aligned to a neoliberal ethos that economist Arvind Subramaniam terms "new welfarism" (quoted in Aiyar 2023). In this new welfarism, welfare as a "moral responsibility of the state to right bearing citizens is underplayed" (Aiyar 2023). Rather, welfare is reframed *within* the neoliberal logic of individual empowerment and patronage—that is, I give you subsidies as gifts that *you* must leverage to empower yourself. This mode of welfare not only moves away from any semblance of state welfare, but it also rewrites the relationship between state and citizen (while of course also obscuring the origins of capital and resources that the state has accumulated). Aiyar argues that this is a transactional approach: "I give you 'X'" for which you do Y to better your lives (2023). This is the

Atmanirbhar Bharat (Self-reliant India) that was proclaimed in Modi's Independence Day speech in 2021. Operationally, it is best captured in Home Minister Amit Shah's comment about toilet construction: "We have made toilets . . . it is up to them to maintain them . . . what we did was to upgrade their lives—this is empowerment" (quoted in Aiyar 2023). Thus, subsidies for toilet construction are to be provided but the poor have to maintain and construct them—and we have seen that these subsidies require top ups from individuals to build a functional toilet (just as gas cylinders are provided to the poor, but when the cylinder is empty they have to buy the refills). This kind of neoliberal rearticulation of welfare divests it of any language of rights and entitlement to infrastructures of well-being and makes it about personal upliftment and upgrade. As this book has repeatedly demonstrated, such neoliberal articulations of individual autonomy and betterment (without attention to structural issues) have been crucial to the way the cleanliness assemblage SBA has come into being. In this kind of "welfare" scheme, toilet subsidies are "given" to citizens to upgrade their lives and "clean" themselves while overall social spending has been drastically cut under the Modi administration. A Bloomberg report notes that in 2022, the food subsidy bill saw a massive 27 percent cut (Pradhan and Srivastava 2022). More than 800 million poor people in India are reliant on this subsidy (Parija 2023), and again we must recall that most of the poor are Dalits, Muslims, and what are known as "other backward classes." Similarly, the rural employment program known as Mahatma Gandhi National Rural Employment Guarantee Scheme (MGNREGS), according to which the government is to guarantee 100 days of paid work to the poor who cannot find it, has been financially choked by the BJP administration, as several independent reports aver.[4] The administration sees the program as a failure of the earlier UPA government.

When there is insecurity regarding employment, food, and land, how can cleanliness through toilet building be the main priority of people, especially when they have to spend their own resources on it? The neoliberal relations dominating economic and political governance in the nation *have everything* to do with cleanliness and the arrangement of the SBA assemblage. If the important thing with an assemblage is not content (essence) but the connections of relations, then the *interplay* between employment, food, land, shelter, bodies, and identities (caste, class, gender, and more) are part of the process of assembling the "clean citizen" that SBA aims for.[5]

I would be remiss if I did not also bring up the issue of water, for it is an important aspect of *any* cleanliness assemblage. Water in India (as elsewhere) has been subject to neoliberal hijack. We need a better understanding of this hijack in order to confront the impossibility of a full national cleanliness project being attempted by programs such as SBA. It is well known that India is one of the most water-stressed nations in the world. Today, there are many private water companies in the market, and the number keeps growing.[6] A study by an NGO that monitors water issues notes that while unlimited access to water resources is enabled by the government to private companies, the livelihoods of the local poor are further hurt as many now have to buy water (cited in Purohit 2016). Water privatization also results in the displacement of communities that are then not allowed to reside near river areas whose resources are extracted by private companies.[7] While the BJP has launched the otherwise commendable Har Ghar Jal (Water in every house) program, which promises to deliver piped water to about 10 crore (100 million) rural households, this does not guarantee *the flow* of water that is needed for cleaning—of one's body, toilets, the home, and so on.[8] Not only is there a lack of adequate water sources connected to taps, but water sources are also not necessarily safe and sustainable in many parts of the country.[9] This problem rarely affects the upper and middle classes and the rich, as they can buy water from water companies. Inadequate access to safe water results in about 200,000 deaths every year.[10] Additionally, given that "the 'flow' of caste is indistinguishable from how water flows through the hydrological cycle" (Waghre 2023), water supply is often denied to Dalit homes in various villages by upper-caste Hindus at will.[11] In alignment with neoliberal logics and the pervasive technocratic ethos that dominates the nation today, the problem of water in India has been reduced "to a technocratic discourse" (Waghre 2023)—as we see in the Har Ghar Jal project—that sees hydrological cycles as disconnected from social, cultural, and political influences. But climate justice scholars Behl and Kashwan (2022, 183) remind us that the focus needs to be on *water equality* instead of *water scarcity*. If the focus is simply on water scarcity, then it provides further justification for huge infrastructural investments that benefit private industries but do not address issues of inequality that keep water from being sufficiently accessed by certain populations.

This is what the government seems to have attempted in the nation: it has followed a water scarcity model that is in sync with the growth model of development that it vigorously promotes. In response to the nation's dwindling water sources—much of which is a result of climate change today—the BJP government has initiated an ambitious project of interlinking rivers. Around sixty of India's rivers will be linked and, when fully completed, the project is expected to transfer 174 trillion tons of water annually (Balachandran 2015). However, protests from ecologists, scientists, activists, and many locals argue that such interlinking upsets the eco systems of rivers and contributes to environmental damage that mostly impacts culturally and economically vulnerable populations who live in forests along rivers. Experts also note that these projects will have deleterious effects on the flora, fauna, and tribal peoples who inhabit forests, who will be displaced by them.[12] Water activists express concern that such ambitious development projects will only "enrich a handful of contractors without addressing the key issue which is that the water tables in our country must be increased" (Sehgal 2019). According to water activists, we need to return to traditional practices of water conservation, which means ceasing encroachments along riverbanks, lakes, and wetlands. All this also calls for strict action against the "land mafia" (Sehgal 2019)—the corporate entities engaged in landgrabs and encroachments, often with government assistance.[13] A nation can expand its water infrastructure, but unless the casteist, classist, privatized (neoliberal), and Hinduized basis of water governance in a nation such as India is challenged, water equality will never be achieved. And cleanliness, too, can never fully be achieved or democratized.

RETHINKING CLEANLINESS THROUGH PLANETARY ETHICS

These discussions understandably lead us to the planetary. No development project today, including national cleanliness projects, can or should be allowed to escape planetary thinking and the responsibilities it calls for. With the recognition of the Anthropocene as a new geological phase— and the assertion that humans have acted as a geophysical force that has destructively intervened in and altered the ecosystem of the planet since the rise of Western modernity and (global) capitalism—planetary talk now dominates many fields and public discourses.[14] Especially influential has been Dipesh Chakrabarty's commanding work, *The Climate of History in a Planetary Age* (2021), in which we see the culmination of his thoughts advanced in a paradigm changing essay (Chakrabarty 2009). Chakrabarty takes great pains to demonstrate how our survival is entangled with the survival of other species and organisms (and vice versa); and if other species (plants, animals, fish, microbes, bacteria, and so on in different living beings) are destroyed, as they are being by anthropocentric development ambitions, we are going to be destroyed as well.[15] Two decades ago, Gayatri Spivak had similarly intimated that if we can "imagine ourselves as planetary subjects rather than global agents," then "alterity remains underived from us" (2003, 73).

Chakrabarty argues that what drives politics in India is not the planet but the "globe" of globalization, "a revolution of aspiration across classes that has been engendered" by "postcolonial development, and the more recent liberalization of the economy and media" (2021, 112). The globe is about global finance capital, multinational corporations, cross-border digital connections, and reckless development in the name of nation building. The planetary, on the other hand, refers to "vast processes of unhuman dimensions" (rock, plants, water, animals, bees, fungi, and so on) and their sustainability, which is entangled with human sustainability (2021, 87). The planet, Spivak reminds us, is "in the species of alterity, belonging to another system; and yet we inhabit it, on loan" (2015, 291), except that we forget that we have borrowed it.

What does all this have to do with cleanliness? The SBA campaign's restrictive vision of cleanliness ignores industrial pollution and damage to nature—accelerated by government-assisted corporate land grabbing that affects forests and their species—and this reflects an anthropocentric interplay of relations that are not accountable to the planet. Planetary thinking forces us to confront that the problem of national cleanliness, along with cleanliness itself, cannot be addressed in isolation from the larger ensemble of ecological/planetary problems that confront us. If one of the goals of the SBA program is to create a "healthy" India (Swasth Bharat) through a "clean" India (Swachh Bharat), as frequently touted by government and the media, then it is imperative to recognize that our health is being damaged by anthropocentric development projects that push planetary concerns to the background, for our health is entangled with the survival of other species.[16] In fact, in health studies today, the emerging notion of planetary health (Baer and Singer 2023) recognizes the importance of natural systems for averting diseases and the potential harm that is caused when such systems are interfered with (Seltenrich 2018). So, if the nation is serious about a Swasth Bharat through Swachh Bharat, then it must foster and emphasize relations with what Joseph Pugliese calls the *other-than-human* (a term that problematizes the lurking anthropocentrism in the term *nonhuman*) in a way that explicitly recognizes the survivalist entanglement of the "human" with the "more than human" (2020, 3). This idea of relationality with the other-than-human calls for a radical restructuring of a cleanliness assemblage—and the reimagining of cleanliness—in a way that is not anthropocentric. Ritwick Dutta, an environmental lawyer in India, noted in an interview that "from 2014 [the year in which the BJP government came to power] onward, you won't find any activity or project stopped on environmental grounds, or even one initiative taken for environment protection" (quoted in Bindra 2018).

Bindra (2018) notes many instances of natural life being disturbed by the development megaprojects planned today. It is worth noting a few to see how "cleanliness" cannot really be achieved in any nation without an attention to the planet and the planetary. In India between 2014 and 2017, 36,500 hectares of forest—the equivalent of sixty-three football fields every single day—were diverted to non-forest purposes such as mining, highways, and industry (Bindra 2018). Habitat destruction and fragmentation of natural habitats to enable megaprojects are splitting animal spaces. The 2016 Wetland Rules further dilute the wetlands "that host waterfowl and rare mammals like fishing cats, recharge ground water, help mitigate floods and support livelihood" (Bindra, quoted in Shah 2017). There are also plans to turn Goa into a coal corridor (CSN 2020). According to Bindra, the Ken Betwa river-linking project mentioned earlier will drown and split the Panna Tiger Reserve (cited in Jha and Sethi 2014). In other words, the other-than-human is being drastically destroyed or endangered, and natural eco systems drastically unsettled, thus endangering the nation's health (*swasth*). This is not a promising picture for a "clean" nation. Unless cleanliness is linked to serious planetary thinking—which also empowers the most disenfranchised populations in the nation (Dalits, tribals, the landless, and the poor, including poor farmers and fisher people, and others), for they are ones on the receiving end of anthropocentric development ambitions (that cause displacement)—egalitarian cleanliness will always be a dream deferred.

FINAL WORDS

As I noted at the outset of this book, there has been no significant resistance to the SBA program. Certainly a few critical journalistic and activist voices, primarily in the nonmainstream, have critiqued elements of the program, but this does not constitute collective resistance. Part of the issue is that most people do not understand cleanliness beyond it simply being a behavioral or aesthetic matter. They do not see cleanliness as being enmeshed with an entire way of life, a democratic life that is in retreat today in India. Yet seeds of resistance needed to reassemble cleanliness exist, though they tend to express resistance to what the nation is becoming under the BJP administration without specific attention to cleanliness. We must nurture these seeds, and extrapolate from them, for that is all that we have today. We find generative resistance in movements such as Bhim Yatra in 2016, when Dalit community activists crisscrossed the nation for 125 days to protest manual scavenging; or in the unrelenting farmer's strike of 2020–2021 that forced the government to roll back its troubled farm laws; or in the Shaheen Bagh protests against the 2019 Citizenship Amendment Act; or in the nationwide labor union strikes in March 2022 that protested the government's anti-labor policies; or even in the 2023 We20: People's Summit—which took place in Delhi just prior to the G20 summit—that protested G20 economic policies and was represented by the working class, Dalits, Adivasis, individuals with disabilities, religious and ethnic minorities, famers and fisher people, informal workers, artisans, and forest workers; or in Adivasi women hugging trees in droves to protect them from coal miners and deforestation; or in forest dwellers taking care of nonhuman species in the forests; and so much more. These pockets of resistance—considered together—provide a ray of hope that perhaps signals the slow coming of a new anti-caste, anti-Hindutva, anti-poverty, and planetary-driven political will in India. Maybe a democratic "clean India" will become a solemn possibility and serious reality if these forces of resistance are themselves not cleansed from the nation, but rather allowed to contribute to new intersectional assemblages of national and planetary cleanliness.

I was not planning on writing a book on cleanliness and the nation. What interested me in the beginning were certain questions: How is Hindu nationalism being revitalized today? How is it working? For working it surely is. Through what logics? What modes of governance have enabled such a violent ordering of the nation under the sign "Hindu"? How are female bodies being mobilized or disciplined in this ordering process? These questions keep so many of us from or in India awake at night as we confront with outrage and fear how successfully democracy has been shredded in India (and unlike many, I am not won over by the idea that a significant move away from a muscular Hindu authoritarianism is demonstrated by the fact that the BJP secured less votes than expected to secure its third term). These questions, which have been intruding on my daily life and imagination since 2014, finally forced me to pay close attention to the various projects of the BJP government, in order to try to comprehend their underlying logics of operation, for you cannot change or challenge what you do not understand. And it is here that I found the SBA campaign—with its almost universal capture of the nation and its mediations—to be an important window through which to examine some of those logics. However, the name that I have given to this constellation of logics and their resulting governmentality—the Hindu modern—far exceeds the singularity of SBA.

In many ways, this book is necessarily an incomplete project because it is only one window through which we have looked at the workings of Hindu modern governmentality. We need more intellectual analyses of the governmentalities of the Hindu modern across various projects, programs, and spaces of the nation. Though such a project is beyond the scope of this book, I hope that this book's foregrounding and exploration of a development project that thus far has failed to incite systemic national or global critique has, in a small way, initiated a conversation about the governmentality of the Hindu modern. While this analysis of SBA will possibly generate anger and outrage among many readers as they peer deeply into the violent workings of Hindu modern governmentality, at the end this is a book about hope. It is about the possibility of reimaging a postcolonial futurity in twenty-first-century India that is unmoored from the violence of Hindu nationalism, destructive neoliberalism, brutal casteism, inhuman class hierarchies, and an aggressive Brahmanical heteropatriarchy. The light (of hope) always emerges from (a plunge into) darkness. This book constitutes such an analytical plunge into a dark period in India that, in my naivete, I never thought would ever come. Finally, while this book is about contemporary India, it also not about it. In a minor way, through the case of India, I hope the book has been able to shed some light on the governmentalities of contemporary authoritarian regimes, especially those that hide under the covers of democracy and developmentalism. For authoritarian regimes, and those leaning toward authoritarianism, learn from each other; they are each other's playbook. That is why it is so crucial to interrogate, critique, and interrupt their assemblages of power, including the national cleansing campaigns that we must radically reconfigure in our pursuit of a cleaner future.

NOTES

CHAPTER 1. CLEANSING THE NATION

Epigraphs: The first quotation is taken from a post on X (formerly Twitter), July 5, 2022. The quote from Narendra Modi, the Indian prime minister, comes from his own account on X, dated September 23, 2017.

1   It bears noting that in 2022 the Supreme Court of India gave Modi a "clean chit," but this judgment has been questioned and criticized by many (Pasha 2022). See also Joseph (2014).

2   See also Chatterji et al. (2019a), Nanda (2011), and Basu (2008).

3   At the time of this writing, I still could not find data about whether the funds had ever been released.

4   For more on the funding of SBA initiatives, see MJS (2017).

5   See Himatsingka (2018), NewsClick (2017) and Singh and Mishra (2019).

6   See Kuchay (2019), Mahaprashasta (2019), and Rukmini (2021).

7   See PM India (n.d.). See also PM India (2014).

8   See esp. Comaroff and Comaroff (1997, 141).

9   For more on the issues mentioned here, see, e.g., Longkumer (2019).

10 See also Nanda (2016) and B. Subramaniam (2019).

11 This reclaiming and remarking of territory as Bharat, and thus Hindu (for Bharat is a mythological Hindu construct, as opposed to India, which reflects a more secular idea) also underpins the Akhand Bharat (Undivided Bharat) movement. Akhand Bharat is the idea that Pakistan, Afghanistan, Tibet, Bangladesh, Nepal, and Sri Lanka were all part of the same Hindu land, but because of British colonial rule they ended up being partitioned into different nation-states. Mother India thus has been divided. So, to recover the wholeness of Mother India, the country needs to reclaim an undivided Bharat. This dangerous idea speaks to Hindu expansionist ambitions.

12 Inaugurating the Swachh Bharat Mission, Modi's speech invoked Mother India and Bharat Mata to refer to the nation's body; see PM India 2014.

13 Recent works have begun attending to how India is operating as a security state, although none wed it to the governmentality of the Hindu modern. See, e.g., Chatterji (2019), and Rai (2019).

14 See also Murty (2022).

15 It is remarkable that in a recent *Forbes* list, Delhi, Chennai, and Mumbai grabbed spots for being some of the most surveilled cities in the world (Inzamam and Qadri 2022).

16 See also Jaffrelot (2019) and Shibli (2019).

17 According to the Stockholm International Peace Research Institute, India was the world's largest arms importer from 2019 to 2023. See FAT (n.d.).

18 The speech was given primarily in Hindi. This quote is from P. Kapur (2018), who offers a translated version. To the view the speech, see ABP Majha (2016).

19 Figure 1.2 shows the image attached to the tweeter's identity when I accessed it in 2020. However, the image has changed as of 2024.

20 I should note that the online handle of the person who tweeted this message had changed when I checked in October 2024, but the tweet remains. I am focused here on the tweet that appeared in 2018 at the height of the SBA campaign.

21 For related discussions, see, e.g., Banaji (2018), Chatterjee (2023), Cook (2019), Hansen (2019), and Jaffrelot (2019).

22 See also A. Basu (2022).

23 The Ujjwala Yojana scheme aims to provide free gas connections to women and families in poor households so they do not have to cook with unclean fuel; Jan Dhan Yojana (National Mission for Financial Inclusion) is a financial services scheme that allows every household to open a bank account, even with zero balance, and access banking services; the Beti Bachao, Beti Padhao: Caring for the Girl Child scheme is aimed at increasing the number of female births through discouraging sex-selective abortion; and the Mahila e-Haat scheme involves an online marketing platform for women entrepreneurs to sell their products.

24 For work that touches on the SBA campaign, see Coffey and Spears (2017), Doron and Jeffrey (2018), Doron and Raja (2015), Gatade (2015), Jack et al. (2020), Jeffrey (2015), Luthra (2018), Singh and Jain (2018), and Teltumbde (2018). One recent article does, however, powerfully call attention to the fact that "the recent religion of sanitation or Swachh Bharat is also born out of the camouflaged avatar of Hindutva" (Bhowmick and Purukayastha 2016, 3). But the article does not explicitly focus on SBA as a nationalist text or address the hetero-gendering of nationalism that occurs in SBA campaigns through Hindu imagery, referents, and logics. These works also do not address how a mediated pedagogy of cleanliness creates the nationalist subject position of a "clean citizen." Coffey and Spears (2017) focus on the problem of open defecation in Indian villages and argue that cultural notions of ritual purity that see in-home latrines as polluting play a role in continuing open defecation.

They also address caste but they do not focus on the relations between cleanliness, nationalism, and gender in the context of the larger Hindutva nationalist climate in the nation.

25 Grosz (1994) has argued how women's menstrual flows have positioned them historically as unclean and inferior to men in ways that men's bodily fluids have not.

26 See also Corbin (1988).

27 See also Smith (2009).

28 See also Corbin (1988) and Thompson (2017).

29 Muecke (2003) has argued that Indigenous people in Australia do not classify waste or filth through anthropocentric logics. Rather, they have an overlapping system of relating to waste where "something maybe useful to humans or to birds [and one can add other nonhuman forms of life] or both, in different ways" (2003, 125). See also Newell (2020), who notes how notions of dirt among residents of Lagos are far removed from the European colonial perception of dirt in West Africa that was projected on to Africans.

30 See, e.g., Chauhan (2017), Dutta and Bhaskar (2017), and Preetika (2023).

31 Esty (1999) discusses how in many postcolonial African fictions, excrement signifies failed postcolonial development and Western colonial underdevelopment in Africa under European colonialism. Similarly, Anderson discusses US colonizers' obsession with Filipino bodies and their "waste" through which an "American sublime" and a Filipino "abject" position was constructed (Anderson 1995, 644).

32 Chacko has discussed how the BJP's notion of female empowerment and protection are intricately tied to the neoliberal ideologies promoted by the Modi government, whereby women's empowerment is tied to a logic of the "market citizen" that simultaneously fuses with Hindutva, or what she terms "marketized Hindutva" (2020, 210).

33 The recent judgment of the Gujarat government in the Bilki Bano case— which concerns a Muslim woman gang-raped and tortured during the infamous 2002 pogrom in Gujarat, and which led to the release of the eleven convicted rapists—made it evidently clear that a Muslim woman's *izzat* (honor) does not figure in the national (Hindu-modern) family/home today, irrespective of whether the family/home has a toilet. Although the Indian Supreme Court fortunately reversed the Gujarat government's judgment and sent the convicts back to prison, the fact that the Gujarat government could even release the rapists of a gang-raped Muslim woman still demonstrates the tenuous and unsafe position that Muslim women hold in the nation.

34 For instance, the 2016 Ujjwala Yojana scheme carries the promotional slogan *Mahilaon ko mila samman.* ("Women receive respect").

CHAPTER 2. PURIFYING BHARAT MATA

Epigraphs: The first epigraph is taken from Media Eye (2014). In the Indian numbering system, one crore equals ten million. The second epigraph is taken from P. Singh (2016).

1   I use articulation in Stuart Hall's sense of the word (in Grossberg 1986).
2   See also Mankekar (1999).
3   Because WhatsApp messaging is encrypted, it was not possible to access content shared across different WhatsApp groups devoted to SBA.
4   See also Jack et al. (2020) and Ramanathan (2019).
5   Abhishek Manu, a Supreme Court lawyer, notes that "the Modi government is the first to create a social media police and make . . . the IT Ministry the principal police station for digital and social media platforms" (*Hindu* 2021a).
6   See Guru (2016) for a good discussion.
7   It is interesting to note also the 2013 Abused Goddesses ad campaign against domestic violence (see Scott 2013). The goddesses Laxmi, Durga, and Saraswati appear in this campaign as bruised and crying. This frequently used way of representing suffering through goddess figures strips real women of any agency, and renders invisible the plights of many minority women who do not identify with these Hindu goddess figures; the violence toward these women seems not to matter.
8   These are my translations of the Hindi dialogue in the short film.
9   *Paan* is betel leaf, in which there are areca nuts and cured tobacco. It is chewed for recreational purposes and often served after a meal.
10 For a thematically similar film, see FFS (2017).
11 Dialogue in the video is spoken in Hindi. All translations of video materials are my own.
12 Mary John, in a speech delivered at JNU, makes an interesting point that the Bharat Mata figure—as a symbol of the nation's women—functions to foreclose any feminist demands because the figure compels obedience to it. See Ali (2016).
13 According to reports, over 11,000 Kashmiri women have been raped by Indian forces since its occupation thirty years ago. See Geo News (2020).
14 This and Bachchan's following dialogue are my translations from Hindi.
15 See also Berlant (2007).
16 For an exception, see Truelove and Ruszczyk (2022).
17 See, e.g., Aishwarya Upadhyay's discussion on NDTV (Upadhyay 2019a).

CHAPTER 3. "WOMEN'S EMPOWERMENT" THROUGH TOILET MODERNITY

Epigraphs: The quote by Nerendra Modi is taken from a speech delivered at Wardha, Maharashtra, in 2019 (*India Today* 2019). The quote by Bezwada Wilson, national convener of the Indian human rights organization Safai Karmachari Andolan, is taken from Us Salam (2016).

1   News items about Neha appeared on many platforms, such as the *Times of India*, the *New Indian Express, Business Standard, OneIndia*, the *Indian Express, NewsTrack, AsiaNet, DesiBlitz*, and *DailyPakistan*; and on various news channels: see, e.g., Aaj Tak News (2016); APN (2016), and Puthi-yaThalaimurai TV (2016).

2   For instance, Modi's Ujjwala Yojana scheme promised gas connections and cylinders to every rural woman so that she would not have to cook in a dirty, smoke-filled atmosphere hunched over a primitive oven fueled by bits of coal. *Mahila ko mila samman* (Women receive dignity) was the tagline that the petroleum and gas minister used to describe this plan. Beyond the fact that these poor rural women cannot afford to refill their gas cylinder (a point that the government did not address), women's dignity was simply linked to an upgrade to a different cooking mode and less smoky environment, but the chores of cooking and household labor in villages are still represented as a woman's responsibility in many images advancing this initiative (*Business Standard* 2017a).

3   Since 2011, the Vishva Hindu Parishad, a Hindu extremist organization, has operated a "Hindu helpline," and in 2022 it announced Hindu protec-tion helplines numbers of Bajrang Dal workers to protect Hindus from love jihad forces (*Times of India* 2022b).

4   See Philipose (2022) and Raha (2022).

5   *Lota* is a round vessel for keeping water, typically used for cleaning one-self after urination or defecation. A *lota* party refers to women's groups in villages engaging in camaraderie while going to the fields to defecate.

6   For instance, in 2015 in Hareva village in Uttar Pradesh, five Dalit women were paraded naked, caned, and put on exhibition on the highway because a son from their family had eloped with an upper-caste girl. See Ghosh (2015).

7   See Kumar (2020). There is an alarming rise of violence toward Dalits and Dalit women, the infamous Hathras gang-rape case in 2020 being a case in point.

8   For a critique of this position, see Rege (1998).

9   For a good discussion of this point, see Dhanaraj (2018).

10   See Arya and Rathore (2020).

11   I thank one of the anonymous reviewers of this book for this point.

12   See, e.g., Gupta et al. (2019b) and Jain et al. (2020).

13   See also Rao (2009).

14   See, e.g., Kowtal (2019).

15 It should also be noted that such assistance often does not find its way to families, an issue that is explored further in chapter 4. See, e.g., Lahariya (2019) and Sumedh (2018).

16 This had been preceded a few months earlier by a similar app, Sulli Deals.

17 My discussion here is influenced by Bhalla (2006), Butalia (2000), Malhotra (2017), Menon and Bhasin (1998), Mookerjea-Leonard (2017), and Zakaria (2015).

18 See, e.g., Sanjai (2018).

19 "Eve-teasing" in Indian parlance refers to sexual teasing.

20 *Ghunghat* is the part of a sari used to cover a woman's face—especially a married woman's face—as a mark of respect to the family, particularly male elders.

21 This is my translation of the Hindi dialogue in the ad.

22 See, e.g., GNI (2020).

23 See also Anand (2011), Jaffrelot (2017), and S. Subramaniam (2019).

24 Bollywood has recently seen a surge of films valorizing this position: *Uri* (2019), *Fighter* (2024), and *Sam Bahadur* (2024) are powerful examples.

25 See also Chakraborty (2022).

26 In the Indian numbering system, one lakh equals one hundred thousand.

27 The initiative initially was launched in a Haryana town by a local man, but Modi, liking it, used it for his own purpose.

28 For example, Sunil Jaglan, who heads the *panchayat* of Bibipur village in Haryana, initiated the Selfie With Daughter campaign, and he encouraged fathers to take selfies and Whatsapp them, as well as upload them to an online museum that he created for this campaign.

29 See Bisht (2021). The government's Sukanya Samriddhi scheme also embodies such contradictions.

30 See, e.g., PTI (2019b).

31 For a discussion of virtuous masculinity and security discourse, see Young (2003).

32 Although a *panchayat* is typically an elected local body, due to deep patriarchal ideologies in rural villages, it is often elderly men who constitute *panchayats*.

33 For other analyses of Brahmanical patriarchy in the film, see Ananya (2021) and Rao (2019).

34 This point is made by many activists and writers. See, e.g., Subrahmaniam (2017) for an interview with Bezwada Wilson. See also Gatade (2015).

CHAPTER 4. SWACHH VIOLENCE

Epigraphs: The first quotation is taken from Srivastav and Khalid (2019). The second is taken from Teltumbde (2018).

1   The phrase "will to punish" is from Fassin (2018), which I discuss in this chapter.

2   I have found helpful here the growing literature that attempts to understand "penal populism"; it has aided some of my thinking in this chapter. See, e.g., Bonner (2019) and Pratt (2007).

3   This was clearly visible during the COVID-19 pandemic in India where the Muslim body became framed as a contagious body, as specters of so-called corona jihad were invoked and corresponding punishment was executed, as with the men from the Islamic movement Tablighi Jamaat, who were wrongly thrown into detention for apparently flouting pandemic guidelines.

4   In a different context, Comaroff and Comaroff (2016) have argued that many of the functions of the state including violence are increasingly being outsourced today to private bodies, thus changing the nature and function of the police.

5   The issues "shadow sovereignties" and "informal sovereignties" have been of particular interest to scholars concerned with the rise of penal populism. See, e.g., Bonner (2019) and Pratt (2007). A comparable example from the Global South is the death squads of Rodrigo Duterte in the Philippines.

6   For a different discussion, see Comaroff (2024).

7   As I finished writing this chapter, Manipur erupted in unforgivable violence. The situation in Manipur, involving the ethnic cleansing of the Kuki (primarily Christian minority) tribes and the central government's silence on this is another example of the pervasiveness of this in India now.

8   See here also Anand (2017) and Larkin (2008).

9   For a parallel discussion of vigilantes as state actors, see Gardenier (2022) and Jaffrelot (2019).

10 The point made by Das (2007) is somewhat similar to Pandey's concept of "routine violence" (2006).

11 For other discussions of violence informed by contemporary Hindutva ideology, see Basu (2022) and Hansen (2021).

12 It should be noted that while the government agreed only late during the 2020–21 farmers' protest to repeal the laws that protected the "minimum support price," in 2024 farmers claimed that the government had betrayed its promise, which led to new protests.

13 This was soon followed by the circulation of an image of an aggressive Ram, a departure from Ram's typical image of kindness and softness.

14 For a similar discussion, in a different context, of the police as vigilantes in Modi's India, see Jaffrelot (2021).

15 See NewsX (2017).

16 I am not inherently opposed to vigilantism, being well aware that when mechanisms of law and justice fail the disempowered or vulnerable, vigi-

lantism can become a means for demanding recognition and justice. The relation between vigilantism and justice/injustice is a complicated one. My interest here is in majoritarian vigilantism.

17   For an interesting exception, see Sen (2018); see also Richards (2016).

18   See S. Jha (2017).

19   See also Chatterjee (2011), Dasgupta (2017), and Gupta et al. (2019a).

20   I am clearly not suggesting here that all Muslim men have beards. Rather, I am suggesting that as they are often stereotyped in the media as having a beard, this image thus seems to invoke a Muslim man.

21   Srivastav and Khalid claim that "village vigilance committees were often dominated by upper caste Hindus" (2019).

22   I should mention here the so-called Pissing Tanker group, a group of citizenly vigilantes who emerged on the streets of Mumbai in 2014, a little before the launch of the SBA campaign. The group took the matter of cleanliness into their own hands. They drove a water tanker, with masks on their faces, and anyone seen publicly urinating was sprayed with a high-pressure water hose. For more on this, see Doron (2016). There are numerous videos of the group on social media. See, e.g., Bharath Autos (2014).

23   See, e.g., Vinayak (2017). The WaterAid India short film on the Dabba Dol Gang that I discuss in this chapter is captioned "See how these young crusaders in the fight against open defecation are inspiring their communities to stop open defecation" (Cherukupalli 2016). See also Bhatia (2016).

24   See Trivedi (2017).

25   See also Govil and Baishya (2018).

26   See also Tiwari (2016).

27   This is my translation of the Hindi dialogue.

28   See also Miller (1998).

29   Indira Gandhi also served as defense minister while she was prime minister, but Sitharam is the first woman to hold this position full-time.

30   Examples of this genre include the films *Phantom* (2015), *Raazi* (2018), *Code Name: Tiranga* (2022), and *Dhaakad* (2022), and the TV series *Special Ops* (2020).

31   See, e.g., Ayub (2016), Bhatia (2020), Mathur (2020), *Mumbai Mirror* (2018), and PTI (2020).

32   See also Ayub (2016), NDTV (2015), and TCI (2015).

33   For one of the best analyses of the problems associated with the SBA program, see Gupta et al. (2019b).

34   See, e.g., Bhowmick (2019), Omjasvin (2021), and Shanmughasundaram (2018).

35   See, e.g., Kumar (2019).

36   "Harijan" is a derogatory term for Dalits. I place it in scare quotes because the article uses this term.

37   See also Mittal and Jafri (2023).

38 Local *swachhagrahis* are called "clean-up marshals" in many states. See Shivadekar (2015).

CHAPTER 5. FROM CLEANSING TO CLEANING

Epigraphs: Amitabh Bachchan is a Bollywood megastar and campaign ambassador for Swachh Bharat Abhiyan; the quotation is taken from Upadhyay (2019b). Prerna Bindra is an eminent Indian environmental journalist, and her words are taken from Shah (2017).

1 For example, while the current administration flags its commitment to renewable energy, it has trampled over existing laws and policies monitoring toxic energy sources by pushing domestic coal production instead of encouraging the import of coal, which has a far lower ash content than domestic coal (Das 2020). Against the earlier mandatory policy that thermal power plants had to use coal with an ash content below 34 percent, thermal power plants now have the ability to change their source of coal without having to seek environmental clearance as long as they simply "inform" the regulators (Das 2020). Reports note that on at least three occasions, coal-related laws were amended to help the Adani coal business empire save at least $1 billion (Shih et al. 2020). It should also be mentioned that as renewable energy is being planned, frequently the land on which solar plants are being envisioned belong to Adivasis (that is, they are historical lands) or the plants displace the poor who work on the land. See, e.g., Chari (2020) and Jairath (2021). Additionally, the toxic waste on Union Carbide premises that created the 1984 Bhopal tragedy is still to be cleared away, and unless that happens, ground water and the soil will continue to be contaminated and the toxicity will keep spreading in the area.

2 For more on how assemblage theory challenges binary thinking, see Puar (2012).

3 For food insecurity data, see Rajalakshmi (2023) and Sen (2023). India's ranking on the Global Hunger Index slipped to 111 out of 125 countries in 2023 (*Business Standard* 2023). There are several reports that document employment insecurity (Ellis-Petersen 2024; Mehrotra 2024; Sharma 2024). For land grabs, see Chandel (2012) and Löw (2020), among many others. It is also claimed that the Modi government accounts for 72 percent of all disinvestment since 1991 (Raghavan 2022).

4 See, e.g., *Hindu* (2024) and Lahariya and Paliath (2018). For instance, the government provides less than the guaranteed days of employment mandated by MGNREGS, and there is delayed payment, as well as the digitization of workers' attendance and payments—all of which hugely disadvantage many workers because of the digital divide.

5   It is to be noted that for the first time since the early 1990s, the number of people living below the poverty line has gone up. In 2021, India added 75 million to the world's poor, and was consequently ranked 132 out of 191 on the Human Development Index for 2021–22 (UNDP 2022, 274). See Prabhakar (2023) for more details. While all this goes on, tax cuts to corporations increase, as does the privatization of many public sector assets such as ports (which hurts workers' benefits and salaries), water, forests, land, and electricity, among others.

6   Among these companies are Veolia Water India Limited, Jamshedpur Utilities and Services Company Limited, Vishwa Infrastructure Limited, MSK Projects India Limited, and Orange City Water Private Ltd.

7   See Chandran (2017). As an example, the controversial Sardar Sarovar Dam displaced three hundred thousand people (Baviskar 2005).

8   While the government claims that it has achieved about 55.62 percent water coverage and the project continues (PIB 2022b), many reports note that reality on the ground is often different. See *Hindu* (2023), Koshy (2023), and Kumar (2022). The Modi government claimed that Goa received the certificate for being the first to have tap water in every household under this program, but residents disagree. See Vohra (2022).

9   For details, see Paliath et al. (2022).

10   See Chaudhary (2024).

11   See, e.g., Behl (2020), BiKa (2023), and Sandhu (2017).

12   The Ken-Betwa link project was approved in December 2021, the first approval in the huge river-linking project. It will result in the removal of 2.3 million trees, submerge nine thousand hectares of land, destroy tiger and forest reserves, and endanger other species that live in this protected area (Perinchery 2021).

13   See, e.g., Chandel (2012) and R. Mohan (2015).

14   I do not wish to address here the debate regarding the appropriateness of the term *Anthropocene* and whether it shores up a human (white European male) exceptionalism. This has been addressed by many others and is beyond the scope of this project.

15   See also Tsing et al. (2017).

16   For an example of the media presence in debates about achieving a "healthy" India through a "clean" India, see *Organiser* (2023).

REFERENCES

Aafaq, Zafar. 2023. "We Have Been Made to Vanish." *Scroll*, September 8. https://scroll.in/article/1055597/we-have-been-made-to-vanish-hidden -by-screens-delhis-poor-feel-pinch-of-g20-curbs.

Aaj Tak. 2016. "No Toilet, No Wedding: Says Kanpur Woman." Aaj Tak, April 18, YouTube, video, 2:49. https://www.youtube.com/user/aajtaktv ?sub_confirmation=1.

ABP Majha. 2016. "PM Narendra Modi Through Video Conference Before Coldplay Concert." YouTube, video, 10:19. https://www.youtube.com /watch?v=97xHKaInZfw.

Abrahams, Ray. 2008. "Some Thoughts on the Comparative Study of Vigilantism." In *Global Vigilantes*, edited by David Pratten and Atreyee Sen, 407–30. New York: Columbia University Press.

Abu-Lughod, Lila. 1998. *Remaking Women: Feminism and Modernity in the Middle East*. Princeton, NJ: Princeton University Press.

Achom, Debanish. 2018. "In This Haryana Village, No Woman Will Marry to Homes Without Toilet." NDTV, June 30. https://www.ndtv.com/india -news/in-this-haryana-village-no-woman-will-marry-to-homes-without -toilet-1875844.

Agamben, Giorgio. 2004. *State of Exception*. Translated by Kevin Attell. Chicago: University of Chicago Press.

Agarwal, Kabir. 2018. "Why Households Are Being Excluded from Modi's Swachh Bharat Scheme." *Wire*, October 9. https://thewire.in/government /swachh-bharat-narendra-modi.

Ahuja, Sonia. 2018. "Women Power Leads the Way Towards a Swachh Bharat." NDTV-Dettol, March 8. https://swachhindia.ndtv.com/women-power -leads-way-towards-swachh-bharat-17986/.

Aiyar, Yamini. 2023. "Citizen vs Labharthi? Interrogating the Welfare State." Centre for Policy Research, January 2. https://cprindia.org /journalarticles/citizen-vs-labharthi-interrogating-the-welfare-state/.

Alarcon, Norma, Caren Kaplan, and Minoo Moallem, eds. 1999. *Between Woman and Nation: Nationalisms, Transnational Feminisms, and the State*. Durham, NC: Duke University Press.

Ali, Asim. 2021. "India's Hindutva Hardliners Treat Religious Conversion as Security Threat." *Diplomat*, July 2. https://thediplomat.com/2021/07/indias-hindutva-hardliners-treat-religious-conversion-as-security-threat/.

Ali, Samim Asgor. 2016. "Mary John's Talk on 'Feminism, Freedom and Bharat Mata' at Freedom Square JNU." YouTube, video, 48: 37. https://www.youtube.com/watch?v=B8Mpf-kJSzA.

Al Jazeera. 2021. "India: Hindu Event Calling for Genocide of Muslims Sparks Outrage." Al Jazeera, December 24. https://www.aljazeera.com/news/2021/12/24/india-hindu-event-calling-for-genocide-of-muslims-sparks-outrage.

Amar, Paul. 2013. *The Security Archipelago: Human-Security States, Sexuality Politics, and the End of Neoliberalism*. Durham, NC: Duke University Press.

Ambedkar, Bhimrao Ramji. 2013. *Against the Madness of Manu: B. R. Ambedkar's Writings on Brahmanical Patriarchy*. Edited by Sharmila Rege. New Delhi: Navayana.

Ambedkar, Bhimrao Ramji. 2014. *Annihilation of Caste*. Edited by S. Anand. London: Verso.

Amudhan, R. P. 2024. "Vande Matram: Shit Version." YouTube, video, 6:03. https://www.youtube.com/watch?v=VwUzWo7xMrI.

Anand, Dibyesh. 2005. "The Violence of Security: Hindu Nationalism and the Politics of Representing 'the Muslim' as a Danger." *Round Table* 94, no. 379: 203–15. https://doi.org/10.1080/00358530500099076.

Anand, Dibyesh. 2007. "Anxious Sexualities: Masculinity, Nationalism and Violence." *British Journal of Politics and International Relations* 9, no. 2: 257–69. https://doi.org/10.1111/j.1467-856X.2007.00282.x.

Anand, Dibyesh. 2011. *Hindu Nationalism in India and the Politics of Fear*. New York: Palgrave Macmillan.

Anand, Nikhil. 2017. *Hydraulic City: Water and the Infrastructures of Citizenship in Mumbai*. Durham, NC: Duke University Press.

Anand, Nikhil, Akhil Gupta, and Hannah Appel, eds. 2018. *The Promise of Infrastructure*. Durham, NC: Duke University Press.

Ananya. 2021. "Male Subjectivity in New India: 'Toilet ek prem katha' (2017) and 'Pad Man' (2018)." *Jump Cut* 60. http://www.ejumpcut.org/archive/jc60.2021/Ananya-NewIndiaGender/index.html.

Anchalia, Vivek, dir. 2018. "Ever Done This to Your Mother?" Facebook, video, 0:40. https://www.facebook.com/watch/?v=1555331771260061.

Anderson, Benedict. 2016. *Imagined Communities*: London: Verso.

Anderson, Edward. 2015. "'Neo-Hindutva': The Asia House M. F. Husain Campaign and the Mainstreaming of Hindu Nationalist Rhetoric in Britain." *Contemporary South Asia* 23, no. 1: 45–66. https://doi.org/10.1080/09584935.2014.1001721.

Anderson, Warwick. 1995. "Excremental Colonialism: Public Health and the Poetics of Pollution." *Critical Inquiry* 21, no. 3: 640–69. https://doi.org/10.1086/448767.

Angad, Abhishek. 2017. "E-Rickshaw Driver Objects to Two Men Urinating in Public Beaten to Death." *Indian Express* (Noida), May 29. https:// indianexpress.com/article/cities/delhi/e-rickshaw-driver-objects-to-two -men-urinating-in-public-beaten-to-death-4678398.

ANI (Asian News International). 2016. "Dabangg Bride Says 'No Toilet No Marriage' to Her Groom." *ANI News*, April 18, YouTube, video, 1:36. https://www.youtube.com/watch?v=JwqxLo3dTpU.

ANI. 2018. "5 Year Old Jannat on Mission to Clean Dal Lake." *Business Standard* (New Delhi), January 23. https://www.business-standard.com/article/news -ani/5-year-old-jannat-on-mission-to-clean-dal-lake-118012300155_1.html.

ANI. 2022. "BJP Govt Restored True Honour of Women in UP: PM Modi." *ANI News*, February 7. https://www.aninews.in/news/national/politics/bjp -govt-restored-true-honour-of-women-in-up-pm-modi20220207141153.

Anima, P. 2023. "Pradeep Mewada: Whistling in Change." *Business Line* (Chennai), May 8. https://www.thehindubusinessline.com/blchangemakers /whistling-in-change/article62222255.ece.

Ansari, Halima Zoha. 2021. "Muslim Women's Rights Day: The BJP's Women Empowerment Farce." *Feminism in India*, August 8. https:// feminisminindia.com/2021/08/13/muslim-womens-rights-day-triple -talaq-bill-bjp/.

APN (APN News Legal). 2016. "Bride Calls Off Wedding After Groom Fails to Build Toilet: Kanpur (UP)." *APN News Legal*, April 18. YouTube, video, 0:24. https://www.youtube.com/watch?v=9mLmDV28LIg.

Appadurai, Arjun. 2001. "Deep Democracy: Urban Governmentality and the Horizon of Politics." *Environment and Urbanization* 13, no. 2: 23–43. https://doi.org/10.1177/095624780101300203.

Appadurai, Arjun. 2004. "The Capacity to Aspire: Culture and the Terms of Recognition." In *Culture and Public Action*, edited by Vijayendra Rao and Michael Walton, 59–84. Stanford, CA: Stanford University Press.

Appadurai, Arjun. 2006. *Fear of Small Numbers: An Essay on the Geography of Anger*. Durham, NC: Duke University Press.

Appadurai, Arjun. 2021. "Modi and His Brand of Hindutva Are Direct Descendants of the British Raj and Its Policies." *Wire*, December 13. https:// thewire.in/politics/narendra-modi-hindutva-british-raj.

Arya, Sunaina, and Aakash Singh Rathore. 2020. "Introduction: Theorizing Dalit Feminism." In *Dalit Feminist Theory: A Reader*, edited by S. Arya and A. Rathore, 1–21. New Delhi: Routledge.

Asad, Talal. 2003. *Formations of the Secular: Christianity, Islam, Modernity*. Stanford, CA: Stanford University Press.

Asthana, N. C. 2022. "Sadhvi Vibhanand's Call to 'Rape' Muslim Women with Impunity Shows Hindutva's Politics of Fear." *Wire*, February 12. https:// thewire.in/communalism/sadhvi-vibhanands-call-to-rape-muslim -women-with-impunity-shows-hindutvas-politics-of-fear.

Ather, Sara. 2023. "India's Bulldozer War on Muslim Neighbourhoods." *Middle East Eye*, February 6. http://www.middleeasteye.net/opinion/india -muslims-undeclared-war-neighbourhoods.

Ayub, Jamal. 2016. "Transgender Turns Swachh Mascot." *Times of India* (Mumbai), August 29. https://timesofindia.indiatimes.com/city/bhopal /transgender-turns-swachh-mascot/articleshow/53903708.cms.

Ayub, Jamal. 2019. "In Madhya Pradesh, If Groom Takes a Loo Selfie, Bride Gets Rs 51,000 from Govt: Bhopal News." *Times of India* (Mumbai), October 10. https://timesofindia.indiatimes.com/city/bhopal/in-madhya -pradesh-a-loo-selfie-ritual-before-wedding-rites/articleshow/71513065 .cms.

Bacchetta, Paola. 1999a. "Militant Hindu Nationalist Women Reimagine Themselves: Notes on Mechanisms of Expansion/Adjustment." *Journal of Women's History* 10, no. 4: 125–47. https://doi.org/10.1353/jowh.2010.0528.

Bacchetta, Paola. 1999b. "When the Hindu Nation Exiles Its Queers." *Social Text* 61: 141–66.

Bacchetta, Paola. 2004. *Gender in the Hindu Nation: RSS Women as Ideologues.* New Delhi: Women Unlimited.

Bacchetta, Paola. 2010. "The (Failed) Production of Hindu Nationalized Space in Ahmedabad, Gujarat." *Gender, Place and Culture* 17, no. 5: 551–72. https://doi.org/10.1080/0966369X.2010.503102.

Bacchetta, Paola. 2019. "Queer Presence in/and Hindu Nationalism." In *Majoritarian State: How Hindu Nationalism Is Changing India*, edited by Angana P. Chatterji, Thomas Blom Hansen, and Christophe Jaffrelot, 375–96. New York: Oxford University Press.

Baer, Hans A., and Merrill Singer. 2023. "Planetary Health: Capitalism, Ecology and Eco-Socialism." *Capitalism Nature Socialism* 34, no. 4: 20–38. https://doi.org/10.1080/10455752.2023.2192953.

Baishya, Anirban. 2015. "#NaMo: The Political Work of the Selfie in the 2014 Indian General Elections." *International Journal of Communication* 9: 1686–1700.

Balachandran, Manu. 2015. "Why India's $168 Billion River-Linking Project Is a Disaster-in-Waiting." *Quartz*, September 18. https://qz.com/india /504127/why-indias-168-billion-river-linking-project-is-a-disaster-in -waiting.

Baluni, Anil. 2019. "Watching Out for the Nation: 'Main Bhi Chowkidar' Is Inspiring People, Rallying Them for a Greater Purpose." *Indian Express* (Noida), March 19. https://indianexpress.com/article/opinion/columns /watching-out-for-the-nation-main-bhi-chowkidar-is-inspiring-people -rallying-them-for-a-greater-purpose-pm-modi-twitter-5634686/.

Bamzai, Kaveree. 2018. "Please, Hanuman Is Rarely Angry." *DailyO* (Noida), May 14. https://www.dailyo.in/politics/hanuman-narendra-modi -hindutva-bjp-karnataka-24111.

Banaji, Shakuntala. 2018. "Vigilante Publics: Orientalism, Modernity and Hindutva Fascism in India." *Javnost—The Public* 25, no. 4: 333–50. https://doi
.org/10.1080/13183222.2018.1463349.

Banaji, Shakuntala, Ramnath Bhat, Anushi Agarwal, Nihal Passanha, and
Mukti Sadhana Pravin. 2019. "WhatsApp Vigilantes: An Exploration of
Citizen Reception and Circulation of WhatsApp Misinformation Linked
to Mob Violence in India." Department of Media and Communications,
London School of Economics and Political Science. https://eprints.lse
.ac.uk/104316/1/Banaji_whatsapp_vigilantes_exploration_of_citizen
_reception_published.pdf.

Banerjee, Biswajeet. 2022. "Thousands Protest 'Bulldozer Justice'
Against Indian Muslims." Associated Press, June 15. https://
apnews.com/article/religion-india-arrests-islam-narendra-modi
-5310432fcdb614beb92d4d195fa19539.

Banerjee, Prathama. 2017. "State (and) Violence." *Seminar* 691: 26–30. https://
www.csds.in/uploads/custom_files/1526966328_State%20(and)%20
violence.pdf.

Banerjee, Sikata. 2005. *Make Me a Man! Masculinity, Hinduism, and Nationalism in India*. Albany: State University of New York Press.

Banerjee, Sikata. 2006. "Armed Masculinity, Hindu Nationalism and Female
Political Participation in India." *International Feminist Journal of Politics* 8,
no. 1: 62–83. https://doi.org/10.1080/14616740500415482.

Banerjee, Sikata, and Rina Verma Williams. 2018. "Making the Nation Manly:
The Case of 'Bhaag Milkha Bhaag' (2013) and India's Search for Regional
Dominance in an Era of Neo-Liberal Globalization." *Studies in South
Asian Film and Media* 10, no. 2: 179–93. https://doi.org/10.1386/safm
_00013_1.

Banerjee, Soumi. 2019. "The New Age Politics of Gender in the Hindutva
Movement and Faith-Based Identity Contestation." *Open Democracy*,
December 16. https://www.opendemocracy.net/en/rethinking-populism
/new-age-politics-gender-hindutva-movement-and-faith-based-identity
-contestation/.

Basnet, Sahara, and Mamudul Hoque. 2022. "Critical Analysis of the Implementation of Clean India Mission in the Rural Areas: A Gender Perspective." *Journal of Women, Politics and Policy* 44, no. 3: 299–318. https://doi
.org/10.1080/1554477X.2022.2115281.

Basu, Amrita. 1993. "Feminism Inverted: The Real Women and Gendered
Imagery of Hindu Nationalism." *Bulletin of Concerned Asian Scholars* 25,
no. 4: 25–37. https://doi.org/10.1080/14672715.1993.10416136.

Basu, Amrita. 2011. "Hindu Women's Activism in India and the Questions
It Raises." In *Appropriating Gender: Women's Activism and Politicized
Religion in South Asia*, edited by Patricia Jeffrey and Amrita Basu, 167–83.
New York: Routledge.

Basu, Amrita. 2021. "Changing Modalities of Violence: Lessons from Hindu Nationalist India." In *Negotiating Democracy and Religious Pluralism: India, Pakistan, and Turkey*, edited by Sudipta Kaviraj, Vatsal Naresh, and Karen Barkey, 277–80. Oxford: Oxford University Press.

Basu, Amrita. 2022. "Normalizing Violence: Lessons from Hindu Nationalist India." In *Saffron Republic: Hindu Nationalism and State Power in India*, edited by Thomas Blom Hansen and Srirupa Roy, 59–71. Cambridge: Cambridge University Press.

Basu, Anustup. 2008. "Hindutva and Informatic Modernization." *Boundary 2* 35, no. 3: 239–50.

Basu, Anustup. 2020. *Hindutva as Political Monotheism*. Durham, NC: Duke University Press.

Basu, Srimati. 2015. *The Trouble with Marriage*. Berkeley: University of California Press.

Bateson, Regina. 2021. "The Politics of Vigilantism." *Comparative Political Studies* 54, no. 6: 923–55. https://doi.org/10.1177/0010414020957692.

Baviskar, Amita. 2003. "Between Violence and Desire: Space, Power, and Identity in the Making of Metropolitan Delhi." *International Social Science Journal* 55, no. 175: 89–98. https://doi.org/10.1111/1468-2451.5501009.

Baviskar, Amita. 2005. *In the Belly of the River: Tribal Conflicts over Development in the Narmada Valley*, 2nd ed. New Delhi: Oxford University Press.

BBC. 2017. "India Top Court Orders Changes In Anti-Dowry Law to Stop Misuse." BBC, July 28. https://www.bbc.com/news/world-asia-india-40749636.

BBC. 2021. "India Paves Way for More Women in Armed Forces." BBC, September 8. https://www.bbc.com/news/world-asia-india-58486771.

BBC. 2023. "Bhopal Gas Tragedy: Supreme Court Rejects More Money for Victims." BBC, March 14. https://www.bbc.co.uk/news/world-asia-india-64899487.

Behl, Vaishnavi. 2020. "Water Politics: Climate Change and Its Impact on Caste." *Goya*, March 17. https://www.goya.in/blog/water-politics-climate-change-and-its-impact-on-caste.

Behl, Vaishnavi, and Prakash Kashwan. 2022. "Intersectional Water Justice in India: At the Confluence of Gender, Caste, and Climate Change." In *Climate Justice in India*, edited by Prakash Kashwan, 183–205. Cambridge: Cambridge University Press.

Berlant, Lauren. 1997. *The Queen of America Goes to Washington City*. Durham, NC: Duke University Press.

Berlant, Lauren. 2007. "Slow Death (Sovereignty, Obesity, Lateral Agency)." *Critical Inquiry* 33, no. 4: 754–80. https://doi.org/10.1086/521568.

Berlant, Lauren. 2016. "The Commons: Infrastructures for Troubling Times." *Environment and Planning D: Society and Space* 34, no. 3: 393–419. https://doi.org/10.1177/0263775816645989.

Bhalla, Alok. 2006. *Partition Dialogues: Memories of a Lost Home*. New Delhi: Oxford University Press.

Bhan, Mona. 2022. "Development: India's Foundational Myth." In *Saffron Republic: Hindu Nationalism and State Power in India*, edited by Thomas Blom Hansen and Srirupa Roy, 275–83. Cambridge: Cambride University Press.

Bhandare, Namita. 2017. "Fire Anti-Romeo Squads." *Mint* (Bengaluru), April 18. https://www.livemint.com/Opinion/CrovfG7kQrZ9hIHaDUZOeK/Fire-antiRomeo-squads.html.

Bharath Autos. 2014. "Fighting Public Urination with Water Canon, the 'Pissing Tanker.'" YouTube, video, 1:22. https://www.youtube.com/watch?v=2ZtugbgxzmM.

Bhatia, Anisha. 2016. "Indore's Swachh Mantra: 'Roko Aur Toko' Whenever You See People Defecating in Open." NDTV-Dettol, November 29. https://swachhindia.ndtv.com/indores-swachh-mantra-roko-aur-toko-whenever-see-people-defecating-open-4119/.

Bhatia, Anisha. 2020. "This Work Has Given Me an Identity: Shalini, a Transgender and a Caretaker of Community Toilets in a Telengana Locality." NDTV-Dettol, November 19. https://swachhindia.ndtv.com/this-work-has-given-me-an-identity-shalini-a-transgender-and-a-caretaker-of-community-toilets-in-a-telangana-locality-53185/.

Bhattacharya, Priyanka. 2017. "Why 'Swachh India' Is the Biggest Women's Movement at the Moment." NDTV-Dettol, March 2. https://swachhindia.ndtv.com/why-swachh-india-is-the-biggest-womens-movement-at-the-moment-5338/.

Bhattacharya, Sabyasachi. 2003. *Vande Mataram: The Biography of a Song*. New Delhi: Primus Books.

Bhowmick, Nilanjana. 2019. "In Uttar Pradesh's Jhansi, Toilets Built Under Swachh Bharat Mission Exist Only on Paper, Open Defecation Continues." *Firstpost*, April 11. https://www.firstpost.com/india/in-uttar-pradeshs-jhansi-toilets-built-under-swachh-bharat-mission-exist-only-on-paper-open-defecation-continues-6429881.html.

Bhowmick, Subhendra, and Anindya Sekhar Purakayastha. 2016. "Scatologising Hindu Eschatology: An (In)Auspicious Journey from Devalaya to Shauchalaya." *History and Sociology of South Asia* 10, no. 2: 1–22. https://doi.org/10.1177/2230807516633589.

BiKa, Haskala. 2023. "They Also Cut the Water Supplies that Comes to Our Tap at Will." Suswa, July 3. https://suswa.org/they-also-cut-the-water-supplies-that-comes-to-our-tap-at-will/.

Billig, Michael. 1995. *Banal Nationalism*. Thousand Oaks, CA: Sage Publications.

Bindra, Prerna Singh. 2018. "We Don't Just Have an Environmental Crisis, but a Govt in Denial as Well." *IndiaSpend*, February 17. https://www

.indiaspend.com/we-dont-just-have-an-environmental-crisis-but-a-govt-in-denial-as-well-61292/.

Bisht, Bhawana. 2018. "50 Women Leave In-Laws' Homes for Lack of Toilets." *SheThePeople.TV*, January 12. https://www.shethepeople.tv/news/no-toilets-grooms-village-50-women-leave-laws-homes/.

Bisht, Bhawana. 2021. "20 Women Die a Day: Dowry Deaths Still a Threatening Reality in India?" *SheThePeople.TV*, June 26. https://www.shethepeople.tv/top-stories/opinion/dowry-deaths-reality-in-india-but-until-when/.

Boehmer, Elleke. 2009. *Stories of Women: Gender and Narrative in the Postcolonial Nation*. Manchester: Manchester University Press.

Bonner, Michelle D. 2019. *Tough on Crime: The Rise of Punitive Populism in Latin America*. Pittsburgh, PA: University of Pittsburgh Press.

Borpujari, Priyanka. 2016. "How 'Pinjra Tod' Spread Its Wings." *Inkl*, December 30. https://www.inkl.com/news/how-pinjra-tod-spread-its-wings.

Bose, Adrija. 2016. "Upper-Caste Villagers Prevent Dalit Family in Gujarat from Building a Toilet." *HuffPost*, July 15. https://www.huffpost.com/archive/in/entry/dalit-family_n_9165140.

Bose, Sugata. 2017. *Nation as Mother: And Other Visions of Nationhood*. Delhi: India Penguin Random House.

Brass, Paul R. 1997. *Theft of an Idol*. Princeton, NJ: Princeton University Press.

Business Standard. 2017a. "Mahilao Ko Mila Samman Yahi Hai Ujjwala Ki Pehchan Says Shri." *Business Standard* (New Delhi), May 4. https://www.business-standard.com/article/government-press-release/mahilao-ko-mila-samman-yahi-hai-ujjwala-ki-pehchan-says-shri-117050500966_1.html.

Business Standard. 2017b. "Modi Govt to States: Call Toilets 'Izzat Ghar' to Instil Pride in Families." *Business Standard* (New Delhi), October 18. https://www.business-standard.com/article/current-affairs/modi-govt-to-states-call-toilets-izzat-ghar-to-instil-pride-in-families-117101800462_1.html.

Business Standard. 2023. "As India's Rank Falls to 111, Here's Everything About Global Hunger Index." *Business Standard* (New Delhi), October 13. https://www.business-standard.com/india-news/as-india-s-rank-falls-to-111-here-s-everything-about-global-hunger-index-123101300136_1.html.

Butalia, Urvashi. 2000. *The Other Side of Silence: Voices from the Partition of India*. Durham, NC: Duke University Press.

Chacko, Priya. 2019. "Marketizing Hindutva: The State, Society, and Markets in Hindu Nationalism." *Modern Asian Studies* 53, no. 2: 377–410. https://doi.org/10.1017/S0026749X17000051.

Chacko, Priya. 2020. "Gender and Authoritarian Populism: Empowerment, Protection, and the Politics of Resentful Aspiration in India." *Critical Asian Studies* 52, no. 2: 204–25. https://doi.org/10.1080/14672715.2020.1711789.

Chakrabarty, Dipesh. 1992. "Of Garbage, Modernity, and the Citizen's Gaze." *Economic and Political Weekly* 27, nos. 10/11: 541–47.

Chakrabarty, Dipesh. 2000. *Provincializing Europe: Postcolonial Thought and Historical Difference.* Princeton, NJ: Princeton University Press.

Chakrabarty, Dipesh. 2009. "The Climate of History: Four Theses." *Critical Inquiry* 35, no. 2: 197–222. https://doi.org/10.1086/596640.

Chakrabarty, Dipesh. 2021. *The Climate of History in a Planetary Age.* Chicago: University of Chicago Press.

Chakraborty, Arpita. 2022. "Tracing the Rise of Ascetic Masculinity in India." In *Women, Gender and Religious Nationalism,* edited by Amrita Basu and Tanika Sarkar, 195–223. Cambridge: Cambridge University Press.

Chakravarti, Uma. 1990. "Whatever Happened to the Vedic Dasi? Orientalism, Nationalism, and a Script for the Past." In *Recasting Women: Essays in Indian Colonial History,* edited by Kumkum Sangari and Sudesh Vaid, 27–87. New Brunswick, NJ: Rutgers University Press.

Chakravarti, Uma, and Maithreyi Krishnaraj. 2018. *Gendering Caste: Through a Feminist Lens.* Los Angeles: Sage Publications.

Chandel, Himani. 2012. "The Tribune India: 'India Among Top Land-Grabbing Nations.'" Rights and Resources Initiative, December 21. https://rightsandresources.org/blog/the-tribune-india-india-among-top-land-grabbing-nations/.

Chandran, Rina. 2017. "Activists Vow Not to Give Up Fight Against Evictions as India's Biggest Dam Opened." Reuters, September 18. https://www.reuters.com/article/us-india-landrights-protests-idUSKCN1BT149.

Chari, Mridula. 2020. "How Solar Farms Fuel Land Conflicts." *Mint* (Bengaluru), September 21. https://www.livemint.com/news/india/how-solar-farms-fuel-land-conflicts-11600612526037.html.

Chatterjee, Liz. 2011. "Time to Acknowledge the Dirty Truth Behind Community-Led Sanitation." *Guardian* (London), June 9. https://www.theguardian.com/global-development/poverty-matters/2011/jun/09/dirty-truth-behind-community-sanitation.

Chatterjee, Manini. 2017. "The Filth Within." *Telegraph* (Kolkata), October 9. https://www.telegraphindia.com/opinion/the-filth-within/cid/1454586.

Chatterjee, Moyukh. 2023. *Composing Violence.* Durham, NC: Duke University Press.

Chatterjee, Partha. 1989. "The Nationalist Resolution of the Women's Question." In *Recasting Women: Essays in Colonial History,* edited by K. Sangari and S. Vaid, 233–53. New Delhi: Kali for Women.

Chatterjee, Partha. 1992. "History and the Nationalization of Hinduism." *Social Research* 59, no. 1: 111–49.

Chatterjee, Partha, Tapati Guha-Thakurta, and Bodhisttva Kar. 2014. *New Cultural Histories of India.* New Delhi: Oxford University Press.

Chatterji, Angana P. 2019. "Remaking the Hindu/Nation: Terror and Impunity in Uttar Pradesh." In *Majoritarian State: How Hindu Nationalism Is*

Changing India, edited by Angana P. Chatterji, Thomas Blom Hansen, and Christophe Jaffrelot, 397–418. New York: Oxford University Press.

Chatterji, Angana P., Thomas Blom Hansen, and Christophe Jaffrelot. 2019a. "Introduction." In *Majoritarian State: How Hindu Nationalism Is Changing India*, edited by Angana P. Chatterji, Thomas Blom Hansen, and Christophe Jaffrelot, 1–16. New York: Oxford University Press.

Chatterji, Angana P., Thomas Blom Hansen, and Christophe Jaffrelot, eds. 2019b. *Majoritarian State: How Hindu Nationalism Is Changing India*. New York: Oxford University Press.

Chaudhary, Monika. 2024. "India's Thirst for Improved Water Security." *East Asia Forum*, February 27. https://eastasiaforum.org/2024/02/27/indias -thirst-for-improved-water-security/#:~:text=Approximately%20600%20 million%20people%20experience,of%20India's%20water%20is%20 contaminated.

Chauhan, Chetan. 2017. "No Water in 60% Toilets Puts Question Mark over Modi Govt's Swachh Bharat Mission." *Hindustan Times* (New Delhi), May 14. https://www.hindustantimes.com/india-news /no-water-in-60-toilets-built-under-swachh-bharat-mission/story -3rdu1Hv1UZbabYQhb68OTP.html.

Cheney-Lippold, John. 2017. *We Are Data: Algorithms and the Making of Our Digital Selves*. New York: New York University Press.

Cherukupalli, Anil, dir. 2016. "The Dabba Dol Gang." YouTube, video, 3:45. https://www.youtube.com/watch?v=rcbzTevEp2I.

Chun, Wendy Hui Kyong. 2016. *Updating to Remain the Same: Habitual New Media*. Cambridge, MA: MIT Press.

Coffey, Diane, and Dean Spears. 2017. *Where India Goes. Abandoned Toilets, Stunted Development and the Costs of Caste*. New York: HarperCollins.

Comaroff, Jean. 2021. "Vigilantism and the Practices of Popular Sovereignty." Keynote address. YouTube, video, 30:38. https://www.youtube.com /watch?v=7CRpMqzmCl4.

Comaroff, Jean. 2024. "Vigilantism and the Paradoxes of Sovereignty." Unpublished manuscript. https://jeancomaroff.com/essays/vigilantism-and-the -paradoxes-of-sovereignty.

Comaroff, John, and Jean Comaroff. 1997. "Postcolonial Politics and the Discourses of Democracy in Southern Africa." *Journal of Anthropological Research* 53: 123–46.

Comaroff, John, and Jean Comaroff. 2016. *The Truth About Crime*. Chicago: University of Chicago Press.

Cook, Ian M. 2019. "Immoral Times: Vigilantism in a South Indian City." In *Majoritarian State: How Hindu Nationalism Is Changing India*, edited by Angana P. Chatterji, Thomas Blom Hansen, and Christophe Jaffrelot, 69–82. New York: Oxford University Press.

Corbin, Alain. 1988. *The Foul and the Fragrant: Odor and the French Social Imagination.* Cambridge, MA: Harvard University Press.

Counterview. 2017. "Rajasthan Labour Activist's Lynching: Swacch Bharat Campaign Blamed for 'Shaming' Women Defecating in Open." *Counterview,* June 19. https://www.counterview.in/2017/06/rajasthan-labour-activists-lynching.html.

Cowie, Sam. 2018. "Bolsonaro Wants to 'Cleanse' Brazil of Left-Wing 'Criminals.'" Al Jazeera, October 23. https://www.aljazeera.com/news/2018/10/23/bolsonaro-wants-to-cleanse-brazil-of-left-wing-criminals.

CSN (Civil Society News). 2020. "Goan Anger over a Dark Coal Corridor." *Civil Society,* January 29. https://www.civilsocietyonline.com/environment/three-projects-and-a-massive-coal-corridor-worry-goa/#:~:text=The%20proposed%20corridor%20will%20cut,coal%20behind%2C%20causing%20air%20pollution.

Das, Ayaskant. 2020. "How Modi Government's Thermal Power Reforms Aggravate Pollution." *NewsClick,* November 20. https://www.newsclick.in/How-Modi-Government-Thermal-Power-Reforms-Aggravate-Pollution.

Das, Veena. 2007. *Life and Words: Violence and the Descent into the Ordinary.* Berkeley: University of California Press.

Dasgupta, KumKum. 2017. "With Stiff Target for Building Toilets Under Swachh Bharat Abhiyan, States Are Flouting Citizens' Rights." *Hindustan Times* (New Delhi), April 3. https://www.hindustantimes.com/india-news/mad-rush-for-toilets-flouting-citizens-rights/story-FootE97suf4Ji8QoCAzZuM.html.

Davis, Richard. 2018. *Picturing the Nation: Iconographies of Modern India.* Hyderabad: Orient Blackswan.

Deccan Chronicle. 2016. "Rajasthan Teachers Told to Click Pictures of Open Defecation." *Deccan Chronicle* (Hyderabad), June 6. https://www.deccanchronicle.com/nation/in-other-news/070616/rajasthan-teachers-told-to-click-pictures-of-open-defecation.html?fromNewsdog=1&utm_source=NewsDog.

Deep, Aroon. 2017. "Swachh Bharat Spent Rs 530 Crore on Publicity in Three Years—but Little on Grassroots Awareness." *Scroll,* November 22. https://scroll.in/article/857030/centre-spent-rs-530-crores-in-3-years-on-swachh-bharat-publicity-but-has-little-to-show-for-it.

De Jong, Wim. 2023. "Goon Squad Democracy? The Rise of Vigilant Citizenship Through Victim Support and Neighborhood Watches in Amsterdam (1980–1990)." *Journal of Urban History* 49, no. 2: 388–410. https://doi.org/10.1177/00961442211010474.

Deleuze, Gilles, and Félix Guattari. 1987. *A Thousand Plateaus.* Minneapolis: University of Minnesota Press.

Dhanaraj, Christina Thomas. 2018. "MeToo and Savarna Feminism: Revolutions Cannot Start with the Privileged, Feminist Future Must Be Equal for All-India News." *Firstpost,* November 13. https://www.firstpost.com

/india/metoo-and-savarna-feminism-revolutions-cannot-start-with-the-privileged-feminist-future-must-be-equal-for-all-5534711.html.

Dhillon, Amrit. 2019. "Tired of Dark Fields and Jeering Men: The Bride Who Led a 'Toilet Revolution.'" *Guardian* (London), January 23. https://www.theguardian.com/global-development/2019/jan/23/tired-dark-fields-jeering-men-bride-led-toilet-revolution.

Doron, Assa. 2016. "Unclean, Unseen: Social Media, Civic Action and Urban Hygiene in India." *South Asia: Journal of South Asian Studies* 39, no. 4: 715–39. https://doi.org/10.1080/00856401.2016.1218096.

Doron, Assa, and Robin Jeffrey. 2018. *Waste of a Nation: Garbage and Growth in India*. Cambridge, MA: Harvard University Press.

Doron, Assa, and Ira Raja. 2015. "The Cultural Politics of Shit: Class, Gender and Public Space in India." *Postcolonial Studies* 18, no. 2: 189–207. https://doi.org/10.1080/13688790.2015.1065714.

Doshi, Vidhi. 2017. "India Turns to Public Shaming to Get People to Use Its 52 Million New Toilets." *Washington Post*, November 5. https://www.washingtonpost.com/world/asia_pacific/india-turns-to-public-shaming-to-get-people-to-use-its-52million-new-toilets/2017/11/03/882166fe-b41c-11e7-9b93-b97043e57a22_story.html.

Douglas, Mary. 2015. *Purity and Danger: An Analysis of Concepts of Pollution and Taboo*. London: Routledge.

Drishti. 2022. "Swachh Survekshan Awards 2022." Drishti, October 4. https://www.drishtiias.com/daily-updates/daily-news-analysis/swachh-survekshan-awards-2022#:~:text=About%3A%20Swachh%20Survekshan%20has%20been,and%20towards%20creating%20cleaner%20cities.

Drolia, Rashmi. 2016. "Man Killed for Buying Time to Build Toilet." *Times of India* (Mumbai), October 8. https://timesofindia.indiatimes.com/city/raipur/Man-killed-for-buying-time-to-build-toilet/articleshow/54742845.cms.

Dumont, Louis. 1981. *Homo Hierarchicus*. Chicago: University of Chicago Press.

Dutta, Aniruddha, and Raina Roy. 2014. "Decolonizing Transgender in India: Some Reflections." *TSQ: Transgender Studies Quarterly* 1, no. 3: 320–36. https://doi.org/10.1215/23289252-2685615.

Dutta, Saptarshi. 2017. "Dance, Music, Plays and Other Ways to Spread the Message of Swachh Bharat at Grassroots Level." NDTV-Dettol, April 25. https://swachhindia.ndtv.com/dance-music-plays-and-other-ways-to-spread-the-message-of-swachh-bharat-at-grassroot-level-6693/.

Dutta, Saptarshi, and Sonia Bhaskar. 2017. "Hyderabad's Public Toilets Reek with Dirt and Lack of Water Supply, Making the City's ODF Certificate Questionable." NDTV-Dettol, August 30. https://swachhindia.ndtv.com/hyderabads-public-toilets-reek-with-dirt-and-lack-of-water-supply-making-the-citys-odf-certificate-questionable-11280/.

Dwivedi, Anju, and Tripti Singh. 2020. "Unlocking Barriers to Inclusive WASH: Learnings from Slums in Bhubaneswar." Center for Policy Research, November 26. https://cprindia.org/briefsreports/unlocking-barriers-to -inclusive-wash-learnings-from-slums-in-bhubaneswar/.

Eck, Diana L. 1998. *Darśan: Seeing the Divine Image in India*. New York: Columbia University Press.

Eck, Diana. 2013. *India: A Sacred Geography*. New York: Harmony/Rodale.

Elias, Norbert. 1978. *The Civilizing Process*. Oxford: Blackwell.

Ellis-Petersen, Hannah. 2019. "'Bhopal's Tragedy Has Not Stopped': The Urban Disaster Still Claiming Lives 35 Years On." *Guardian* (London), December 8. https://www.theguardian.com/cities/2019/dec/08/bhopals-tragedy -has-not-stopped-the-urban-disaster-still-claiming-lives-35-years-on.

Ellis-Petersen, Hannah. 2024. "Modi Builds Highways but Where Are Our Jobs?" *Guardian* (London), May 19. https://www.theguardian.com/world /article/2024/may/20/india-election-rising-inequality-unemployment -narendra-modi.

Enloe, Cynthia. 1990. *Bananas, Beaches and Bases: Making Feminist Sense of International Politics*. Berkeley: University of California Press.

Enloe, Cynthia. 2018. "Cynthia Enloe Discusses Gender and the Rise of the Global Right with Agnieszka Graff, Ratna Kapur, and Suzanna Danuta Walters." *Signs: Journal of Women in Culture and Society*, podcast, 1:17:42. http://signsjournal.org/podcast/cynthia-enloe-discusses-gender-and-the -rise-of-the-global-right-with-agnieszka-graff-ratna-kapur-and-suzanna -danuta-walters/.

Escobar, Arturo. 2004. "Development, Violence and the New Imperial Order." *Development* 47, no. 1: 15–21.

Esty, Joshua D. 1999. "Excremental Postcolonialism." *Contemporary Literature* 40, no. 1: 22–59.

Farris, Sara R. 2017. *In the Name of Women's Rights: The Rise of Femonationalism*. Durham, NC: Duke University Press.

Fassin, Didier. 2018. *The Will to Punish*. Edited by Christopher Kutz. New York: Oxford University Press.

Ferguson, James. 1994. *The Anti-Politics Machine: "Development," Depoliticization and Bureaucratic Power in Lesotho*. Minneapolis: University of Minnesota Press.

FFS (Flyingstar Film Studio). 2017. "Maa. . . . A Short Film on Swachh Bharat." YouTube, video, 2:29. https://www.youtube.com/watch?v=Z8J-yZF9hjM.

Firstpost. 2018. "Dalit Youth Beaten with Sticks in Uttar Pradesh's Muzzafarnagar, Made to Chant 'Jai Mata Di.'" *Firstpost*, January 17. https://www .firstpost.com/india/dalit-youth-beaten-with-sticks-in-uttar-pradeshs -muzaffarnagar-made-to-chant-jai-mata-di-4306541.html.

FAT (Forum on the Arms Trade). n.d. "US Arms Sales to India." Forum on the Arms Trade. https://www.forumarmstrade.org/usindia.html.

Gale, Jason, and Bibhudatta Pradhan. 2018. "India's Women Want a Toilet Revolution." *Bloomberg News*, October 31. https://www.bloomberg.com /news/features/2018-10-31/india-s-toilet-revolution-unleashes-women-s -earning-potential.

Ganesh, Kamala. 2010. "In Search of the Great Indian Goddess: Motherhood Unbound." In *Motherhood in India*, edited by Maithreyi Krishnaraj, 73–105. New Delhi: Routledge.

Gardenier, Matthijs. 2022. *Towards a Vigilant Society: From Citizen Participation to Anti-Migrant Vigilantism*. Oxford: Oxford University Press.

Gatade, Subhash. 2015. "Silencing Caste, Sanitising Oppression: Understanding Swachh Bharat Abhiyan." *Economic and Political Weekly* 50, no. 44: 29–35.

Geo News. 2020. "Indian Forces Have Raped, Molested More than 11,000 Kashmiri Women in 3 Decades: Report." Geo News, November 25. https://www.geo.tv/latest/320584-indian-forces-raped-molested-more -than-11000-women-in-kashmir-kms.

Ghertner, Asher. 2018. "Hindu Extrastatecraft? Coding the Future Hindu, or the Infrastructural Inertia of Indian Urbanism." In *Urban Asias: Essays on Futurity Past and Present*, edited by Tim Bunnell and Daniel Goh, 97–108. Berlin: Jovis.

Ghosh, Bishnupriya. 2002. "Queering *Hindutva*: Unruly Bodies and Pleasures in Sadhavi Rithambara's Performances." In *Right-Wing Women: From Conservatives to Extremists Around the World*, edited by Paola Bacchetta and Margaret Power, 259–72. London: Routledge.

Ghosh, Bishnupriya. 2020. "Big Bad Social Media: Distributed Affects and Popular Politics." *Culture Machine* 19. https://culturemachine.net/vol-19 -media-populism/big-bad-social-media-bishnupriya-ghosh/.

Ghosh, Pallavi. 2015. "Five Women Stripped and Paraded on the Street." *Youth Ki Awaaz*, May 21. https://www.youthkiawaaz.com/2015/05/violence -against-dalit-women/.

Ghoshal, Devjyot. 2019. "Amit Shah Vows to Throw Illegal Immigrants into Bay of Bengal." Reuters, April 13. https://www.reuters.com/article/india -election-speech-idUSKCN1RO1YD.

Ghouse, Mike. 2018. "Whitewashing India's Religious Freedom." *Muslim Mirror*, August 12. https://muslimmirror.com/whitewashing-indias-religious -freedom/.

Gitelman, Lisa. 2014. "Holding Electronic Networks by the Wrong End." *Amodern* 2. https://amodern.net/article/holding-electronic-networks-by -the-wrong-end/.

Gitelman Lisa, and Virginia Jackson. 2013. "Introduction." In *"Raw Data" Is an Oxymoron*, edited by Lisa Gitelman, 1–14. Cambridge, MA: MIT Press.

GNI (Go News Inida). 2020. "8 Dalit Women Get Raped in India Every Day, UP Has Most Victims." Go News India, November 25. https://www

.gonewsindia.com/latest-news/news-and-politics/8-dalit-women-get
-raped-in-india-every-day-up-has-most-victims-19156.

Gökarıksel, Banu, Christopher Neubert, and Sara Smith. 2019. "Demographic Fever Dreams: Fragile Masculinity and Population Politics in the Rise of the Global Right." *Signs* 44, no. 3: 561–87. https://doi.org/10.1086/701154.

Gosavi, Akanksha, dir. 2018. "Bharat Mata ke is roop ko dekh kar har Hindustani ki ruh kaap uthegi." YouTube, video, 9:10. https://www.youtube .com/watch?v=p1zoeDWEWCs.

Gotinga, J. C. 2018. "Thousands of Street Loiterers Arrested in the Philippines." Al Jazeera, June 28. https://www.aljazeera.com/news/2018/6/28 /thousands-of-street-loiterers-arrested-in-the-philippines.

Govil, Nitin, and Anirban Kapil Baishya. 2018. "The Bully in the Pulpit: Autocracy, Digital Social Media, and Right-Wing Populist Technoculture." *Communication, Culture and Critique* 11, no. 1: 67–84. https://doi.org/10 .1093/ccc/tcx001.

Gowda, Chandan. 2015. "The Mirage of Purity." *Bangalore Mirror*, September 11. https://bangaloremirror.indiatimes.com/opinion/views/raja-ram -mohan-roy-sir-syed-ahmed-khan-ishwar-chandar-vidyasagar-swami -vivekananda-tagore-gandhi-periyar-nehru-ambedkar-lohia/articleshow /48918491.cms.

Graff, Agnieszka, Ratna Kapur, and Suzanna Danuta Walters. 2019. "Introduction: Gender and the Rise of the Global Right." *Signs* 44, no. 3: 541–60. https://doi.org/10.1086/701152.

Gray, Herman. 2015. "The Feel of Life: Resonance, Race, and Representation." *International Journal of Communication* 9: 1108–19.

Greenpeace. 2010. "Greenpeace Points Spotlight at Potential Bhopal-Type Disaster at Dow Plants in the US." Greenpeace, July 6. https://www .greenpeace.org/usa/news/greenpeace-points-spotlight-at.

Gregory, Derek. 2017. "Dirty Dancing: Drones and Death in the Borderlands." In *Life in the Age of Drone Warfare*, edited by Lisa Parks and Caren Kaplan, 25–58. Durham, NC: Duke University Press.

Grewal, Inderpal. 2017a. *Saving the Security State: Exceptional Citizens in Twenty-First-Century America*. Durham, NC: Duke University Press.

Grewal, Inderpal. 2017b. "Drone Imaginaries: The Technopolitics of Visuality in Postcolony and Empire." In *Life in the Age of Drone Warfare*, edited by Lisa Parks and Caren Kaplan, 343–66. Durham, NC: Duke University Press.

Grewal, Inderpal. 2020. "Authoritarian Patriarchy and Its Populism." *English Studies in Africa* 63, no. 1: 179–98. https://doi.org/10.1080/00138398.2020 .1784554.

Grossberg, Lawrence. 1986. "On Postmodernism and Articulation." *Journal of Communication Inquiry* 10, no. 2: 45–60. https://doi.org/10.1177 /019685998601000204.

Grossberg, Lawrence. 2019. "Cultural Studies in Search of a Method, or Looking for Conjunctural Analysis." *New Formations* 96/97: 38–68. https://doi .org/10.3898/newf:96/97.02.2019.

Grosz, Elizabeth. 1994. *Volatile Bodies: Toward a Corporeal Feminism.* Bloomington: Indiana University Press.

Guha-Thakurta, Tapati. 2016. "Bharat Mata: The Nation as a Goddess." *India Today,* May 30. https://www.indiatoday.in/magazine/guest-column /story/20160530-bharat-mata-the-nation-as-a-goddess-828923-2016-05-18.

Gulankar, Akash Chandrashekhar. 2020. "Swachh Bharat: One Sweep for Modi, ₹67,000 Crore for Country." *Federal,* October 2. https://thefederal .com/analysis/swachh-bharat-one-sweep-for-modi-%E2%82%B967000 -crore-for-country/?infinitescroll=1.

Gupta, Aashish, Nazar Khalid, Devashish Desphande, et al. 2019a. "Changes in Open Defecation in Rural North India: 2014–2018." IZA Discussion Paper No. 12065. IZA,—Institute of Labor Economics. https://docs.iza .org/dp12065.pdf.

Gupta, Aashish, Nazar Khalid, Payal Hathi, Nikhil Srivastav, Sangita Vyas, and Diane Coffey. 2019b. "Coercion, Construction, and 'ODF Paper Pe': Swachha Bharat According to Local Officials." *India Forum,* March 5. https://www.theindiaforum.in/article/swachh-bharat-mission-according -local-government-officials#:~:text=We%20find%20that%20local%20 officials,different%20places%3B%20that%20the%20ODF.

Gupta, Akhil. 1998. *Postcolonial Developments: Agriculture in the Making of Modern India.* Durham, NC: Duke University Press.

Gupta, Charu. 2000. "Hindu Women, Muslim Men: Cleavages in Shared Spaces of Everyday Life, United Provinces, c. 1890–1930." *Indian Economic and Social History Review* 37, no. 2: 121–49. https://doi.org/10.1177 /001946460003700201.

Gupta, Charu. 2002. *Sexuality, Obscenity, Community: Women, Muslims, and the Hindu Public in Colonial India.* London: Palgrave.

Gupta, Smita. 2021. "The Dalit-Hindutva Paradox." *Hindu* (Chennai), December 4. https://www.thehindu.com/opinion/op-ed/The-Dalit-Hindutva -paradox/article62115057.ece.

Guru, Gopal. 1995. "Dalit Women Talk Differently." *Economic and Political Weekly* 30, nos. 41/42: 2548–50. http://www.jstor.org/stable/4403327.

Guru, Gopal. 2009. "Archaeology of Untouchability." *Economic and Political Weekly* 44, no. 37: 49–56. http://www.jstor.org/stable/25663543.

Guru, Gopal. 2016. "Nationalism as the Framework for Dalit Self-Realization." *Brown Journal of World Affairs* 23, no. 1: 239–52. https://www.jstor.org /stable/26534721.

Haggarty, Kevin, and Richard Ericson. 2003. "The Surveillant Assemblage." *British Journal of Sociology* 51, no. 4: 605–22. https://doi.org/10.1080 /00071310020015280.

Hall, Stuart. 1992. "Cultural Studies and Its Theoretical Legacies." In *Cultural Studies*, edited by Lawrence Grossberg, Cary Nelson, and Paula A. Treichler, 277–94. New York: Routledge.

Hansen, Thomas Blom. 1994. "Controlled Emancipation: Women and Hindu Nationalism." *European Journal of Development Research 6*, no. 2: 82–94.

Hansen, Thomas Blom. 1999. *The Saffron Wave. Democracy and Hindu Nationalism in Modern India*. Princeton, NJ: Princeton University Press.

Hansen, Thomas Blom. 2019. "Democracy Against the Law: Reflections on India's Illiberal Democracy." In *Majoritarian State: How Hindu Nationalism Is Changing India*, edited by Angana P. Chatterji, Thomas Blom Hansen, and Christophe Jaffrelot, 19–40. New York: Oxford University Press.

Hansen, Thomas Blom. 2021. *The Law of Force: The Violent Heart of Indian Politics*. New Delhi: Aleph Book Company.

Hansen, Thomas Blom, and Srirupa Roy. 2022. "What Is New about 'New Hindutva'?" In *Saffron Republic: Hindu Nationalism and State Power in India*, edited by Thomas N. Hansen and Srirupa Roy, 1–24. Cambridge: Cambridge University Press.

Hansen, Thomas Blom, and Finn Stepputat, eds. 2005. *Sovereign Bodies: Citizens, Migrants, and States in the Postcolonial World*. Princeton, NJ: Princeton University Press.

Harriss, John, Craig Jeffrey, and Trent Brown. 2020. *India: Continuity and Change in the Twenty-First Century*. Cambridge: Polity.

Hawkins, Gay. 2006. *The Ethics of Waste: How We Relate to Rubbish*. Landham, MD: Rowman and Littlefield.

Himatsingka, Anuradha. 2018. "Swachh Bharat Mission: Getting People to Use Toilets Is Next Big Challenge." *Economic Times*, February 17. https:// economictimes.indiatimes.com/news/politics-and-nation/swachh-bharat -mission-getting-people-to-use-toilets-is-next-big-challenge/articleshow /62955975.cms?from=mdr.

Hindu. 2021a. "Modi Govt First to Create Social Media Police: Congress." *Hindu* (Chennai), May 26. https://www.thehindu.com/news/national/modi-govt -first-to-create-social-media-police-congress/article34650086.ece.

Hindu. 2021b. "Treat Murder of Youth in Belagavi as Religious Honour Killing: Fact Finding Team." *Hindu* (Chennai), October 28. https://www .thehindu.com/news/national/karnataka/treat-murder-of-youth-in -belagavi-as-religious-honour-killing-fact-finding-team/article37207695 .ece.

Hindu. 2023. "Clearing the Water: On Piped, Potable Water to Rural Households." *Hindu* (Chennai), July 4. https://www.thehindu.com /opinion/editorial/clearing-the-water-on-piped-potable-water-to-rural -households/article67037710.ece.

Hindu. 2024. "Modi Government Trying to End MGNREGS Says Jairam Ramesh." *Hindu* (Chennai), February 3. https://www.thehindu.com

/news/national/narendra-modi-government-trying-to-end-mgnrega-says
-jairam-ramesh/article67807972.ece.

History Place. 2001. "The Triumph of Hitler: Dachau Opens." History Place.
https://www.historyplace.com/worldwar2/triumph/tr-dachau.htm.

Hobsbawm, Eric. 1983. "Inventing Traditions." In *The Invention of Tradition*,
edited by Eric Hobsbawm and Terrence Ranger, 1–14. Cambridge: Cambridge University Press.

IAC (Indian Advertising Company). 2020. "Tanishq Ad: Hindu Muslim
Marriage." YouTube, video, 0:45. https://www.youtube.com/watch?v
=UYDNSxhSQNc.

IANS (Indo-Asian News Service). 2012. "Runaway Bride Returns Home to
New Toilet in Uttar Pradesh." *New Indian Express* (Chennai), June 28.
https://www.newindianexpress.com/nation/2012/jun/28/runaway-bride
-returns-home-to-new-toilet-in-uttar-pradesh-381602.html.

ICJ (International Commission of Jurists). 2021. "India: Authorities Must
Stop Suppressing Peaceful Protests by Farmers and Their Allies." International Commission of Jurists, February 11. https://www.icj.org/india
-authorities-must-stop-suppressing-peaceful-protests-by-farmers-and
-their-allies/.

ICJB (International Campaign for Justice in Bhopal). n.d. "Compensation and
the Injustice of the 1989 Settlement." International Campaign for Justice
in Bhopal. Accessed January 21, 2025. https://www.bhopal.net/what
-happened/the-immediate-aftermath-1984-1989/compensation-injustice
-1989-settlement/.

Ilaiah, Kancha. 2018. "Dalit Spring in the Hindi Heartland." *India Today*,
April 16. https://www.indiatoday.in/magazine/cover-story/story
/20180416-dalit-protest-bharat-bandh-kancha-ilaiah-shepherd-sc-st-act
-1206285-2018-04-05.

Ilaiah, Kancha. 2019. *Why I Am Not a Hindu: A Sudra Critique of Hindutva
Philosophy, Culture and Political Economy*. New Delhi: Sage Publications.

Independent. 2010. "Indian Leather Hub Targeted in Ganges Clean-Up."
Independent (London), March 9. https://www.independent.co.uk/climate
-change/news/indian-leather-hub-targeted-in-ganges-cleanup-5527101.html.

Indian Express. 2019. "PM Modi Launches #MainBhiChowkidar Campaign,
Says Everyone Working for Progress Is Chowkidar." *Indian Express*
(Noida), March 16. https://indianexpress.com/elections/everyone
-working-for-progress-is-a-chowkidar-says-pm-narendra-modi-5629366/.

India Today. 2016a. "New Generation Must Be Told to Say 'Bharat Mata Ki
Jai': RSS Chief." *India Today*, March 3. https://www.indiatoday.in/india
/story/new-generation-must-be-told-to-say-bharat-mata-ki-jai-rss-chief
-311648-2016-03-03.

India Today. 2016b. "No Toilet, No Marriage!" Facebook, April 18. https://
www.facebook.com/watch/?v=10154593870242119.

India Today. 2019. "I'm Chowkidar of Toilets: PM Modi Hits Campaign Trail in Maharashtra's Wardha." *India Today*, April 1. https://www.indiatoday.in /elections/lok-sabha-2019/story/pm-modi-in-maharashtra-chowkidar-of -toilets-1491143-2019-04-01.

India Tomorrow. 2019. "Poverty in India: Every Second Tribal, Every Third Dalit and Muslim Are Poor, Says UN Report." *India Tomorrow*, July 17. https://indiatomorrow.net/2019/07/17/poverty-in-india-every-second -tribal-every-third-dalit-and-muslim-are-poor-says-un-report/.

India TV. 2017. "Good News: 'No Toilet, No Bride,' Says UP Village." YouTube, video, 2:55. https://www.youtube.com/watch?v=lXj9uiul3LE.

Indiyanesan. 2018. "Replying to @narendramodi." X (formerly Twitter), November 17. https://twitter.com/indiyanesan/status/1711200440585765170.

Inglehart, Ronald, and Pippa Norris. 2019. *Cultural Backlash: Trump, Brexit, and Authoritarian Populism.* Cambridge: Cambridge University Press.

Inzamam, Qadri, and Haziq Qadri. 2022. "This Part of India Is on the Verge of Becoming a Complete Surveillance State." *Slate*, July 13. https://slate.com /technology/2022/07/telangana-india-surveillance-state.html.

Isalkar, Umesh. 2013. "Census Raises Stink over Manual Scavenging." *Times of India* (Mumbai), April 30. https://timesofindia.indiatimes.com /city/pune/Census-raises-stink-over-manual-scavenging/articleshow /19794299.cms.

Jack, Tullia, Manisha Anantharaman, and Alison L Browne. 2020. "'Without Cleanliness We Can't Lead the Life, No?' Cleanliness Practices, (In)Accessible Infrastructures, Social (Im)Mobility and (Un)Sustainable Consumption in Mysore, India." *Social and Cultural Geography* 23, no. 6: 814–35. https://doi.org/10.1080/14649365.2020.1820561.

Jacob, Suraj, Balmurli Natrajan, and T. G. Ajay. 2021. "'Why Don't They Use the Toilet Built for Them?': Explaining Toilet Use in Chhattisgarh, Central India." *Contributions to Indian Sociology* 55, no. 1: 89–115. https://doi .org/10.1177/0069966720972565.

Jaffrelot, Christophe. 2015. "The Modi-Centric BJP 2014 Election Campaign: New Techniques and Old Tactics." *Contemporary South Asia* 23, no. 2: 151–66. https://doi.org/10.1080/09584935.2015.1027662.

Jaffrelot, Christophe. 2017. "Over to the Vigilante." Carnegie Endowment for International Peace. https://carnegieendowment.org/2017/05/13/over-to -vigilante-pub-70028.

Jaffrelot, Christophe. 2019. "A De Facto Ethnic Democracy? Obliterating and Targeting the Other, Hindu Vigilantes, and the Ethno-State." In *Majoritarian State: How Hindu Nationalism Is Changing India*, edited by Angana P. Chatterji, Thomas Blom Hansen, and Christophe Jaffrelot, 41–68. New York: Oxford University Press.

Jaffrelot, Christophe. 2021. *Modi's India: Hindu Nationalism and the Rise of Ethnic Democracy.* Princeton, NJ: Princeton University Press.

Jaffrelot, Christophe, and Laurent Gayer. 2010. *Armed Militias of South Asia: Fundamentalists, Maoists and Separatists.* Oxford: Oxford University Press.

Jain, Anoop, Ashley Wagner, Claire Snell-Rood, and Isha Ray. 2020. "Understanding Open Defecation in the Age of Swachh Bharat Abhiyan: Agency, Accountability, and Anger in Rural Bihar." *International Journal of Environmental Research and Public Health* 17, no. 4: 1384. https://pubmed.ncbi.nlm.nih.gov/32098057/.

Jain, Kajri. 2007. *Gods in the Bazaar: The Economies of Indian Calendar Art.* Durham, NC: Duke University Press.

Jain, Kajri. 2021. *Gods in the Time of Democracy.* Durham, NC: Duke University Press.

Jain, Mayank. 2014. "Indian Women Are Loitering to Make Their Cities Safer." *Scroll,* December 17. https://scroll.in/article/695586/indian-women-are-loitering-to-make-their-cities-safer.

Jain, Shruti. 2017. "Dirty Backstory to 'Swachch Bharat' Lynching: No Toilets, No Water and the Threat of Eviction." *Wire,* June 22. https://thewire.in/politics/conspiracy-masquerades-swachh-bharat-mission-cpi-ml-activists-lynching.

Jairath, Vasundhara. 2021. "Indigeneous Land Grabbed for Solar Power Plant in Assam." *Countercurrents,* December 4. https://countercurrents.org/2021/04/adivasi-land-grabbed-for-solar-power-plant/.

Jansatta. 2017. "Punished for Defecating in the Open; Removed Pants in Front of Everyone, Sit Ups Were Held." YouTube, video, 0:36. https://www.youtube.com/watch?v=EtCRzYB9AWY&list=PLeNldlpJuGwCn7WbBp6StjifbNE7dxm8D&index=7.

Javaid, Maham. 2015. "How India's 'Untouchable' Women Are Fighting Back Against Sexual Violence." *Refinery 29,* October 15. https://www.refinery29.com/en-us/2015/10/95759/dalit-untouchable-women-india-sexual-violence.

Jayawardena, Kumari. 2016. *Feminism and Nationalism in the Third World.* London: Verso.

Jeffrey, Robin. 2015. "Clean India! Symbols, Policies and Tensions." *South Asia: Journal of South Asian Studies* 38, no. 4: 807–19. https://doi.org/10.1080/00856401.2015.1088504.

Jenkins, Henry. 2015. "Affective Publics and Social Media: An Interview with Zizi Papacharissi (Part Two)." *Pop Junctions,* January 21. http://henryjenkins.org/blog/2015/01/affective-publics-and-social-media-an-interview-with-zizi-papacharissi-part-two.html.

Jenkins, Henry, Sam Ford, and Joshua Green. 2013. *Spreadable Media: Creating Value and Meaning in a Networked Culture.* New York: New York University Press.

Jha, Dhirendra K. 2017. *Shadow Armies: Fringe Organizations and Foot Soldiers of Hindutva.* New Delhi: Juggernaut Books.

Jha, Sanjeev. 2017. "'Halla Bol Lungi Khol' Drive Offensive: RMC." *Pioneer* (India), September 29. https://www.dailypioneer.com/2017/state -editions/halla-bol-lungi-khol-drive-offensive-rmc.html.

Jha, Somesh, and Nitin Sethi. 2014. "Ken-Betwa River Link to Hit Panna Tiger Reserve." *Business Standard* (New Delhi), August 23. https://www .business-standard.com/article/economy-policy/ken-betwa-river-link-to -hit-panna-tiger-reserve-114082300811_1.html.

Jha, Vijay Deo. 2017. "ODF: Open Deception Fiasco—Capital's Urban Slums Bare Poop Posers." *Telegraph* (Kolkata), October 4. https://www .telegraphindia.com/jharkhand/odf-open-deception-fiasco-capital-s -urban-slums-bare-poop-posers/cid/1660852.

Jitendra, Verma, Rashmi, Goswami, Subhojit, and Sengupta Shushmita. 2018. "Swachh Bharat Mission: Other Name for Coercion and Deprivation." *Down to Earth*, April 28. https://www.downtoearth.org.in/coverage /governance/swachh-bharat-mission-the-other-name-for-coercion-and -deprivation-60351.

Joseph, Manu. 2014. "Questioning a Rising Star's Exoneration." *New York Times*, February 27. https://www.nytimes.com/2014/02/27/world/asia /27iht-letter27.html.

Kandiyoti, Deniz. 1991. *Women, Islam and the State.* London: Palgrave Macmillan.

Kaplan, Caren. 2013. "Drone Sight." In "Soldier Exposures and Technical Publics," edited by Zoe Wool. Public Books, February 14. https://www .publicbooks.org/soldier-exposures-and-technical-publics/.

Kapur, Avani, and Devashish Deshpande. 2019. "Swacch Bharat Mission-Gramin, GOI 2019–20." Budget Briefs 11, no. 6, Accountability Initiative, Centre for Policy Research. https://accountabilityindia.in/sites/default /files/pdf_files/Swachh_Bharat_Gramin.pdf.

Kapur, Prerna. 2018. "Of Indian Ideals/Idols." *Lacanian Review*, December 15. https://www.thelacanianreviews.com/of-indian-ideals-idols/.

Kapur, Ratna. 2005. *Erotic Justice: Law and the New Politics of Postcolonialism.* Abingdon, UK: Routledge.

Karelia, Gopi. 2017a. "5 Women Who Inspired Us with Their Innova-tive Fight for a Swachh India." NDTV-Dettol, February 28. https:// swachhindia.ndtv.com/5-women-inspired-us-innovative-fight-swachh -india-5268/.

Karelia, Gopi. 2017b. "Drones Deployed in This Town of Telangana to End Open Defecation." NDTV-Dettol, November 17. https:// swachhindia.ndtv.com/drones-deployed-town-telangana-end-open -defecation-14866/.

Karelia, Gopi. 2017c. "Karva Chauth with a Difference: Husbands Take Pledge to Build Toilets for Wives in Uttar Pradesh." NDTV-Dettol, October 9. https://swachhindia.ndtv.com/karva-chauth-difference-husbands-take -pledge-build-toilets-wives-uttar-pradesh-13257/.

Karelia, Gopi. 2017d. "Swachhta Bandhan: Brothers in Varanasi District to Gift Toilets to Sisters This #Rakshabandhan." NDTV-Dettol, August 7. https://swachhindia.ndtv.com/swachhta-bandhan-brothers-varanasi-district-gift-toilets-sisters-rakshabandhan-10505/.

Kaul, Suvir Dar. 2017. *Of Gardens and Graves: Kashmir, Poetry, Politics.* Durham, NC: Duke University Press.

Kaviraj, Sudipta. 1997. "Filth and the Public Sphere." *Public Culture* 10, no. 1: 83–113.

Kedia, Mohnish. 2022. "Sanitation Policy in India—Designed to Fail?" *Policy Design and Practice* 5, no. 3: 307–25.

Khetarpal, Lakshay, dir. 2016. "Swachh Bharat Abhiyan." YouTube, video, 3:00. https://www.youtube.com/watch?v=Dqw_r17zkNA.

Khosla, Saksham, and Aidan Milliff. 2021. "India's Farm Protests Turned Violent Last Week. But Why Are Farmers Protesting in the First Place?" *Washington Post*, February 5. https://www.washingtonpost.com/politics/2021/02/05/indias-farm-protests-turned-violent-last-week-why-are-farmers-protesting-first-place/.

Kidwai, Naina. 2021. "Women's Needs Are Key to Swachh Bharat Success." *Indian Express* (Noida), March 6. https://indianexpress.com/article/opinion/columns/womens-needs-are-key-to-swachh-bharat-success-7216123/.

Kislaya, Kelly. 2017. "Ranchi Civic Body Disrobes Those Defecating in the Open." *Times of India* (Mumbai), September 25. https://timesofindia.indiatimes.com/city/ranchi/ranchi-civic-body-disrobes-those-defecating-in-the-open/articleshow/60820903.cms.

Koonz, Claudia. 2005. *The Nazi Conscience.* Cambridge, MA: Belknap Press.

Koshy, Jacob. 2023. "Jal Jeevan Mission Remains a Pipe Dream." *Hindu* (Chennai), September 16. https://www.thehindu.com/news/national/the-missing-link-in-the-jal-jeevan-scheme-water/article67311157.ece.

Kowtal, Asha. 2019. "Building a Feminism that Centres the Voices of the Oppressed." *Wire*, February 15. https://thewire.in/caste/building-a-feminism-that-centres-the-voices-of-the-oppressed.

Kuchay, Bilal. 2019. "Modi Declares India Open Defecation Free, Claim Questioned." Al Jazeera, October 2. https://www.aljazeera.com/news/2019/10/2/modi-declares-india-open-defecation-free-claim-questioned.

Kumar, D. S. 2019. "Swachh Bharat Abhiyan: What Are the Barries for Toilet Construction." *Down to Earth*, September 10. https://www.downtoearth.org.in/blog/waste/swachh-bharat-abhiyan-what-are-the-barriers-for-toilet-construction-66656.

Kumar, Priyanka, and Shubham Preet. 2020. "Manual Scavenging: Women Face Double Discrimination as Caste and Gender Inequalities Converge." *Economic and Political Weekly* 55, nos. 26–27. https://www.epw.in/engage/article/manual-scavenging-women-face-double-discrimination-caste-gender.

Kumar, Rajiv. 2020. "On an Average, India Reported 10 Cases of Rape of Dalit Women Daily in 2019, NCRB Data Shows." *News18*, October 3. https://www.news18.com/news/india/on-an-average-india-reported-10 -cases-of-rape-of-dalit-women-daily-in-2019-ncrb-data-shows-2930179 .html.

Kumar, Satyam. 2022. "Taps Run Dry Under the Government's Har Ghar Jal Scheme." *IndiaSpend*, June 6. https://www.indiaspend.com/cover-story /taps-run-dry-under-governments-har-ghar-jal-scheme-in-uttarakhand -821009.

Kumar, Sunaina. 2015. "Revolution of the Runaway Brides." *Open*, November 25. https://openthemagazine.com/features/living/revolution-of-the -runaway-brides/.

Kuntsman, Adi. 2017. "Introduction: Whose Selfie Citizenship?" In *Selfie Citizenship*, edited by Adi Kuntsman, 20–27. Cham, Switzerland: Palgrave Macmillan.

Kuntsman, Adi, and Rebecca Stein. 2015. *Digital Militarism: Israel's Occupation in the Social Media Age*. Stanford, CA: Stanford University Press.

Lahariya, Khabar. 2019. "MP: Villagers Forced to Repay Loans as They Await Swachh Bharat Funds." *Wire*, June 28. https://thewire.in/government /swachh-bharat-abhiyan-funds-vilages-loans.

Lahariya, Khabar, and Shreehari Paliath. 2018. "Amid Agri Crisis, Pain for Rural India as Modi Govt Chokes MGNREGS Funding." *Business Standard* (New Delhi), May 4. https://www.business-standard.com/article /economy-policy/amid-agri-crisis-pain-for-rural-india-as-modi-govt -chokes-mgnregs-funding-118050400103_1.html.

Laporte, Dominique. 2002. *History of Shit*. Translated by Nadia Benabid and Rodolphe El-Khoury. Cambridge, MA: MIT Press.

Larkin, Brian. 2008. *Signal and Noise: Media, Infrastructure, and Urban Culture in Nigeria*. Durham, NC: Duke University Press.

Larkin, Brian. 2013. "The Politics and Poetics of Infrastructure." *Annual Review of Anthropology* 42, no. 1: 327–43. https://doi.org/10.1146/annurev-anthro -092412-155522.

Leung, Scarlett. 2016. "Indian Bride Rejects Groom with No Toilet." *DESIblitz*, April 20. https://www.desiblitz.com/content/indian-bride-rejects -groom-with-no-toilet.

Longkumer, Arkotong. 2019. "Playing the Waiting Game: The BJP, Hindutva, and the Northeast." In *Majoritarian State: How Hindu Nationalism Is Changing India*, edited by Angana P. Chatterji, Thomas Blom Hansen, and Christophe Jaffrelot, 281–97. New York: Oxford University Press.

Löw, Christine. 2020. "Under Cover of the Pandemic, Stealth Landgrabs Area Ongoing in India" *Open Democracy*, July 6. https://www.opendemocracy .net/en/oureconomy/under-cover-pandemic-stealth-land-grabs-are -ongoing-india/.

Luthra, Aman. 2018. "'Old Habits Die Hard': Discourses of Urban Filth in Swachh Bharat Mission and the Ugly Indian." *Journal of Multicultural Discourses* 13, no. 2: 120–38. https://doi.org/10.1080/17447143.2018.1467917.

Mahaprashasta, Ajoy. 2019. "Claiming that Rural India Is 'Open Defecation Free' Is Blatant Exaggeration." *Wire*, October 2. https://thewire.in/health/the-claim-that-india-is-odf-is-blatant-exaggeration.

Mahaprashasta, Ajoy Ashirwad. 2022. "As Kanpur Tanneries Face Extinction, Adityanath's (Mis)Rule Dominates Poll Talk." *Wire*, February 19. https://thewire.in/labour/as-kanpur-tanneries-face-extinction-adityanaths-misrule-dominates-poll-talk.

Malhotra, Aanchal. 2017. *Remnants of a Separation: A History of the Partition Through Material History.* Noida: HarperCollins India.

Mali, Vikram, dir. 2016. "Swachh Bharat Abhiyan—Bharat Mata Short Films." YouTube, video, 3:00. https://www.youtube.com/watch?v=wueIMaNoHTA.

Mamdani, Mahmood. 2005. *Good Muslim, Bad Muslim: America, the Cold War, and the Roots of Terror.* New York: Penguin Random House.

Mandavilli, Apoorva. 2018. "The World's Worst Industrial Disaster Is Still Unfolding." *Atlantic*, July 10. https://www.theatlantic.com/science/archive/2018/07/the-worlds-worst-industrial-disaster-is-still-unfolding/560726/.

Mankekar, Purnima. 1999. *Screening Culture, Viewing Politics: An Ethnography of Television, Womanhood, and Nation in Postcolonial India.* Durham, NC: Duke University Press.

Mankekar, Purnima, and Hannah Carlan. 2019. "The Remediation of Nationalism: Viscerality, Virality, and Digital Affect." In *Global Digital Cultures*, edited by Aswin Punathembekar and Sriram Mohan, 203–22. Ann Arbor: University of Michigan Press.

Mann, Steve, and Joseph Ferenbok. 2013. "New Media and the Power Politics of Sousveillance in a Surveillance-Dominated World." *Surveillance and Society* 11, nos. 1/2: 18–34. https://doi.org/10.24908/ss.v11i1/2.4456.

Manorama, Ruth. n.d. "Background Information on Dalit Women in India." In *India—Dalit Women in India.* Women's UN Report Network. https://wunrn.com/2006/12/india-dalit-women-in-india/.

Manral, Anvisha. 2018. "Transgender Individuals Demand Safer Gender-Neutral Bathrooms in India Post-Section 377 Verdict." *Firstpost*, November 21. https://www.firstpost.com/india/transgender-individuals-demand-safer-gender-neutral-bathrooms-in-india-post-section-377-verdict-5414801.html.

Matfess, Hilary. 2015. "Rwanda and Ethiopia: Developmental Authoritarianism and the New Politics of African Strong Men." *African Studies Review* 58, no. 2: 181–204. https://doi.org/10.1017/asr.2015.43.

Mathur, Barkha. 2020. "Swachh Bharat Mission: Transngender Community of Ujjain Becomes a Changemaker as it Leads the Cleanliness Awareness Initiative." NDTV-Dettol, January 21. https://swachhindia.ndtv.com/swachh-bharat-mission-transgender-community-of-ujn-becomes-a-changemaker-as-it-leads-the-way-to-cleaner-lifestyle-41095/.

Mazumdar, Sucheta. 1995. "Women on the March: Right-Wing Mobilization in Contemporary India." *Feminist Review* 49, no. 1: 1–28. https://doi.org/https://doi.org/10.1057/fr.1995.1.

Mbembe, Achille. 2003. "Necropolitics." *Public Culture* 15, no. 1: 11–40. https://doi.org/10.1215/08992363-15-1-11.

McClintock, Anne. 1995. *Imperial Leather: Race, Gender and Sexuality in the Colonial Contest.* New York: Routledge.

Media Eye. 2014. "Modi Urges Youth to Join Clean India Mission." *Media Eye,* October 1. https://www.mediaeyenews.com/national/modi-urges-youths-to-join-clean-india-mission/34977.html.

Mehrotra, Santosh. 2024. "Some Proof Required: Modi Government's Abysmal Record of No Jobs." *Wire,* May 8. https://thewire.in/labour/some-proof-required-modi-government-abysmal-record-no-jobs.

Mekaad, Salil. 2016. "Villager Forced to Clean His Feces with Hands in Ujjain as Part of Swachh Bharat Abhiyan." *Times Of India* (Mumbai), December 29. https://timesofindia.indiatimes.com/city/indore/villager-forced-to-clean-his-feces-with-hands-in-ujjain-as-part-of-swachh-bharat-abhiyan/articleshow/56240660.cms.

Menon, Aditya. 2019. "Truth of 'Beti Bachao Beti Padhao': 56% Funds Spent on Publicity." *Quint,* January 21. https://www.thequint.com/news/india/truth-of-beti-bachao-beti-padhao-funds-spent-on-publicity.

Menon, Nivedita. 2004. *Recovering Subversion: Feminist Politics Beyond the Law.* Urbana: University of Illinois Press.

Menon, Nivedita. 2017. "Bharat Mata and Her Unruly Daughters." *Wire,* July 18. https://thewire.in/featured/bharat-mata-unruly-daughters.

Menon, Nivedita. 2020. "A Critical View on Intersectionality" In *Dalit Feminist Theory: A Reader,* edited by Sunaina Arya and Singh Rathore, 22–37. New York: Routledge.

Menon, Ritu, and Kamla Bhasin. 1998. *Borders and Boundaries: How Women Experienced the Partition of India.* New Brunswick, NJ: Rutgers University Press.

Mihelj, Sabina. 2022. "Platform Nations." *Nations and Nationalism* 29, no. 1: 10–24. https://doi.org/10.1111/nana.12912.

Miller, William. 1998. *The Anatomy of Disgust.* Cambridge, MA: Harvard University Press.

Mirchandani, Maya. 2018. "Digital Hatred, Real Violence: Majoritarian Radicalisation and Social Media in India." Occasional Paper, Observer Research Foundation. https://www.orfonline.org/public/uploads/posts/pdf/20230811130128.pdf.

Misra, Deepti. 2014. *Beyond Partition: Gender, Violence, and Representation in Postcolonial India*. Urbana: University of Illinois Press.

Mittal, Tusha, and Alishan Jafri. 2023. "Driving Muslims Out of 'Devbhoomi: The Sangh's Quest for a Hindu Holy Land.'" *Caravan*, July 31. https://caravanmagazine.in/politics/bjp-rss-create-hindu-holy-land-dev-bhoomi-uttarakhand-muslim-ethnic-cleansing.

MJS (Ministry of Jal Shakti). 2017. "Complete Guidelines for Swachh Bharat Mission (Gramin) 2017." Ministry of Jal Shakti, Department of Drinking Water and Sanitation, Government of India. https://swachhbharatmission.gov.in/sbmcms/writereaddata/images/pdf/Guidelines/Complete-set-guidelines.pdf.

Modi, Narendra [@narendramodi]. 2014. "Tributes to Veer Savarkar on His Birth Anniversary. We Remember & Salute His Tireless Efforts towards the Regeneration of Our Motherland." X (formerly Twitter), May 28. https://twitter.com/narendramodi/status/471512471690170368.

Mohan, Rohini. 2015. "Modi's Seized Earth Campaign." *Foreign Policy*, May 26. https://foreignpolicy.com/2015/05/26/narendra-modi-land-law-acquisition-india/.

Mohan, Sriram. 2015. "Locating the 'Internet Hindu.'" *Television and New Media* 16, no. 4: 339–45. https://doi.org/10.1177/1527476415575491.

Mookerjea-Leonard, Debali. 2017. *Literature, Gender, and the Trauma of Partition: The Paradox of Independence*. London: Routledge.

Moore, Molly. 1994. "Kashmir Fighting Speeds Pollution of India's Idyllic Dal Lake." *Washington Post*, November 1. https://www.washingtonpost.com/archive/politics/1994/11/01/kashmir-fighting-speeds-pollution-of-indias-idyllic-dal-lake/1f3f2dcb-1cb8-42ee-a6fc-e7ff390048a6.

MPBC (Manjunath P. B. Creations). 2018. "Sorry Bharath Mata." YouTube, video, 8:16. https://www.youtube.com/watch?v=PybaXzHeXGU.

Muecke, Stephen. 2003. "Devestation." In *Culture and Waste: The Creation and Destruction of Value*, edited by Gay Hawkins and Stephen Muecke, 117–28. Lanham, MD: Rowman and Littlefield.

Mukherjee, Rahul. 2020. "Mobile Witnessing on WhatsApp: Vigilante Virality and the Anatomy of Mob Lynching." *South Asian Popular Culture* 18, no. 1: 79–101. https://doi.org/10.1080/14746689.2020.1736810.

Mukhopadhyay, Bhaskar. 2006. "Crossing the Howrah Bridge." *Theory, Culture and Society* 23, nos. 7/8: 221–41. https://doi.org/10.1177/0263276406073224.

Mulvey, Laura. 1975. "Visual Pleasure and Narrative Cinema." *Screen* 16, no. 3: 6–18. https://doi.org/10.1093/screen/16.3.6.

Mumbai Mirror. 2018. "Transgenders Educate Villagers About Cleanliness, Build 7500 Toilets." *Mumbai Mirror*, March 16. https://mumbaimirror.indiatimes.com/mumbai/civic/transgenders-educate-villagers-about-cleanliness-build-7500-toilets-in-palghar/articleshow/63334233.cms.

Murty, Madhavi. 2022. *Stories That Bind: Political Economy and Culture in New India*. New Brunswick, NJ: Rutgers University Press.

Nail, Thomas. 1997. "What Is an Assemblage." *Substance* 46, no. 1: 21–37. https://doi.org/10.1353/sub.2017.0001.

Nair, Nithya. 2016. "Win Rs 500 by Clicking Selfie with People Defecating in Open." *India.com*, December 28. https://www.india.com/news/india/win-rs-500-by-clicking-selfie-with-people-defecating-in-open-1728477/.

Najmabadi, Afsaneh. 1997. "The Erotic Vaṭan [Homeland] as Beloved and Mother: To Love, to Possess, and to Protect." *Comparative Studies in Society and History* 39, no. 3: 442–67. https://doi.org/10.1017/s0010417500020727.

Nanda, Meera. 2011. *The God Market: How Globalization Is Making India More Hindu*. New York: Monthly Review Press.

Nanda, Meera. 2016. *Science in Saffron: Skeptical Essays on History of Science*. New Delhi: Three Essays Collective.

Naqash, Rayan. 2019. "After Hindu Group Rally to Support Man Accused of Muslim Child's Rape and Murder, Jammu Rift Widens." *Scroll*, June 11. https://scroll.in/article/869164/hindu-groups-rally-for-accused-in-a-muslim-childs-rape-and-murder-sparks-communal-tension-in-jammu.

Nath, Anjali. 2017. "Stoners, Stones, and Drones: Transnational South Asian Visuality from Above and Below." In *Life in the Age of Drone Warfare*, edited by Lisa Parks and Caren Kaplan, 241–58. Durham, NC: Duke University Press.

NDTV. 2015. "Transgenders Bring Government and Villages Together to Build Toilets." NDTV, November 19, video, 2:30. https://www.ndtv.com/video/transgenders-bring-government-and-villages-together-to-build-toilets-391425.

NDTV. 2019. "No Coercion Under Swachh Bharat, Centre After Dalit Children's Killing." NDTV, September 28. https://www.ndtv.com/india-news/no-coercion-under-swachh-bharat-centre-after-dalit-childrens-killing-2108481.

Neelakandan, Aravindan. 2019. "Toilet, Ek 'Hindutva' Katha: How Modi's Swachh Bharat Draws from the Oldest Upanishads." *Swarajya*, April 8. https://swarajyamag.com/ideas/toilet-ek-hindutva-katha-how-modis-swachh-bharat-draws-from-the-oldest-upanishads.

New Indian Express. 2015. "Selfie with Daughter: Ehsan Jafri's Daughter Shares Picture to 'Haunt' Modi?" *New Indian Express* (Chennai), June 30. https://www.newindianexpress.com/nation/2015/Jun/30/selfie-with-daughter-ehsan-jafris-daughter-shares-picture-to-haunt-modi-776598.html.

Newell, Stephanie. 2020. *Histories of Dirt: Media and Urban Life in Colonial and Postcolonial Lagos*. Durham, NC: Duke University Press.

News18. 2019. "A Pre-Wedding Shoot to Forget: Why 'Selfie with Loo' Has Become a Marriage Ritual in MP." *News18*, October 10. https://www.news18

.com/news/india/a-pre-wedding-shoot-to-forget-why-selfie-with-loo-has
-become-a-marriage-ritual-in-mp-2339961.html.

NewsClick. 2017. "Glaring Corruption in Implementation of Swachh Bharat Abhiyan in UP." *NewsClick*, November 30. https://www.newsclick.in/glaring
-corruption-implementation-swachh-bharat-abhiyan.

News Minute. 2017. "No Toilet at Home Akin to 'Cruelty,' Rajasthan Court Says
While Granting Divorce to Woman." *News Minute*, August 20. https://
www.thenewsminute.com/news/no-toilet-home-akin-cruelty-rajasthan
-court-says-while-granting-divorce-woman-67090.

News Minute. 2018. "Hyd Corporator's Insensitive Selfie, Posts a Pic of Lorry
Driver Defecating in Open." *News Minute*, January 23. https://www
.thenewsminute.com/article/hyd-corporators-insensitive-selfie-posts-pic
-lorry-driver-defecating-open-75233.

NewsX. 2017. "Halla Bol Lungi Khol: Ranchi Municipal Corporation to Punish
Defecators." YouTube, video, 2:13. https://www.youtube.com/watch?v
=mCKZ5tZ7cnE.

Nixon, Rob. 2011. *Slow Violence and the Environmentalism of the Poor*. Cambridge, MA: Harvard University Press.

Nizaruddin, Fathima. 2022. "Institutionalized Riot Networks in India and
Mobile Instant Messaging Platforms." *Asiascape: Digital Asia* 9, nos. 1/2:
71–94. https://doi.org/10.1163/22142312-bja10028.

Omabm Productions. 2016. "Swachh Bharat Abhiyan—Thank You." YouTube,
video, 2:59. https://www.youtube.com/watch?v=H17VdfMui34.

Omjasvin, M. D. 2021. "Toilets Look 'Swachh' on Paper but Dirty Deals
Keep Open Defecation Rampant near Chennai." *New Indian Express*
(Chennai), July 19. https://www.newindianexpress.com/cities/chennai
/2021/Jul/19/toilets-look-swachh-on-paper-but-dirty-deals-keep-open
-defecation-rampant-near-chennai-2332122.html.

Organiser. 2023. "Swachh Bharat: Paving the Way for Swasth Bharat." *Organiser*, October 2. https://organiser.org/2023/10/02/198907/bharat/swachh
-bharat-paving-the-way-for-swasth-bharat/.

Outlook. 2022a. "'Bulli Bai' App Row: BSP MP Accuses Modi Govt of Being
'Apathetic' Towards Muslim Women." *Outlook*, January 4. https://www
.outlookindia.com/website/story/india-news-bulli-bai-app-row-bsp-mp
-accuses-modi-govt-of-being-apathetic-towards-muslim-women/408264.

Outlook. 2022b. "India Needs to Be Self-Reliant: RSS Chief Mohan Bhagwat."
Outlook, August 15. https://www.outlookindia.com/national/india-needs
-to-be-self-reliant-rss-chief-mohan-bhagwat-news-216475.

Oxford Poverty and Human Development Initiative (OPHI). 2018. *Global Multidimensional Poverty Index 2018: The Most Detailed Picture to Date of the
World's Poorest People*. Report. OPHI, University of Oxford.

Paliath, Shreehari, Geeta Devi, and Meera Devi. 2022. "In UP, Centre's Hope
to Provide Safe Tap Water to All by 2024 May Remain a Pipe Dream."

Scroll, September 28. https://scroll.in/article/1033672/in-up-centres
-hope-to-provide-safe-tap-water-by-2024-may-remain-a-pipe-dream.

Pande, Mrinal. 2018. "Angry Hanuman: This Viral Image That Won Modi's
Praise Symbolises Today's Aggressive, Macho India." *Scroll*, May 26.
https://scroll.in/article/879108/angry-hanuman-this-viral-image-that
-won-modis-praise-symbolises-todays-aggressive-macho-india.

Pandey, Gyanendra. 2006. *Routine Violence: Nations, Fragments, Histories.*
Stanford, CA: Stanford University Press.

Papacharissi, Zizi. 2014. *Affective Publics: Sentiment, Technology, and Politics.*
New York: Oxford University Press.

Pareek, Shreya. 2015. "How Children Blew the Whistle to Make this MP
Village Open Defecation Free." *Better India*, July 14. https://www
.thebetterindia.com/28845/how-children-blew-the-whistle-to-make-this
-mp-village-open-defecation-free/.

Parija, Pratik. 2023. "India to Slash Spending on Food Subsidy for 800 Million
People." *Bloomberg News*, February 1. https://www.bloomberg.com/news
/articles/2023-02-01/india-to-slash-spending-on-food-subsidy-for-800
-million-people.

Parks, Lisa, and Caren Kaplan, eds. 2017. *Life in the Age of Drone Warfare.*
Durham, NC: Duke University Press.

Parmar, Sarubh. 2020. "Swachch Bharat Abhiyan—Clean INDIA Initiative:
Objectives, Targets and Progress Report." *Indian Wire*, April 25. https://
www.theindianwire.com/politics/swachch-bharat-abhiyan-207010/.

Pasha, Nizam. 2022. "Supreme Court Judgment in Zakia Jafri Case Missed
both the Woods and the Trees." *Wire*, July 13. https://thewire.in/law
/supreme-court-judgment-in-zakia-jafri-case-missed-both-the-woods
-and-the-trees.

Patel, Sujata, D. Parthasarathy, and George Jose. 2022. *Mumbai/Bombay: Majoritarian Neoliberalism, Informality, Resistance, and Wellbeing.* New York:
Routledge.

Peralta, Eyder. 2018. "The Dark Side of Keeping the Streets Clean in Rwanda's
Capital." NPR, June 25. https://www.npr.org/2018/06/25/623114826/the
-dark-side-of-keeping-the-streets-clean-in-rwanda-s-capital.

Perinchery, Aathira. 2021. "Ken-Betwa Interlink Means 'Bundelkhand Will
Suffer for Decades to Come.'" *Wire*, December 10. https://thewire.in
/environment/ken-betwa-interlink-means-bundelkhand-will-suffer-for
-decades-to-come.

Philipose, Pamela. 2022. "Backstory: Framing a Monstrous Crime of Passion
Through the Lens of 'Love Jihad.'" *Wire*, November 19. https://thewire.in
/media/backstory-mehrauli-murder-reportage.

PIB (Press Information Bureau). 2022a. "Toilets Built Under Swachh Bharat
Mission." Press Information Bureau, Government of India, February 10.
https://pib.gov.in/Pressreleaseshare.aspx?PRID=1797158.

PIB. 2022b. "Year End Review 2022: Department of Drinking Water and Sanitation, Ministry of Jal Shakti." Press Information Bureau, Government of India, December 27. https://pib.gov.in/pib.gov.in/Pressreleaseshare.aspx ?PRID=1886953.

Pinney, Christopher. 2004. *Photos of the Gods: The Printed Image and Political Struggle in India*. London: Reaktion Books.

PM India. 2014. "English Rendering of PM's Address at the Launch of 'Swachh Bharat Mission' at Rajpath." PM India, October 2. https://www.pmindia .gov.in/en/news_updates/english-rendering-of-pms-address-at-the -launch-of-swachh-bharat-mission-at-rajpath/.

PM India. n.d. "Major Initiatives: Swachh Bharat Abhiyan." PM India. https:// www.pmindia.gov.in/en/major_initiatives/swachh-bharat-abhiyan/.

Prabhakar, Parakala. 2023. *The Crooked Timber of New India: Essays on a Republic in Crisis*. New Delhi: Speaking Tiger Books.

Pradhan, Bibhudatta, and Shruti Srivastava. 2022. "India's Modi Cuts Social Spending Even with Local Polls Nearing." *Bloomberg News*, February 4. https://www.bloomberg.com/news/articles/2022-02-04/india-s-modi -cuts-social-spending-even-with-local-polls-nearing.

Pratt, John. 2007. *Penal Populism*. London: Routledge.

Preetika, P. 2023. "Swachh Bharat Mission Toilets Remain Locked in Southern Suburbs." *Times of India* (Mumbai), September 24. https://timesofindia .indiatimes.com/city/chennai/swachh-bharat-mission-toilets-remain -locked-in-southern-suburbs/articleshow/103899242.cms?from=mdr.

PTI (Press Trust of India). 2016a. "Nation Will Not Tolerate Insult to Mother India: Irani." *Daijiworld*, February 12. https://www.daijiworld.com/news /newsDisplay?newsID=380392.

PTI. 2016b. "No Toilet in Groom's House, Kanpur Woman Refuses to Tie Knot." *Indian Express* (Noida), April 17. https://indianexpress.com /article/trending/trending-in-india/no-toilet-in-grooms-house-kanpur -woman-refuses-to-tie-knot-2757870/.

PTI. 2017a. "Hindutva and Development Complementary to Each Other: Yogi Adityanath." *Deccan Chronicle* (Hyderabad), November 15. https:// www.deccanchronicle.com/nation/current-affairs/151117/hindutva-and -development-complementary-to-each-other-yogi-adityanath.html.

PTI. 2017b. "Modi Praises Akshay's 'Toilet Ek Prem Katha' Trailer." *Hindu* (Chennai), June 13. https://www.thehindu.com/news/national/modi -praises-akshays-toilet-ek-prem-katha-trailer/article18970513.ece.

PTI. 2018a. "Inspired by Cleanliness Drive, Maharashtra Couple Names Baby 'Swachhata.'" *Indian Express* (Noida), March 31. https://indianexpress .com/article/india/inspired-by-cleanliness-drive-maharashtra-couple -names-baby-swachhata-5118459/.

PTI. 2018b. "Maharashtra Baby Named 'Swachhata' as Parents Inspired by Cleanliness Drive: Mumbai News." *Times of India* (Mumbai), March 31.

https://timesofindia.indiatimes.com/city/mumbai/maharashtra-baby
-named-swachhata-as-parents-inspired-by-cleanliness-drive/articleshow
/63557862.cms.

PTI. 2018c. "Swachh Bharat: Maharashtra Constructs Most Toilets; BJP-Ruled
States Shine." *Business Standard* (New Delhi), January 21. https://
www.business-standard.com/article/economy-policy/swachh-bharat
-maharashtra-constructs-most-toilets-bjp-ruled-states-shine-118012100236
_1.html.

PTI. 2019a. "Defecating Kids Lynched." *Telegraph* (Kolkata), September 26.
https://www.telegraphindia.com/india/defecating-kids-lynched/cid
/1707553.

PTI 2019b. "Modi Govt Synonymous with National Security, Development:
Shah." *Business Standard* (New Delhi), September 8. https://www.
business-standard.com/article/pti-stories/modi-govt-synonymous-with-
national-security-development-shah-119090800229_1.html.

PTI. 2020. "Kinnars of Ujjain Lead the Way to Cleaner Lifestyle." *Business
Standard* (New Delhi), January 19. https://www.business-standard.com
/article/pti-stories/kinnars-of-ujjain-lead-the-way-to-cleaner-lifestyle
-120011900537_1.html.

PTI. 2021a. "Build Toilets to Tackle Rape: Sulabh Founder to Modi."
Hindu (Chennai), December 4. https://www.thehindu.com/news
/national/build-toilets-to-tackle-rape-sulabh-founder-to-modi
/article6078958.ece.

PTI. 2021b. "Muslim Men Attacked in Assam's Barpeta, Forced to Say Jai Shri
Ram." *Quint*, June 21. www.thequint.com/news/india/muslim-men
-attacked-in-assam-barpeta-forced-to-say-jai-shri-ram#read-more.

PTI. 2022. "Criminalising Marital Rape Will End Institution of Marriage: BJP's
Sushil Modi." *India Today*, February 2. https://www.indiatoday.in/india
/story/criminalising-marital-rape-will-end-institution-of-marriage-bjp
-sushil-modi-1907791-2022-02-02.

PTI. 2023. "India Climbs Eight Places to 127 in Global Gender Index, Says WEF
Report." *Hindu* (Chennai), June 21. https://www.thehindu.com/news
/national/india-climbs-eight-places-to-127-in-global-gender-index-says
-wef-report/article66994156.ece.

Puar, Jasbir K. 2007. *Terrorist Assemblages: Homonationalism in Queer Times*.
Durham, NC: Duke University Press.

Puar, Jasbir K. 2012. "I Would Rather Be a Cyborg than a Goddess: Becoming-
Intersectional in Assemblage Theory." *Philosophia: A Journal of Transconti-
nental Feminism* 2, no. 1: 49–66. https://doi.org/10.1353/phi.2012.a486621.

Puar, Jasbir K. 2013. "Homonationalism as Assemblage: Viral Travels, Affective
Sexualities." *Jindal Global Law Review* 4, no. 2: 23–43.

Pugliese, Joseph. 2020. *Biopolitics of the More-than-Human: Forensic Ecologies
of Violence*. Durham, NC: Duke University Press Books.

Purohit, Makarand. 2016. "Privatising India's Water Is a Bad Idea." *Wire*, October 17. https://thewire.in/politics/water-privatisation.

PuthiyaThalaimurai TV. 2016. "'No Toilet No Marriage': A Bride from Kanpur Rejected to Marry." PuthiyaThalaimurai TV, April 18. YouTube, video, 0:59. https://www.youtube.com/watch?v=91teHF9xnl8.

Raghavan, Sharad. 2022. "Govt Not in Business: Modi Govt Accounts for 72% of All Disinvestment Since 1991, Data Shows." *The Print*, October 31. https://theprint.in/economy/govt-not-in-business-modi-govt-accounts -for-72-of-all-disinvestment-since-1991-data-shows/1185450/.

Raha, Shuma. 2022. "Shraddha's Murder and the Pernicious Bogey of 'Love Jihad.'" *Deccan Herald* (Bengaluru), November 20. https://www .deccanherald.com/opinion/shraddhas-murder-and-the-pernicious -bogey-of-love-jihad-1164270.html.

Rai, Mridu. 2019. "Kashmiris in the Hindu Rashtra." In *Majoritarian State: How Hindu Nationalism Is Changing India*, edited by Angana P. Chatterji, Thomas Blom Hansen, and Christophe Jaffrelot, 259–80. New York: Oxford University Press.

Rajagopal, Arvind. 2001. *Politics After Television: Religious Nationalism and the Reshaping of the Indian Public*. Cambridge: Cambridge University Press.

Rajgopal, Arvind. 2015. "Indian Democracy and Hindu Populism: The Modi Regime." *Social Text Online*, February 27. https://socialtextjournal.org /periscopearticle/indian-democracy-and-hindu-populism-the-modi -regime/.

Rajagopal, Divya. 2017. "World Bank Yet to Release Fund for Swachh Bharat." *Economic Times* (Mumbai), January 10. https://economictimes .indiatimes.com/industry/banking/finance/world-bank-yet-to-release -fund-for-swachh-bharat/articleshow/56429289.cms?from=mdr.

Rajalakshmi, T. K. 2023. "Despite India's Low Ranking in the Global Hunger Index, Modi Government Is Hesitant to Address the Issue." *Frontline*, November 16. https://frontline.thehindu.com/the-nation/public-health /india-red-flags-over-global-hunger-index-ranking-expose-narendra-modi -government-duplicity/article67460978.ece.

Ramanathan, Usha. 2019. "Foreword." In *The Right to Sanitation in India: Critical Perspectives*, edited by Philippe Cullet, Sujith Koonan, and Lovleen Bhullar, xv–xviii. Delhi: Oxford University Press.

Ramaswamy, Sumathi. 2010. *The Goddess and the Nation: Mapping Mother India*. Durham, NC: Duke University Press.

Rancière, Jacques. 2004. *The Politics of Aesthetics: The Distribution of the Sensible*. Translated by Gabriel Rockhill. New York: Continuum.

Ranhotra, Sanbeer Singh. 2020. "Feminists Are No Holy Cows, Amit Shah's Direct Attack on Pinjra Tod Is a Clear Cut Sign of It." TFI Post, May 24. https://tfipost.com/2020/05/feminists-are-no-holy-cows-amit-shahs -straight-attack-on-pinjra-tod-is-a-clear-cut-sign-of-it/.

Rao, Anupama. 2009. *The Caste Question: Dalits and the Politics of Modern India*. Berkeley: University of California Press.

Rao, Pallavi Rao. 2019. "Soch Aur Shauch: Reading Brahmansm and Patriarchy in 'Toilet Ek Prem Katha.'" *Studies in South Asian Film and Media* 9, no. 2: 79–96. https://doi.org/ https://doi.org/10.1386/safm.9.2.79_1.

Rao, Shakuntala. 2018. "Making of Selfie Nationalism: Narendra Modi, the Paradigm Shift to Social Media Governance, and Crisis of Democracy." *Journal of Communication Inquiry* 42, no. 2: 166–83. https://doi.org /10.1177/0196859917754053.

Ratnu, Omendra. 2022. "From the US to UP, Hindus Are Awakening: Of Hope and Caution Because the Task for Our Generation Is Cut Out." *OpIndia*, September 28. https://www.opindia.com/2022/09/from-the-usa-to-up -hindus-are-awakening-hope-caution/.

Rege, Sharmila. 1998. "Dalit Women Talk Differently: A Critique of Difference and Towards a Dalit Feminist Standpoint Position." *Economic and Political Weekly* 33, no. 44: WS39–WS46.

Rege, Sharmila. 2005. "A Dalit Feminist Standpoint." In *Gender and Caste: Issues in Contemporary Indian Feminism*, editd by Anupama Rao, 90–101. London: Zed Books.

Reuters. 2019a. "Amit Shah Vows to Throw Illegal Immigrants into Bay of Bengal." *Open View*, April 1. https://theopenview.in/2019/04/13/amit-shah -vows-to-throw-illegal-immigrants-into-bay-of-bengal/.

Reuters. 2019b. "France Needs 'Society of Vigilance' Against Islamist 'Hydra': Macron." October 8. https://reuters.com/article/world /france-needs-society-of-vigilance-against-islamist-hydra-macron -idUSKBN1WN16o/.

Richards, Matthew S. 2016. "The Gulabi Gang, Violence, and the Articulation of Counterpublicity." *Communication, Culture and Critique* 9, no. 4: 558–76. https://doi.org/10.1111/cccr.12139.

Rodgers, Dennis, and Bruce O'Neill. 2012. "Infrastructural Violence: Introduction to the Special Issue." *Ethnography* 13, no. 4: 401–12. https://journals .sagepub.com/doi/10.1177/1466138111435738.

Roy, Arundhati. 2020. *Azadi: Freedom, Fascism, Fiction*. Chicago: Haymarket Books.

Roy, Srila. 2016. "Breaking the Cage." *Dissent*, Fall 2016. https://www.dissentmaga zine.org/article/breaking-cage-india-feminism-sexual-violence-public-space.

Rukmini, S. 2021. "Survey Data Again Casts Doubt over Reality of Open Defecation-Free India." *Mint* (Bengaluru), January 13. https://www .livemint.com/news/india/survey-data-again-casts-doubt-over-reality-of -open-defecation-free-india-11610516625786.html.

Russell, Bertie, Andre Pusey, and Paul Chatterton. 2011. "What Can an Assemblage Do?" *City* 15, no. 5: 577–83. https://doi.org /10.1080/13604813.2011.609024.

Sabrang. 2015. "Stop Killing Us." *Sabrang*, December 21. https://sabrangindia
.in/stop-killing-us-bhim-yatra-indias-manual-scavengers-tells-indian
-government/.

Sachdev, Chhavi. 2017. "Watch Women Shame Men Who Pee in Public."
NPR, May 29. https://www.npr.org/sections/goatsandsoda/2017/05/29
/530244262/watch-women-shame-men-who-pee-in-public.

Sandhu, Kulwinder. 2017. "Dalits Allege Bias, Say Water Supply Cut." *Tribune*
(Chandigarh), June 3. https://www.tribuneindia.com/news/archive
/punjab/dalits-allege-bias-say-water-supply-cut-416691.

Sanjai, P. R. 2018. "World's Biggest Nationwide Toilet Building Campaign
Is Creating New Markets in India." *The Print*, July 31. https://theprint
.in/economy/worlds-biggest-nationwide-toilet-building-campaign-is
-creating-new-markets-in-india/90875/.

Sanjiv, Deepthi. 2019. "Viral Art: Chowkidar Sher Hai Poster." *Times of India*,
March 28. https://timesofindia.indiatimes.com/elections/lok-sabha
-elections-2019/karnataka/news/latest-viral-art-chowkidar-sher-hai
-poster/articleshow/68609098.cms.

Sarkar, Pradeep, dir. 2016. "#DontLetHerGo." YouTube, video, 2:45. https://
www.youtube.com/watch?v=jezSduqsRjs.

Sarkar, Tanika. 1987. "Nationalist Iconography: Image of Women in
19th Century Bengali Literature." *Economic and Political Weekly* 22, no. 47:
2011–15.

Sarkar, Tanika. 2001. *Hindu Wife, Hindu Nation: Community, Religion, and
Cultural Nationalism*. Bloomington: Indiana University Press.

Sarkar, Tanika. 2002. "Semiotics of Terror: Muslim Children and Women in
Hindu Rashtra." *Economic and Political Weekly* 37, no. 28: 2872–76.

Sarkar, Tanika, and Urvashi Butalia, eds. 1995. *Women and Right-Wing Movements: Indian Experiences*. London: Zed Books.

Savarkar, Vinayak Damodar. 2022. *Hindutva: Who Is a Hindu?* Edited by Jagath
Jayaprakash. Independently published.

Sax, Boria. 2013. *Animals in the Third Reich*. London: Continuum Press.

Sayeed, Vikhar Ahmed. 2021. "Unmasking Hindutva." *Hindu* (Chennai),
September 24. https://frontline.thehindu.com/the-nation/unmasking
-hindutva-looking-back-on-dismantling-global-hindutva-online
-conference-september-2021/article36628499.ece.

SBM (Swachh Bharat Mission). 2016a. "Amitabh Bachchan as 'Jadugar'- Swachh
Bharat Mission." YouTube, video, 1:06. https://www.youtube.com/watch
?v=ENFqgP6J6nY.

SBM. 2016b. "Khyora Katri Village in Kalyanpur Block of District Kanpur is
Adopting New-Age Technology to Stop People from Defecating in the
Open." Facebook, August 28. https://www.facebook.com/SBMGramin
/photos/khyora-katri-village-in-kalyanpur-block-of-district-kanpur-is
-adopting-new-age-t/1774094492861956/.

SBM. 2016c. "ODF War Room Is Cooch Behar's Winning Strategy." Swachh Bharat Mission (Grameen), December 21. https://sbmgramin.wordpress.com/2016/12/21/odf-war-room-is-cooch-behars-winning-strategy/.

Scott, Linda. 2013. "Abused Indian Goddesses: Controversial Ad Campaign Against Gender Violence." Double X Economy, September 12. https://www.doublexeconomy.com/post/abused-indian-goddesses-controversial-ad-campaign-against-gender-violence.

Sedgwick, Eve Kosofsky. 1985. *Between Men: English Literature and Male Homosocial Desire*. New York: Columbia University Press.

Sehgal, Rashme. 2019. "Is 'Nal Se Jal' Just a Pipe Dream?" *Wire*, June 9. https://thewire.in/environment/nal-se-jal-water-scarcity.

Seltenrich, Nate. 2018. "Down to Earth: The Emerging Field of Planetary Health." *Environmental Health Perspectives* 126, no. 7: 072001. https://ehp.niehs.nih.gov/doi/10.1289/ehp2374.

Sen, Amartya. 1999. *Development as Freedom*. Oxford: Oxford University Press.

Sen, Atreyee. 2007. *Shiv Sena Women: Violence and Communalism in a Bombay Slum*. Bloomington: Indiana University Press.

Sen, Atreyee. 2018. "Security and Purity: Female Surveillance, Child Vigilantism, and the Moral Policing of Deviant Women in Two Radicalized Indian Slums." *Current Anthropology* 59, no. 5: 549–71. https://doi.org/10.1086/699898.

Sen, Geeti. 2002. "Iconising the Nation: Political Agendas." *India International Centre Quarterly* 29, nos. 3/4: 154–75. http://www.jstor.org/stable/23005824.

Sen, Suhit K. 2023. "Hunger Stalks India, Modi Government in Denial." *Deccan Herald* (Bengaluru), October 16. https://www.deccanherald.com/opinion/hunger-stalks-india-modi-government-in-denial-2728345.

Shah, Shreya. 2017. "India's Wildlife Crisis, and Why Hope Is So Important." *IndiaSpend*, July 8. https://www.indiaspend.com/indias-wildlife-crisis-and-why-hope-is-so-important-19304/.

Shanmughasundaram, J. 2018. "Toilets Constructed Under Swachh Bharat Mission Hardly Fit for Purpose." *Times of India* (Mumbai), January 8. https://timesofindia.indiatimes.com/city/chennai/toilets-constructed-under-swachh-bharat-mission-hardly-fit-for-purpose/articleshow/62407335.cms.

Shantha, Sukanya. 2017. "Demolitions, Evictions and Toilets for Show: How Indore Won Swachh Bharat's Top Rank." *Wire*, October 2. https://thewire.in/politics/indore-swachh-bharat-abhiyan.

Sharma, Abhishek. 2024. "PM Modi Continues to Face Unemployment Crisis, Poverty in His Third Working Tenure Too." *BW People*, June 5. https://bwpeople.in/article/pm-modi-continues-to-face-unemployment-crisis-poverty-in-his-third-working-tenure-too-522158.

Sharma, Hemender. 2017. "Swachh Bharat Mission: Death for Those Defecating in the Open in Madhya Pradesh." *India Today*, January 5. https://www.indiatoday.in/india/story/swachh-bharat-mission-madhya-pradesh-death-defecating-meghnagar-nagar-panchayat-ujjain-jhabua-953379-2017-01-05.

Sharma, Saurabh. 2019. "PM Modi Wants to Replace Constitution with Manusmriti: Savitri Phule." *NewsClick*, March 5. https://www.newsclick.in/pm-modi-wants-replace-constitution-manusmriti-savitri-phule.

Sharma, Saurabh. 2020. "'Friends of Coronavirus': Police in North India Shame Those Defying Lockdown." Reuters, March 24. https://www.reuters.com/article/us-health-coronavirus-india-police-idUSKBN21B23Z.

Sharma, Shalini. 2017. "Narendra Modi: Women Empowered." *Sulabh Swachh Bharat*, July 31–August 6. https://issuu.com/sulabhindia/docs/31-06_august-2017_english.

Shekhar, Sudsanshu. 2023. "Sanitising India or Cementing Injustice? Scrutinising the Swachh Bharat Mission in India." *Caste* 4, no. 1: 130–43. https://doi.org/ https://doi.org/10.26812/caste.v4i1.418.

Shibli, Murtaza 2019. "Hindutva Vigilantism and Muslims: Institutionalization of Violence." *Policy Perspectives* 16, no. 1: 137–48. https://doi.org/10.13169/polipers.16.1.0137.

Shih, Gerry, Niha Masih, and Anant Gupta. 2020. "How Political Will Often Favors a Coal Billionaire and His Dirty Fossil Fuel." *Washington Post*, December 9. https://www.washingtonpost.com/world/2022/12/09/india-coal-gautam-adani-godda/.

Shivadekar, Sanjeev. 2015. "Clean-Up Marshalls Will Patrol Streets Once More, Says BMC." *Mumbai Mirror*, December 17. https://mumbaimirror.indiatimes.com/mumbai/civic/clean-up-marshals-will-patrol-streets-once-more-says-bmc/articleshow/50211422.cms.

Shome, Raka. 2014. *Diana and Beyond: White Femininity, National Identity, and Contemporary Media Culture*. Champaign: University of Illinois Press.

Shome, Raka. 2019. "When Postcolonial Studies Interrupts Media Studies." *Communication, Culture and Critique* 12, no. 3: 305–22. https://doi.org/10.1093/ccc/tcz020.

Simone, A. M. 2004. "People as Infrastructure: Intersecting Fragments in Johannesburg." *Public Culture* 16, no. 3: 407–29. https://muse.jhu.edu/article/173743.

Singh, Ananya, and Pooja Jain. 2018. "Significance of Political Advertisements in Indian Society: A Critical Analysis on 'Swachh Bharat Mission.'" *Journal of Management Practices, Humanities and Social Sciences* 2, no. 2: 35–41. https://doi.org/10.33152/jmphss-2.2.2.

Singh, Atyasha, and Ramashankar Mishra. 2019. "Swachh Bharat Mission in Bihar Stumbling Due to Government Corruption and Slow Construction of Toilets, Says Villagers." *Firstpost,* January 10. https://firstpost .com/india/swachh-bharat-mission-in-bihar-stumbling-due-to-govt -corruption-and-slow-construction-of-toilets-say-villagers-5864481 .html.

Singh, Neha. 2017. "Mother India and Ambedkar's India." *Forward Press,* September 28. https://www.forwardpress.in/2017/09/mother-india-and -ambedkars-india/.

Singh, Poonam. 2016. "Bharat Mata and the Ideal Indian Woman." *Feminism in India,* April 29. https://feminisminindia.com/2016/04/29/bharat-mata -indian-womanhood-2/.

Singh, Shree Narayan, dir. 2017. *Toilet: Ek Prem Katha* (Toilet: A love story). Viacom 18 Motion Pictures. 155 mins.

Sinha, Indra. 2009. "Bhopal: 25 Years of Poison." *Guardian,* December 3. https://www.theguardian.com/environment/2009/dec/04/bhopal-25 -years-indra-sinha.

Sircar, Oishik. 2021. "A Deep and Ongoing Dive into the Brutal Humanism that Undergirds Liberalism: An Interview with Jasbir Puar." *Humanity Journal* 11, no. 3: 332–51 https://humanityjournal.org/issue11-3/a-deep -and-ongoing-dive-into-the-brutal-humanism-that-undergirds-liberalism -an-interview-with-jasbir-k-puar/.

Sivakami, P. 2021. "Gender and Sexual Politics of Hindutva." Paper presented at the "Dismantling Global Hindutva" conference, September 10–12, 2021.

SKS (Shri Krishna Studio). 2017. "Woman Caught Defecating in the Open." YouTube, video, 0:50. https://www.youtube.com/watch?v=o7H4q6Rh88E&list =PLeNldlpJuGwCn7WbBp6StjifbNE7dxm8D&index=9.

Smith, Virginia. 2009. *Clean: A History of Personal Hygiene and Purity.* Oxford: Oxford University Press.

Spivak, Gayatri Chakravorty. 2003. *Death of a Discipline.* New York: Columbia University Press.

Spivak, Gayatri Chakravorty. 2009. "Nationalism and the Imagination." *Lectora* 15: 75–98.

Spivak, Gayatri Chakravorty. 2015. "Planetarity." *Paragraph* 38, no. 2: 290–92.

SRC (Sambodhi Research and Communications). n.d. "Access to Toilets and the Safety, Convenience and Self-Respect of Women in India." Report, Swachh Bharat Mission. https://swachhbharatmission.ddws.gov.in /sites/default/files/Studies-and-surveys/Safety-security-and-dignity-of -women.pdf.

Srinivas, Tulasi. 2002. "Flush with Success." *Space and Culture* 5, no. 4: 368–86. https://doi.org/10.1177/1206331202005004004.

Srivastav, Nikhil, and Nazar Khalid. 2019. "What India's Next Sanitation Policy Can Learn from the Swachh Bharat Mission." *Wire,* October 2. https://

thewire.in/government/what-indias-next-sanitation-policy-can-learn
-from-the-swachh-bharat-mission.

Srivastava, Rajiv. 2017. "PM Narendra Modi: 'Izzat Ghar' Will Protect
Dignity of the House." *Times of India* (Mumbai), September 23.
https://timesofindia.indiatimes.com/city/varanasi/pm-narendra-modi
-izzat-ghar-will-protect-dignity-of-the-house/articleshow/60806440
.cms.

Srivastava, Ritesh. 2014. "PM Modi Launches 'Swachh Bharat Abhiyan,' Says
It's Patriotism Not Politics." *Zee News*, May 6. https://zeenews.india
.com/news/india/pm-modi-launches-swachh-bharat-abhiyan-says-its
-patriotism-not-politics_1479062.html.

Srivastava, Sanjay. 2015. "Modi-Masculinity: Media, Manhood, and 'Traditions' in a Time of Consumerism." *Television and New Media* 16, no. 4:
331–38. https://doi.org/10.1177/1527476415575498.

Srivastava, Sanjay. 2019. "The Making of Toxic Hindu Masculinity." *Firstpost*,
March 18. https://www.firstpost.com/india/the-making-of-toxic-hindu
-masculinity-6266861.html.

Stallybrass, Peter, and Allon White. 1986. *The Politics and Poetics of Transgression*. Ithaca, NY: Cornell University Press.

Star, Susan Leigh. 1999. "The Ethnography of Infrastructure." *American Behavioral Scientist* 43, no. 3: 377–91. https://doi.org
/10.1177/00027649921955326.

Suares, Coreena. 2017. "Telangana: Saying It with a Toilet This Raksha
Bandhan." *Deccan Chronicle* (Bengaluru), August 5. https://www
.deccanchronicle.com/nation/current-affairs/060817/telangana-saying-it
-with-a-toilet-this-raksha-bandhan.html.

Subrahmaniam, Vidya. 2017. "There Can Be No Swachh Bharat Without
Ending Institutional Discrimination Against Dalits." *Wire*, October 31.
https://thewire.in/caste/can-no-swachh-bharat-without-ending
-institutional-discrimination-dalits.

Subramaniam, Banu. 2019. *Holy Science: The Biopolitics of Hindu Nationalism*.
Seattle: University of Washington Press.

Subramaniam, Sujatha. 2019. "Is Hindutva Masculinity on Social Media Producing a Culture of Violence Against Women and Muslims?" *Economic
and Political Weekly* 54, no. 15. https://www.epw.in/engage/article
/hindutva-masculinity-social-media-producing-violence-against-women
-muslims.

Sulabh Swachh Bharat. 2017. "Narendra Modi: Women Empowered." *Sulabh
Swachh Bharat* 1, no. 33 (July 31–August 6).

Sumedh, M. K. 2018. "ODF Status—Claims vs Reality of the Swachh Bharat
Mission." Observer Research Foundation, October 6. https://www
.orfonline.org/expert-speak/odf-status-claims-vs-reality-swachh-bharat
-mission.

Sundaram, Ravi. 2020. "Hindu Nationalism's Crisis Machine." HAU: *Journal of Ethnographic Theory* 10, no. 3: 734–41. https://doi.org/10.1086/712222.

Suraj, Sagar. 2017. "Union Minister Caught Urinating in Public, Says There Was No Urinal Nearby." *Hindustan Times* (New Delhi), June 29. https://www.hindustantimes.com/india-news/minister-radha-mohan-singh-caught-urinating-in-public-says-there-was-no-urinal-nearby/story-tC2O8TPWYeZbFE8UmaV1aP.html.

Suta Dogra, Chander. 2023. "Kashi Vishwanath Corridor Project Done, Varanasi Holds Its Breath for Bigger Changes." *Wire*, January 15. https://thewire.in/religion/kashi-vishwanath-corridor-varanasi-gyanvapi.

Swachhata Darshan. 2016. "Women's Safety." YouTube, video, 0:40. https://www.youtube.com/watch?v=d9ny3-IPfqs.

Talukdar, Joyeeta. 2019. "Only Team Effort to 'Clean Up Our Act' Can Make Swachh Bharat Successful." *Youth Ki Awaaz*, October 15. https://www.youthkiawaaz.com/2019/10/bharatiyas-and-swachh-bharat-abhiyan-healthandlife/.

Tan, Rebecca. 2018. "President Duterte Waged a War Against Drug Suspects. Next Up? Street Loiterers." *Washington Post*, July 3. https://www.washingtonpost.com/news/worldviews/wp/2018/07/03/president-duterte-waged-a-war-against-drug-suspects-next-up-street-loiterers/.

Taneja, Richa. 2018. "Kathua Rape Case: From Kaskhay Kumar to Karan Johar, Celebs Demand Justice." NDTV, April 14. https://www.ndtv.com/india-news/kathua-rape-case-from-akshay-kumar-to-karan-johar-celebs-demand-justice-1836772.

Tapscott, Rebecca. 2020. "Militarized Masculinity and the Paradox of Restrain: Mechanisms of Social Control Under Modern Authoritarianism." *International Affairs* 96, no. 6: 1565–84. https://doi.org/10.1093/ia/iiaa163.

Tata Steel. 2019. "Swachh Bharat and Ezynest." Tata Steel. https://www.tatasteel.com/corporate/our-organisation/campaigns/swachh-bharat-and-ezynest/.

Taussig, Michael T. 1999. *Defacement: Public Secrecy and the Labor of the Negative.* Stanford, CA: Stanford University Press.

TCI (Think Change India). 2015. "This Transgender Is Using Her Skills to Spead the Message of Cleanliness and Hygiene Among Villagers." *YourStory*, November 21. https://yourstory.com/2015/11/sanjana-singh.

Team Divine. 2020. "New Bharat Mata—A Short Documentary for Swachh Bharat Abhiyan." YouTube, video, 5:12 . https://www.youtube.com/watch?v=ts_bSCA6b4Q.

Teltumbde, Anand. 2018. *Republic of Caste: Thinking Equality in the Time of Neoliberal Hindutva.* New Delhi: Navayana.

Tewari, Ruhi, and Abhishek Mishra. 2019. "Every Second ST, Every Third Dalit and Muslim in India Poor, Not Just Financially: UN Report." *The*

Print, July 12. https://theprint.in/india/every-second-st-every-third-dalit
-muslim-in-india-poor-not-just-financially-un-report/262270/.

Thompson, Michael. 2017. *Rubbish Theory*. Cambridge: Pluto.

Times of India. 2016. "Drones to Shame Haryana Villagers into Toilets." *Times
of India* (Mumbai), September 19. https://timesofindia.indiatimes
.com/city/chandigarh/drones-to-shame-haryana-villagers-into-toilets
/articleshow/54399670.cms.

Times of India. 2018a. "Rape-Murder in Kathua Meant to Drive Out Muslim Tribe." *Times of India* (Mumbai), April 12. https://timesofindia
.indiatimes.com/india/rape-murder-in-kathua-meant-to-drive-out
-muslim-tribe/articleshow/63721581.cms.

Times of India. 2018b. "Singapore and India: A Shared Vision for a Clean
Future." *Times of India* (Mumbai), October 2. https://timesofindia
.indiatimes.com/india/singapore-india-a-shared-vision-for-a-clean-future
/articleshow/66035768.cms.

Times of India. 2021. "Dabur's Karwa Chauth Ad Row: Company Takes Down Ad
with Lesbian Couple After MP Minister's Warning." *Times of India* (Mumbai), October 26. https://timesofindia.indiatimes.com/business/india
-business/daburs-karwa-chauth-ad-row-company-takes-down-ad-with
-lesbian-couple-after-mp-ministers-warning/articleshow/87274601.cms.

Times of India. 2022a. "To Condemn Every Man as Rapist Not Advisable."
Times of India (Mumbai), February 3. https://timesofindia.indiatimes
.com/india/to-condemn-every-man-as-rapist-not-advisable-smriti-irani
/articleshow/89311448.cms.

Times of India. 2022b. "VHP's Helpline to 'Protect Hindus from Jihadi Forces.'"
Times of India (Mumbai), July 9. https://timesofindia.indiatimes.com
/india/vhps-helpline-to-protect-hindus-from-jihadi-forces/articleshow
/92758627.cms.

Times Now. 2022. "Full Text of PM Modi's Independence Day Speech 2022."
Times Now, August 15. https://www.timesnownews.com/india/full-text
-of-pm-modis-independence-day-speech-2022-article-93572730.

Tiwari, Abhishek Kumar. 2016. "Dabba Dol Gang Is Fighting Against Open
Defecation." *Dainik Jagran Inext* (Kanpur, India), May 5. https://www
.inextlive.com/dabba-dol-gang-is-fighting-against-open-defecation
-201605050033.

Tomar, Shruti. 2017. "In Gwalior, Win Rs 100 for Every Photo You Click of
People Defecating in the Open." *Hindustan Times* (New Delhi), September 15. https://www.hindustantimes.com/india-news/in-gwalior-win-rs
-100-for-every-photo-you-click-of-people-defecating-in-the-open/story
-R30OuZqNAKLQbqSQlVCNtI.html.

Trivedi, Divya. 2019. "Officials Under Pressure to Meet Toilet Construction
Targets." *Frontline*, October 1. https://frontline.thehindu.com/dispatches
/article29565664.ece.

Trivedi, Vivek. 2017. "Officials Force Man to Get Naked, Do Sit-Ups for Defecating in Open." *News18*, February 23. https://www.news18.com/news/india/officials-force-man-to-get-naked-do-sit-ups-for-defecating-in-open-1352431.html.

Truelove, Yaffa, and Kathleen O'Reilly. 2021. "Making India's Cleanest City: Sanitation, Intersectionality, and Infrastructural Violence." *Environment and Planning E: Nature and Space* 4, no. 3: 718–35. https://doi.org/10.1177/2514848620941521.

Truelove, Yaffa, and Hanna A. Ruszczyk. 2022. "Bodies as Urban Infrastructure: Gender, Intimate Infrastructures and Slow Infrastructural Violence." *Political Geography* 92: 102492. https://www.sciencedirect.com/science/article/pii/S0962629821001529.

Tsing, Anna, Bubandt Nils, Gan Elaine, and Swanson Heather, eds. 2017. *Art of Living on a Damaged Planet*. Minneapolis: University of Minnesota Press.

Turner, Elen. 2012. "Empowering Women? Feminist Responses to Hindutva." *Intersections: Gender and Sexuality in Asia and the Pacific* 28. http://intersections.anu.edu.au/issue28/turner.htm.

Tyler, Imogen. 2013. *Revolting Subjects*. London: Zed Books.

Udupa, Sahana. 2015. "Archiving as History-Making: Religious Politics of Social Media in India." *Communication, Culture and Critique* 9, no. 2: 212–30. https://doi.org/10.1111/cccr.12114.

Udupa, Sahana. 2019. "Nationalism in the Digital Age: Fun as a Metapractice of Extreme Speech." *International Journal of Communication* 13: 3143–63.

UNDP (United Nations Development Programme). 2022. "Human Development Report 2021/2022: Uncertain Times, Unsettled Lives." United Nations Development Programme. https://hdr.undp.org/system/files/documents/global-report-document/hdr2021-22reportenglish_0.pdf.

Upadhyay, Aishwarya. 2019a. "Demeaning, Illegal, Lethal yet Prevalent: Manual Scavenging Continues Despite Being Banned 25 Years Ago." NDTV, March 8. https://swachhindia.ndtv.com/manual-scavenging-india-2018-status-swachh-bharat-abhiyan-32161/.

Upadhyay, Aishwarya. 2019b. "Only a Swacch India Can Become a Swasth Bharat: Amitabh Bachchan on Supporting the Clean India Cause." NDTV-Dettol, October 11. https://swachhindia.ndtv.com/this-is-how-campaign-ambassador-amitabh-bachchan-leading-cause-swasth-swachh-india-39184/.

Upadhyay, Nishant. 2020. "Hindu Nation and Its Queers: Caste, Islamophobia, and De/Coloniality in India." *Interventions* 22, no. 4: 464–80. https://doi.org/10.1080/1369801X.2020.1749709.

Us Salam, Ziya. 2016. "The Focus Has to Be on the Safai Karamchari Women." *Frontline*, August 17. https://frontline.thehindu.com/the-nation/the-focus-has-to-be-on-the-safai-karamchari-women/article8986010.ece.

Vashisht, Mahima. 2018. "Swachh Shakti: Why More Women Must Come Forward to Spearhead the Sanitation Revolution." *Swarajya*, February 25.

https://swarajyamag.com/ideas/swachh-shakti-why-more-women-must
-come-forward-to-spearhead-the-sanitation-revolution.

Venugopal, Vasudha. 2014. "Swachh Bharat Mission: Government Makes
Toilet Photos Must to End Bogus Claims." *Economic Times* (Mumbai),
November 12. https://economictimes.indiatimes.com/news/politics-and
-nation/swachh-bharat-mission-government-makes-toilet-photos-must
-to-end-bogus-claims/articleshow/45116352.cms.

Verma, Lalmani. 2017. "Anti-Romeo and Love Jihad: Experiments in Moral
Policing in Uttar Pradesh." *Indian Express* (Noida), March 23. https://
indianexpress.com/article/explained/anti-romeo-love-jihad-experiments
-in-moral-policing-in-uttar-pradesh/.

Vinayak, Gayatri. 2017. "Towards an ODF India: The Women Sanitation
Crusaders of India." *Yahoo News*, April 11. https://www.yahoo.com
/news/towards-an-odf-india-the-women-sanitation-crusaders-of-india
-034802730.html.

Vohra, Supriya. 2022. "Government Claims Every Household in Goa Has
Piped Water; Records, Residents Disagree." *Mongabay*, October 27.
https://india.mongabay.com/2022/10/government-claims-every
-household-in-goa-has-piped-water-records-residents-disagree/.

Wacquant, Loïc. 2009. *Punishing the Poor: The Neoliberal Government of Social
Insecurity*. Durham, NC: Duke University Press.

Waghre, Abhijit. 2023. "Caste's Role in Shaping Water Access Is Missing
from Indian Environmental Discourse." *Wire*, August 14. https://
thewire.in/caste/caste-water-access-missing-india-environmental
-discourse.

Walsh, James P. 2014. "Watchful Citizens: Immigration Control, Surveillance
and Societal Participation." *Social and Legal Studies* 23, no. 2: 237–59.
https://doi.org/10.1177/0964663913519286.

Wells, Corin. 2017. "No Loo? No I Do!" Tushy, October 5. https://hellotushy
.com/blogs/the-posterior/no-loo-no-i-do.

Willis, Graham Denyer. 2015. *The Killing Consensus: Police, Organized Crime,
and the Regulation of Life and Death in Urban Brazil*. Berkeley: University
of California Press.

Wire. 2017. "Ranchi Civic Body Resorts to Public Shaming, Fining Open
Defecators." *Wire*, September 26. https://thewire.in/government/ranchi
-civic-body-resorts-public-shaming-fining-open-defecators.

Wire. 2019. "Swachh Bharat Unable to Popularise Safest Type of Toilets:
Report." *Wire*, January 11. https://thewire.in/government/twin-pit-toilet
-swachh-bharat.

Withnall, Adam. 2019. "Bhopal Gas Leak." *Independent* (London), February 14.
https://www.independent.co.uk/news/world/asia/bhopal-gas-leak
-anniversary-poison-deaths-compensation-union-carbide-dow-chemical
-a8780126.html.

Xu, Yuhan. 2018. "China's 'Toilet Revolution' Is Flush with Lavish Loos." NPR, February 3. https://www.npr.org/sections/goatsandsoda/2018/02/03/579283921/chinas-toilet-revolution-is-flush-with-lavish-loos.

Yadav, Anumeha. 2018. "Swachh Bharat Abhiyan: Four Years On, Ground Visits Show Many Targets Were Met Through Coercion and Exclusion." *HuffPost*, January 31. https://www.huffpost.com/archive/in/entry/swachh-bharat-abhiyan-four-years-on-ground-visits-show-many-targets-were-met-through-coercion-and-exclusion_in_5c11fed9e4b0508b21371cff.

Yadavar, Swagata, 2017. "World Bank Rates Swachh Bharat Abhiyan as 'Moderately Unsatisfactory.'" NDTV-Dettol, May 24. https://swachhindia.ndtv.com/world-bank-rates-swachh-bharat-abhiyan-moderately-unsatisfactory-7873/.

Yengde, Suraj. 2023. "71% Dalits Are Landless Labourers, Dalits Want the Land." *Ambedkarite Today*, March 28. https://www.ambedkaritetoday.com/2019/06/Article-71-percent-Dalits-are-landless-labourers-Suraj-Yengde.html.

YFI (Yes Foundation India). 2017. "The Real Picture: Yes! I Am the Change 2016—Open Challenge." YouTube, video, 2:59. https://www.youtube.com/watch?v=TTNEKaImfto.

Young, Iris. 2003. "The Logic of Masculinist Protection." *Signs* 29, no. 1: 1–25.

Yuval-Davis, Nira. 1993. "Gender and Nation." *Ethnic and Racial Studies* 16, no. 4: 621–32. https://doi.org/10.1080/01419870.1993.9993800.

Yuval-Davis, Nira. 1997. *Gender and Nation.* London: Sage Publications.

Yuval-Davis, Nira. 2003. "Nationalist Projects and Gender Relations." *Narodna Umjetnost: Croatian Journal of Ethnology and Folklore Research* 40, no. 1: 9–36.

Zakaria, Anam. 2015. *The Footprints of Partition: Narratives of Four Generations of Pakistanis and Indians.* Noida: HarperCollins India.

INDEX

Hall, Stuart, 30–31
Halla Bol, Lungi Khol (HBLK), 171–76
Hansen, Thomas Blom, 2, 47–48, 159
Har Ghar Jal program, 214
Hawkins, Gay, 33
Hindu Brahmanical order. *See* casteism
Hindu heteropatriarchal order, 10, 13–14,
    23, 39, 42–48, 73, 93, 99, 109–12, 119–21,
    124–25, 130–32, 134–42, 154, 160, 165–66,
    187–88, 206. *See also* Hindutva
Hinduism: and cleanliness, 92–93, 210;
    imagery of, 2, 17, 28, 83–84; and mod-
    ernization, 11, 146–47; and purity, 34;
    signifiers of, 60, 71–72, 79–80, 149–51;
    visual foregrounding of, 148–49; and
    women's honor, 96–97
Hindu majoritarian neoliberal culture, 161,
    165–66, 168–71, 175
Hindu modern: as an assemblage, 211;
    and the common man, 140–47; and
    disappearing populations, 192–93; and
    gender, 9, 22; governmentality of, 8–9,
    20–21, 26, 72, 78, 86–87, 155, 158, 161, 176,
    188–89, 202–3, 219; and intimacy, 148–49;
    logics of, 3, 8–27, 63, 125, 144, 180–81;
    and masculinity, 134–41; and mediation,
    18–19, 153–54; and sacralization of land,
    11–13; and security, 13–18; and violence,
    19–21, 119–20, 159–60, 162–63; and
    young girls, 92. *See also* modernization;
    Modi, Narendra; violence
Hindu modernity, 8–9
Hindu nationalism. *See* Hindutva
Hindu supremacists. *See* Hindutva
Hindutva: and censorship, 103; and
    corporate power, 15; and gender, 26,
    46–48; normalization of, 2–3, 29–30;
    and online spaces, 18–19, 49–52, 77,
    153–54; perceptions of, 64, 166; and
    purifying the national family, 110, 120;
    rise of, 2, 11–12, 62, 153–54; and violence,
    65, 83, 89, 159–60, 168, 185–86, 195–96;
    women's role in, 185–86. *See also* Hindu
    heteropatriarchal order; India
Hitler, Adolf, 33

Hitler Youth, 51
homonationalism, 46
homophily, 69–70
honor, 44–45, 54, 65–66, 96, 98–99, 107–9,
    112, 122–34, 142–44, 156–57, 175. *See also*
    women
Human Rights Watch, 55

Ilaiah, Kancha, 57, 85
immigrants, 159–61
imperialism, 36–37
India: farmers' movements in, 164; gender
    equity in, 10, 186; as Hindu mother,
    57, 59–62, 222n12; independence
    movement, 3–4, 61–62, 65, 151–52, 160;
    international perceptions of, 8, 40, 106,
    184; and national honor, 122–23; and pa-
    triotism, 7, 66, 71–72; pre-independence
    era, 34, 58; and vertical logic of power,
    86; water access in, 213–14, 230n8; weap-
    ons and defense programs, 15, 222n17.
    See also Bharat Mata; Hindutva; na-
    tional identity; Partition; *punyabhoomi;*
    Swachh Bharat Abhiyan (SBA)
Indian Congress Party, 1–2, 61, 146
Indian National Congress, 71
Indore Municipal Corporation, 192
infantilization, 176–77
informal Hindutva, 153–54
informational Hindutva, 18
infrastructural abandonment, 193
infrastructures, 29, 94, 98, 101–2, 190–94
Inglehart, Ronald, 15
internet freedom, 19
invisibility, xii, 7, 16, 102–3, 120, 164–65
Irani, Smriti, 66, 120
Islam, Kazi Nazrul, 61
izzat. See honor

Jadugar campaign, 183
Jaffrelot, Christophe, 2, 19, 159
Jafri, Ehsan, 139
Jain, Ashok, 194
Jain, Kajri, 12
Jan Dhan Yojana, 206, 222n23

national identity, xiii, 1–2, 29, 206–7. *See also* India; patriotism

National Rally party, 46

National Register of Citizens (NRC), 14, 22, 160–61, 192

Nazis, 33, 51

NDTV, 25, 43

necropolitics, 32, 65, 156, 161, 195, 197

Nehru, Jawaharlal, 27, 61, 124, 134

neo-Hindutva, 29

neoliberalism, 15, 54, 99, 126, 131, 159–63, 165–66, 184, 188, 195, 203, 206, 212–17, 223n33

Nirbhaya rape case, xiii

Nirmal Bharat Abhiyan, 25

Nixon, Rob, 101–2

Norris, Pippa, 15

No Toilet, No Bride (NTNB) campaign: dominance of Hindu marriage, 148–51; and masculinity narratives, 136–37, 141–43; and Muslims, 152–53; spread of, 44, 53; and surveillance, 52, 153–54; and women's honor, 44–45, 112–22, 143–44. *See also* Swachh Bharat Abhiyan (SBA); toilet construction

Ogilvy and Mather, 183

open defecation, 5, 18, 32, 39, 53, 82–83, 108–9, 112, 117, 126, 129, 142–43, 145, 171–73, 176–77, 181–82, 185, 193–94, 197–200. *See also* toilet construction; urination

othering, 2, 82, 174–75, 177–79, 203–4, 216

Pakistan, 16, 123–24, 221n11. *See also* Partition

Palli, Sudhakar, 198

Pandey, Gyanendra, 21

Papacharissi, Zizi, 68

Partition, xiii, 16, 48, 61, 122–24, 134, 174. *See also* India; Pakistan

paternalism, 131

patriotism, 7, 17, 72. *See also* national identity

Pednekar, Bhumi, 109

penal populism, 227n2

personal protective equipment, 101–3

Philippines, 55–56

Phule, Savitri, 71, 146

Pinjra Tod movement, 131–32

Pissing Tanker group, 228n22

planetary ethics, 215–17

Plant a Tree challenge, 42

poverty, 68, 165–66, 171–85, 193–94, 203–4, 230n5

prostitution, 37

Puar, Jasbir, 46, 209–10

Pugliese, Joseph, 216

punitive populism, 54

punyabhoomi, 12, 22, 59, 78, 85, 87, 161, 193, 207. *See also* India; sacralization of land

purity, 1, 29, 31, 34, 47, 72, 79, 89, 102, 117, 122, 124, 145. *See also* cleanliness

Quill Studio, 78–80

Rahman, A. R., 103

Raja, Ira, 39–40

Rajagopal, Arvind, 28, 62, 83

Raksha Bandhan, 141–43

Ramaswamy, Sumathy, 75

Ramayana, 12, 62, 83–84

Ram Rajya, 18, 167

Ram Sene, 66

Ranaut, Kangana, 95

Ranchi Municipal Corporation (RMC), 171

Rao, Anupama, 34, 115–16

rape: and caste, 118, 133; and honor, 129–30; as motivation for toilet construction, 113–14; prevalence of, 19, 92, 115–16, 121, 123, 133, 224n13; promotion of, 14, 35, 119; silence surrounding, xii–xiii

Rashtriya Swayamsevak Sangh (RSS), 1, 19, 30, 48–51, 61, 72, 146. *See also* Bhartiya Janata Party (BJP)

"Real Picture, The" (Yes Foundation), 73–78

Redmond, Sean, 38

religious conversion, 14, 148–49

R. G. Kar Medical Hospital case, xiii

Rohingya refugees, 16, 43

Roy, Srirupa, 2
Rwanda, 55

Sabarimala protests, 34–35
sacralization of land, 11–12, 57–58, 61,
    221n11. See also *punyabhoomi*
Safai Karmachari Andolan, 32, 103, 157
Sangh Parivar, 29, 62
sanitation work, 5–6, 29, 53, 101, 156
Saraswati, 95, 224n7
Sarkar, Pradeep, 95
Sarkar, Tanika, 60, 121–23
Savarkar, Vinayak Damodar, 11–12, 19, 48, 85
Savarna feminism, 117
school curricula, 162
Scroll, 68
secularism, 27, 29, 34, 61, 207
security logics, 14–16, 21, 49, 58, 64–65,
    73, 90, 95, 109–10, 119–20, 125, 140–41,
    147–54, 163–64, 200
Sedgwick, Eve, 173
selfies, 76–77, 139–40, 153–55, 180
Selfie With Daughter initiative, 139–40
Sen, Geeti, 62, 65
sexuality: and deviance, 16; and the Hindu
    modern, 10; homosexual children,
    120; and purity, 122, 124; regulation of,
    110–12, 128, 133; state recognitions of,
    189. See also gender
shadow sovereignties, 161, 227n5
Shah, Amit, 16, 132, 159
Sharma, Mahesh, 12
Shri Krishna Studios, 185
Signs, 45
Singapore, 55
Singh, C. P., 173
Singh, Jyoti, 118
Singh, Manmohan, 134–35
Singh, Neha, 61
Singh, Poonam, 57
Sitharam, Nirmala, 186
slow violence, 101
soap, 36–37
social media: everyday use of, 13, 24–25,
    51–52, 63, 75–77; as Hindu nationalist

space, 18–19, 49–51, 58, 77; and looking
    relations, 86; regulation of, 19, 69, 196;
    and spreadability, 63–64, 67, 73, 78–79;
    and vigilante virality, 179–80. See also
    virality
sousveillance, 196
sovereignty, 161–62, 169
Spivak, Gayatri, 216
Srinivas, Tulasi, 34
Srivastav, Nikhil, 158
stripping, 171–74
Subramaniam, Banu, 49
Sulabh International, 113
Sulabh Swachh Bharat, 24
Sundaram, Ravi, 18
Swachhata Hi Seva campaign, 33
Swachh Bharat Abhiyan (SBA): assess-
    ment of cleanliness, 171–72, 184, 190;
    and caste, 85–86, 102, 157; coercive
    tactics of, 20, 23–24, 54, 82–83, 165,
    176–79, 184–85, 187, 199; and the com-
    mon man, 141–47; critiques of, 68;
    culture of violence, 15–16, 158–60, 162,
    168–71, 194–95; and *darshan*, 84–85;
    funding models of, 4–5, 118–19, 122,
    190; goals of, 7–8, 216–17; influence of,
    107, 209–10; international perception
    of, 8, 40–41, 108–9; and masculiniza-
    tion, 20; as mode of governmentality,
    9, 20–21, 30; popularity of, 25, 217–18;
    and privatization of cleanliness, 42,
    206; promotion of, 6, 15–16, 19, 24–25,
    49, 51–52, 67–70; scholarly attention
    to, 26, 222n24; slogans of, 73–74; as
    supposedly apolitical, 82, 105; and
    war mentality, 201–2; and women's
    empowerment, 23, 43, 47–48, 149.
    See also Bharat Mata; Bhartiya Janata
    Party (BJP); cleanliness; India; No
    Toilet, No Bride (NTNB) campaign;
    toilet construction
Swachh Survekshan, 172, 184, 192
Swaraj, Sushma, 32
Swarajya, 27
Syria, 56